Anthropologies of Cancer in Transnational Worlds

Cancer is a transnational condition involving the unprecedented flow of health information, technologies and people across national borders. Such movement raises questions about the nature of therapeutic citizenship, how and where structurally vulnerable populations obtain care, and the political geography of blame associated with this disease. This volume brings together cutting-edge anthropological research carried out across North and South America, Europe, Africa and Asia, representing low-, middle- and high-resource countries with a diversity of national health care systems. Contributors ethnographically map the varied nature of cancer experiences and articulate the multiplicity of meanings that survivorship, risk, charity and care entail. They explore institutional frameworks shaping local responses to cancer and underlying political forces and structural variables that frame individual experiences. Of particular concern is the need to interrogate underlying assumptions of research designs that may lead to the naturalizing of hidden agendas or intentions. Running throughout the chapters, moreover, are considerations of moral and ethical issues related to cancer treatment and research. Thematic emphases include the importance of local biologies in the framing of cancer diagnosis and treatment protocols, uncertainty and ambiguity in definitions of biosociality, shifting definitions of patienthood, and the sociality of care and support.

Holly F. Mathews is Professor of Anthropology at East Carolina University.

Nancy J. Burke is an Associate Professor in the Department of Anthropology, History and Social Medicine and the Helen Diller Comprehensive Cancer Center at the University of California, San Francisco.

Eirini Kampriani is adjunct lecturer at IST/University of Hertfordshire and the National School of Public Health, Greece.

Routledge Studies in Anthropology

Anthropologies of Cancer in Transnational Worlds

Edited by Holly F. Mathews,
Nancy J. Burke, and
Eirini Kampriani

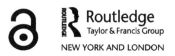

Routledge
Taylor & Francis Group

NEW YORK AND LONDON

First published 2015
by Routledge
605 Third Avenue, New York, NY 10017

and by Routledge
4 Park Square, Milton Park, Abingdon, Oxon OX14 4RN

First issued in paperback 2017

*Routledge is an imprint of the Taylor & Francis Group,
an informa business*

Library of Congress Cataloging-in-Publication Data
Anthropologies of cancer in transnational worlds / edited by Holly F.
    Mathews, Nancy J. Burke, and Eirini Kampriani.
        pages cm. — (Routledge studies in anthropology ; 23)
    Includes index.
    1. Cancer—Social aspects. 2. Cancer—Patients—Care—Moral and
ethical aspects. 3. Medical anthropology. I. Mathews, Holly F.
II. Burke, Nancy Jean. III. Kampriani, Eirini.
    RC262.A665 2015
    362.19699'4—dc23
    2015005841

ISBN 13: 978-0-8153-4647-0 (pbk)
ISBN 13: 978-1-138-77693-7 (hbk)

Typeset in Sabon
by Apex CoVantage, LLC

Contents

Foreword
The Emperor of All Terrors: Forging an Alternative Biography of Cancer

When my colleague, Eirini Kampriani, who also conducts research on cancer in Greece, contacted me about becoming involved with this volume on cancer transnationally, I was intrigued by the idea. I previously participated in a seminar entitled "Confronting Cancer" at the School of Advanced Research with another of the editors, Holly Mathews. I knew that we shared an interest in understanding the lived experience of cancer in specific cultural contexts. I am pleased to write the foreword for this important volume, which extends the work of that conference to look beyond US borders to the experience of cancer globally. Specifically, the authors bring anthropological methods to bear on studies of cancer in different geographical regions of the world and within a diversity of national health care systems. Central to this comparative effort is an attempt to use fine-grained ethnographic data to construct an alternative and more nuanced conceptualization of cancer that will ultimately aid in global efforts to understand and address this persistent and complex disease.

My own thoughts on the importance of this endeavor began in October of 2012, when I joined a packed auditorium at Harvard University Medical School to hear the 37th Joseph Garland Lecture, sponsored by the Boston Medical Library and presented by Siddhartha Mukherjee. "A society's narrative of cancer often evolves based on the technologies of its time . . ." the *Harvard Gazette* reported him saying in their Friday, October 19, 2012, electronic issue (Koch, 2012). The inspiration for Mukherjee's award winning book, *The Emperor of All Maladies: A Biography of Cancer* (2010), came from a patient who needed to know "what he was fighting." The patient's uncertainty led Mukherjee, a Boston-based oncologist and bench cancer researcher, to morph into a medical historian in order to search for "cancer's roots."

In his book, Mukherjee weaves a persuasive story of the disease's *biography*: a voyage that begins with early *Homo sapiens*; continues through ancient Egypt, Persia, Greece and Rome; and ends with Western biomedicine's discoveries and therapeutic promises. Although it provides a lucid history of the scientific war against cancer and the development of chemotherapy, the biography is limited because it is based solely on a "Western journey" rather than one stretching to all the corners of the world. In reality, Mukherjee's book is a biography of oncology not of cancer as a whole; it is a history of how technologies of detection and treatment came into being in the West. Although it tells the story of the professionalization of oncology, it does not show how this process brought about the very Western conceptualization of cancer as an individualized disease with a long evolutionary history based upon the phenomenological, embodied Western notions of warfare.

Cancer's journey to Western modernity is more than a controversial mention in an Egyptian papyrus or the Hippocratic recognition of its clinical manifestations. Cancer has a multifaceted history and needs anthropological and ethnographic representations that offer alternative conceptualizations to biomedicine's universalizing and hegemonic tendencies. My own research on the "cultures of cancer" took me to the island of Crete, where we researched the local discourse on fertilizers and cancer, and 10 years ago to the provinces of Sichuan and Yunnan in China, where I collected similar narratives on chemical agriculture and the rise of cancer incidence. The reply of a traditional Chinese doctor to the question of what causes cancer serves as an indication of what the majority of the people I talked with believe about cancer pathogenesis. He responded:

> Bad environment, both internal and external. Illness comes when the functional balance of the body's organs is upset or destroyed. Modernization and pollution speed up disruptive forces and increase imbalance. The destruction of the natural environment, pollution, and depression are causing cancer. Yin and yang are out of balance.

The impetus behind this volume and the conference that produced it was to use detailed, cross-cultural ethnographic data to demonstrate the importance of similarly neglected components of the Western cancer story. To develop a global, multicultural biography of cancer we need to know more about the voices that are not heard. What are the multiple possible stories of the disease's biography? How do non-Western peoples explain carcinogenesis? What are the moral reasonings and cultural explanations of the disease in other parts of the world?

The message of biomedical superiority and monopoly in the diagnosis and treatment of cancer travels quickly around the world and is tied to national and transnational material practices that involve public health decisions about how health resources should be invested, what treatments can be adopted and which innovations must be prioritized. According to the World Health Organization (WHO), between a 5 and 10% yearly increase in cancer incidence is now observed in non-Western countries. Over the next two decades, WHO expects cancer incidence to increase by 70% with new yearly cases hitting 25 million. The new global patient looks toward the West for treatment and hope for survival. Yet ethnographic studies of the experience of cancer transnationally, such as the ones included in this volume, demonstrate that these technologies and the priorities they generate are not necessarily the best choices for alleviating suffering and improving health in the West where they originate much less in other parts of the world where many are being tested for the first time.

Unfortunately, biomedical discourse tends to lead experts and lay people alike to shift attention away from analyzing the origins of carcinogenesis and cancer causality to focus, instead, on a collective dream of finding *the cure* by encouraging patients to take personal responsibility for doing everything possible to *fight* the disease with science. Through well-crafted narratives, like Mukherjee's, an evolutionary *telos* is inserted in our collective consciousness: humanity traveled from magic to rationality, from cancer terror to survivorship, and biomedicine made this possible. Mukherjee confidently asserts that scientists now know that cancer is an "organismal" and a "pathway disease," and these views will lead to the development of new drugs, new chemical bullets and new potent radiation waves to morph cancer into a chronic disease. Yet these claims are far from established, and many critics contest their validity, pointing out the fallacious basis of the metaphorical assumptions upon which they are based.

Many in the West marginalize the efforts of environmentalists to argue that cancer and its proliferation in the industrial and post-industrial era is due to chemical modernity. For example, the 2008–2009 report of the US President's Cancer Panel documents over 80,000 chemicals in daily use in the United States. Yet of these, only a few hundred have been tested for carcinogenicity and physicians rarely ask cancer patients about past exposures to pollutants. Even though US rates of cancer remain higher than those of other industrial nations, claims that such chemicals contribute to cancer causation have been dismissed in part because of the blinders imposed by the warfare rhetoric, which looks solely at the individual somatic level of carcinogenesis and neglects the systemic components, both environmental and socioeconomic, which shape the contexts of exposure to toxins for whole communities in the United States and elsewhere.

Yet, despite much collective and individual wishful thinking in the West, cancer does not seem to bow to human will, neither does it get defeated with fancy imaging, genetic knowledge, radioactive burning and chemical bullets. The voices of scientific biomedicine are always optimistic, prompting an almost religious belief that research will save humans from cancer, sending millions of Americans to the streets walking, running, hiking, jumping from airplanes, with colors and ribbons, with fun and games, to raise those funds that will put the scientists to war in this collective warfare effort to "face up" to cancer. Today, more than 12 million Americans live with cancer, with breast and prostate cancers counting for more than one third of all cases. According to the American Cancer Society over 1.5 million cases are newly diagnosed every year, and the numbers are increasing rapidly. Recently, the International Agency for Research on Cancer, part of the World Health

Organization, reported that the global cancer burden rose to 14.1 million new cases in 2012 and is projected to increase to 19.3 million cases by the year 2025. The proliferation of the disease among peoples of all ages, ethnicities and socioeconomic classes suggests that more than individualized biology and lifestyle choices are involved in its cause.

The warfare metaphor has given rise to a *conspiracy of silence* that diverts our attention from the crucial question of carcinogenesis. Somewhere, sometime, something triggers normal growth cells to become cancerous, and starts the genetic pathway of carcinogenesis. We understand much about the pathway of carcinogenesis, but we ignore its starting point.

It is time now to give renewed consideration to just how integral the role of the environment is in cancer pathogenesis. Cancer is something that develops within the body, but interactions with our environment ("the air we breathe, the food we eat," as one Chinese doctor told me) as well as our socioeconomic position in society can dictate how, where and if cancer develops. In casting miasmatic theory aside, we are left with no choice, except to internalize the biomedical explanation for cancer. It is time to reexamine how we as organisms maintain our homeostasis within our environment in a more holistic manner.

Environmental citizenship means the international spread of localized problems. Cancer citizenship, on the other hand, is the international spread of Western problems. Cancer has become a global vernacular, a sign of modernism that through narratives of conformity, like Mukherjee's, maintains its subaltern status and allows the global democracy of glamour to sidetrack discussions of danger. The millions of women who undergo the rite of passage of breast cancer diagnosis and treatment are congratulated for their cultural heroism. But, survivorship and survival are two different things, and anthropology can offer a new perspective on how cancer should be represented. The essays in this volume provide rich ethnographic data from diverse cultural contexts that allow us to hear alternative and often unvoiced views of the social and environmental influences shaping the experience of this disease. While cancer still remains the emperor of all terrors, attempts to dislodge some of the master narratives of cancer from the global north is our best hope for the development of more effective global public health practice.

Anastasia Karakasidou
Wellesley, MA
November 2014

Acknowledgments

This volume emerged from a November 2010 conference organized by Jeannine Coreil and Holly Mathews in New Orleans, LA, entitled "Cancer Narratives in Global Perspective." We wish to acknowledge the lead role Jeannine played in conceiving of the idea for the initial conference and planning for its execution. She was a guiding spirit for all of us in preparing this volume. Special thanks go to Karen Dyer for her help in organizing the conference. The Wenner Gren Foundation provided the funding to bring scholars from Argentina, Brazil, France, Hong Kong, India, Kenya, Greece, Scotland and Slovenia together with colleagues in the United States. A subset of the papers presented are included herein. Thanks to all the contributors for their collegiality, insight, originality and commitment to critical engagement. Others who participated and made valuable contributions to the development of the ideas in this volume include Amarasira De Silva, Deborah Gordon, Wendy Lam, Mojca Ramšak, Ayşecan Terzioğlu and Fouzieyha Towghi. Appreciation is owed to three anonymous reviewers who offered wise and constructive comments. Michell Gilman assisted in the preparation of the manuscript. Without her help and careful eye for detail we would possibly still be checking bibliographies. We also thank our Routledge editor, Max Novick, for his support, patience and guidance through this process.

Introduction
Mapping the Landscape of Transnational Cancer Ethnography

Holly F. Mathews and Nancy J. Burke

Cancer is a global epidemic. While incidence and mortality rates for most cancers are decreasing in countries in the global north, they are increasing in less developed and economically transitioning nations, where the proportion of new cancer cases diagnosed is projected to grow from about 56% of the world total in 2008 to more than 60% in the year 2030 (Jemal, Center, DeSantis & Ward, 2010). The biomedical model of cancer and its treatment as expressed within the specialty of oncology in the global north still informs most international health initiatives. It remains the norm for how specialists and lay people alike conceptualize and respond to the disease worldwide even though many scholars have pointed out the ethnocentric and culture-bound parameters of this model, which asserts that cancer is a natural illness in which the individual patient alone is responsible for prevention through control of lifestyle choices and for cure by pursuing biomedical treatments aggressively.

The contributors to this volume ask how we might go about constructing an alternative conceptualization of cancer. They draw upon empirically rich, cross-cultural ethnographic data to add complexity to our understanding of the fundamental nature of cancer itself and the shifting contexts of suffering and uncertainty that the increasing burden of this disease evokes. This volume brings together cutting-edge anthropological research carried out across countries in North and South America, Europe, Africa and Asia representing the full range of economies from low-, middle- and high-resource countries with a diversity of national health care systems. The insights emerging from these detailed ethnographic studies challenge some of the basic concepts that undergird the standard view of cancer and the practices accepted in oncology.

Specifically, contributors to this volume argue that:

- Cancer is a multitude of conditions with varying sets of causes and symptoms that shape the possibilities for successful treatment and prevention in different localities.
- Cancer is not solely a biological phenomenon but a politics with which people engage and struggle within the context of national health systems, volunteer and charity organizations and local institutions.

- Cancer is an economic disorder rooted in material practices, which vary among nations arrayed along a continuum from resource rich to resource poor.
- Cancer is a profoundly social disease that requires a reexamination of the boundaries of patienthood in an era of biosocial identity making.
- Cancer today is a transnational condition involving the unprecedented flow of health information and technologies as well as people across national borders, raising issues about the nature of therapeutic citizenship, about how and where structurally vulnerable populations obtain care, and about the political geography of blame associated with this disease.

SITUATING THIS VOLUME

This collection grew out of a Wenner-Gren funded workshop held in November of 2010, in New Orleans, LA, on the topic "Cancer Narratives in Global Perspective." The organizers brought together anthropologists researching cancer in the developing world to exchange ideas and information with their colleagues in the United States and Europe in order to promote broader perspectives on the manifestations and consequences of the disease globally and collaborative theorizing on its emerging transnational nature. The chapters in this volume are an outgrowth of that initial and fruitful conference. As a group, we share a commitment to the importance of globalizing the discourse on cancer both as a way to inform and combat the paternalism at the heart of many international health practices and also as a way to deconstruct some of the implicitly ethnocentric assumptions about the nature of cancer and the practice of oncology in the global north (Comaroff & Comaroff, 2012). The comparative, cross-cultural perspective employed by the authors in this volume aims to unfold the multiplicity of meanings and forms that concepts such as survivorship, risk, charity and care entail.

In 1999, Lenore Manderson edited a special issue of *Anthropology & Medicine* offering new perspectives on cancer control, disease and palliative care cross-culturally. She called attention to the emerging importance of cancer globally and argued that anthropological research had an important role to play in addressing its etiology, epidemiology, prevention, detection, management and care (1999a). Despite this pioneering effort, anthropologists have been slow to take up her challenge. Almost 10 years afterward, Juliet McMullin and Diane Weiner (2008) published an important edited collection that featured anthropological studies of cancer in US populations. In their introduction, they noted that research over the past few decades focused primarily on exploring, deciphering and analyzing the metaphors surrounding cancer in order to understand their impacts on and meanings in individual and social lives. Cancer, they wrote, is itself a common metaphor for lack of control and degeneration as well as a signifier of difference, being "something that is part of our body and world and yet an unacceptable occurrence" (p. 3). Wherever it strikes, cancer has common properties. It attacks the physical, social and emotional body and is frequently described across cultures as dangerous and dreaded, understood biologically as cells growing out of control, and perceived locally by many as an evil force, an outside enemy, or a thief that robs one of the life force. Yet metaphor, in particular, influences and often constrains thought (Lakoff & Johnson, 1980). As a result, McMullin and Weiner pointed out that the particular ways we conceptualize cancer can also lead us to stigmatize certain individuals and groups and may shift attention away from the social inequalities that hasten the death of some while prolonging the lives of others (2008, p. 14).

Until recently, most anthropological research on cancer continued to be conducted primarily on US populations and to a lesser extent in Australian, Canadian and European contexts; as a result, our theoretical perspectives have been shaped by the relatively narrow slice of the historical, sociocultural and intellectual contexts analyzed in these studies. For example, a number of scholars document the ubiquity of war metaphors in the rhetoric of cancer in the global north. Sontag (1979) pointed out the overriding conceptualization of cancer in the United States as an enemy invading the body, which evoked responses of fear and dread and led logically to the idea of a battle against a hostile invader. Garrison (2007) traced the history of war metaphors for cancer back to the early 1930s, noting that the American Society for the Control of Cancer adopted uniforms, observed rank and adopted the *Sword of Hope* as its emblem and appropriated military language in its rhetoric about health and cancer prevention. When cancer is depicted as invading the body and the body becomes a battleground, then patients logically become soldiers or warriors who are charged to aggressively search and destroy the enemy within. As a result, McMullin and Weiner write that men and women *battling* testicular and breast cancer in the United States become *survivors, warriors* and *thrivers*, not merely patients (2008, p. 10). To the extent that such metaphors are used in biomedical practice, they may shape the judgments clinicians make about patients who are good and deserving of help and those who are not.

Mary-Jo Delvecchio Good and colleagues (1990) were the first to examine systematically the metaphors and shared assumptions that guided the practice of oncology. They found that US oncologists varied in their ideas about just when and what should be disclosed to patients in part because they perceived their mission to be one of instilling, not dashing, patients' hopes (Delvecchio-Good, Good, Schaffer & Lind, 1990). Many oncologists embrace this mission, they argue, not because they believe as some Americans do that the mind can really influence disease, but rather because they believe that hope helps patients adopt a positive attitude that makes forging a partnership with them in the healing process easier. The oncologists that Good and colleagues studied attempted to do this by encouraging patients to develop a *fighting spirit* and to join the *team* with health personnel in order to *beat* the disease. In such a depiction, the cancer patient is portrayed as being locked in mortal combat with the *enemy* disease and is encouraged to become a *hero-survivor*, not a *victim* (see Saillant, 1990, for a similar discussion about oncology in French Canada). In such a context, survivorship becomes a *transformative* experience where biographical disruption and socioeconomic hardships are minimized and heroic struggles against an enemy disease are valorized (Coreil, Wilke & Pintado, 2004).

Mathews, Lannin & Mitchell (1994) and Mathews (2000) reported that African American breast cancer patients in the United States who followed oncologists' recommendations unquestioningly, pursued treatment aggressively, and maintained a positive and uncomplaining attitude, were labeled as *good patients* and praised for their efforts. However, those women who were uncomfortable with the prevailing military imagery and voiced alternative ideas about spirituality and harmony were sometimes ridiculed by clinicians and risked being labeled as *fatalistic*. Indeed, as Weiner and McMullin point out, fatalistic beliefs are viewed in the United States and elsewhere as the reason why certain ethnic and minority groups do not seek care for cancer (2008, p. 15). Yet investigators continue to document the importance of alternative conceptions of cancer in communities within the United States. Many Native American groups, for instance, emphasize social interdependence and family imagery in formulating a more group-oriented alternative to the "individual alone on the battlefield scenario" characteristic of modern oncology (Burhansstipanov, Gilbert, LaMarca & Krebs, 2001) and Filipina immigrants attribute a variety of meanings to survivorship (Burke, Villero & Guerra, 2012).

Similarly, Gordon and Paci (1997) document an alternative cultural narrative of "social-embeddedness," in Tucsany, Italy. This narrative emphasizes social unity and hierarchy and works to promote a sense of family and group protection. In the past, this narrative served to frame the common practice of the nondisclosure of a cancer diagnosis. Gordon (1990) also documents how this narrative contributed to the ways that oncologists avoided naming the disease or disclosing it to their patients and how patients in turn avoided disclosing their diagnoses to family members. Gordon and Paci (1997) further report that nondisclosure and the larger narrative from which it derives is being challenged as it confronts other medical narratives such as the US model discussed previously.

Bennett's (1999) study of truth telling regarding cancer diagnosis and prognosis in rural northeast Thailand provided an early example of how an alternative cultural perspective could help forge broader understandings of this phenomenon. Despite rapid cultural change and the prevalence of aspects of Western biomedical practice in Thailand, Bennett found that disclosures of terminal illness were rarely made to patients. Much like their counterparts in Italy, physicians and family members alike believed that telling the truth to a person with cancer robbed them of hope and the strength needed to cope with the disease (p. 400). If disclosure was made at all, it was to family members. Because those with terminal cancers were sent home to die, they had close family support and the actions of relatives often signaled implicitly the reality of impending death. Yet end-stage illness and dying were never discussed, and the tears of family members were shed privately (p. 401).

These brief examples demonstrate that regional perspectives matter in understanding the complexity of the disease experience and the tensions arising when global health paradigms are introduced and appropriated in specific contexts. This volume documents the efforts of anthropologists working and residing in many different countries to bring innovative methods and perspectives to bear on broadening the base of our understandings about cancer and the ways in which this disease impacts individuals, expert activist and lay groups, and national health policies around the world. Contributors move beyond the ubiquitous study of explanatory narratives and metaphors to explore both the institutional frameworks shaping local responses to cancer and the underlying political forces and structural variables that frame individual experiences. Of particular concern is the need to interrogate the underlying assumptions of research designs that may lead to the naturalizing of hidden agendas or intentions. Running throughout all of the chapters in this volume, moreover, are considerations of the moral and ethical issues related to cancer treatment and research. Authors implicitly question the appropriateness of a global bioethics based in the Western values of individuality and autonomy, and in touching on the importance of these questions to cancer care at the end of life, they also question the ethics of research conducted under the auspices of these values. Taken together, these chapters begin to provide a framework for researching and engaging with cancer transnationally.

POSITIONING OURSELVES

The contributors to this volume are united by a shared anthropological perspective and a commitment to field-based ethnographic research, which distinguishes their work from other types of research in the social sciences and in public health. The importance of this approach is highlighted in several recent publications extolling the value of long- term, inductive, reflexive ethnography (Adams, Burke & Whitmarsh, 2014; Beihl & Petryna, 2013). Stacy Pigg, in a 2013 article, utilizes her research on HIV/AIDS education and outreach strategies in 1990s Nepal to show how the path toward decisions in international health research is never entirely clear, nor is it obvious who benefits or loses from different approaches. Detailing the inadequacy of USAID's implementation in Nepal of interventions developed elsewhere (Uganda) and the subtle ways in which Nepalese health workers resisted the dissemination of them, Pigg shows how the "in between times" she spent sitting, talking informally, listening and actively observing informed her ability to understand and describe the previously unrecognized problem. She also argues that the critical thinking and thick description anthropologists bring to global health problems, including the study of cancer, is one form of doing something relevant to, but often unrecognized in, the action-oriented field of global health. Biehl and Petryna qualify ethnography as *an early warning system* (2013, p. 18). They state that:

> Ethnographers are uniquely positioned to see what more categorically minded experts may overlook: namely, the empirical evidence that emerges when people express their most pressing and ordinary concerns, which then open up to complex human stories in time and space.
>
> (2013, p. 19)

Contributors to this volume engage ethnography in this way—they give rigorous attention to the lived, embodied experiences of people in specific locations—and chapters serve as "cases to think with" (Geertz, 2007).

For example, Mulemi's chapter explores the dynamics of cancer care in Kenya, where the disease has remained largely invisible due to the priority placed nationally on communicable diseases. He immersed himself in the life of a cancer ward in the main hospital in Nairobi. He observed and interviewed patients and health care personnel. He also followed patients from the hospital back to their home villages to find out how they fared after treatment and to chart the difficulties they and their family members faced. In this case study, Mulemi documents the prevalence of late-stage disease in Kenya, where patients and their families must follow long referral chains to obtain diagnoses. The lack of cancer specialists and hospital treatment centers means that screening services are virtually nonexistent and, as Livingston (2012) also reports for Botswana, in situ and early stage cancers do not exist. Moreover, once patients with advanced cancers are diagnosed, the initiation of treatment does not guarantee the restoration of health or a better quality of life. Thus, as Mulemi (2008) has written, cancer patients and their families do not view cancer as an especially significant disruption to their lives as do patients in the global north. Rather, he reports that life during hospital treatment is a microcosm of the larger society where treatment ambiguity depicts not only the present physical suffering, but also a wider spectrum of daily life struggles. Cancer is one more burden in the trajectories of misfortune that characterize the lives of the poor.

The implications of his findings are important in two ways. First, the availability of advanced medical technologies drives many global health initiatives. Thus programs to address cancer often seek to export cancer surveillance and screening guidelines and technologies from the global north to the developing world. Yet resource shortages and a lack of facilities may render these efforts meaningless except for the wealthiest of patients.

Second, Mulemi's observations about the suffering engendered by the lack of access to care is very applicable to particular populations within the global north, but it is a problem that often remains invisible to the medical establishment because standard biomedical assumptions underlie categorization of disease independent of patient experiences. Mathews (2014), for example, documents several public health initiatives during the 1990s in North Carolina that emphasized the importance of early detection of breast cancer through improved access to mammography screening. Although these efforts dramatically increased the rates of poor African American women having mammograms, there were no corresponding steps taken to ensure that women for whom the results were abnormal or suspicious had access to follow-up care and treatment. As the majority was uninsured, these women often had to live with the knowledge that they had a tumor for which nothing could be done, causing them great fear and anguish.

In her chapter for this volume, Alison Macdonald immerses herself in the ethnographic study of patient volunteer groups for breast cancer in a hospital in Mumbai, India. She begins to realize that the ways women view their roles as survivors and the kinds of aid they provide to others vary greatly from those reported from the United States and parts of Europe and Australia. Newly diagnosed women fear stigma and ostracism and engage in strenuous acts of concealment both within and outside of the family. There are no support groups where people meet publicly to obtain information and share feelings. Instead, the role of survivor volunteers is deeply shaped by the Hindu emphasis on the aesthetics of vision as a vital mode of communion. Volunteer survivors *reveal* themselves privately to newly diagnosed women as symbols of hope—visible manifestations that women can live beyond the diagnosis. This revelation is the means by which patients, their families and the volunteers reckon with the uncertainty of suffering. Macdonald's ethnographic analysis suggests that attempts to export a Euro-American model of cancer survivorship to Indian public health initiatives would likely fail. Alternatively, her nuanced ethnography demonstrates that the very concept of survivorship is itself context bound and shows how the changing oncological and patient activist arena in India is giving rise to novel forms of volunteer activism.

None of these insights would have emerged without detailed ethnographic research, and they remind social scientists to be open to possibilities and to imagine new ways of thinking about what might appear too familiar to be worthy of in-depth consideration. The chapters that follow seek to expand the very ways that we think about cancer in light of cross-cultural evidence. At base, anthropology is a comparative discipline. Contributions to this book provide an overview of cancer experiences, treatment and medical practices in different countries. Based upon individual ethnographic research, the authors analyze themes of uncertainty, suffering and meaning as they emerge in the varied contexts they explore. These include meanings of patienthood and survivorship; variable understandings of resources and research; cultures of risk, susceptibility, and responsibility; as well as meanings of documentation and access to care, and biological versus ethnic identities. In the process they highlight the convergence of globalizing healthcare agendas and local moral worlds of practice, and trace a very different biography of cancer than the one which underlies oncological practice in the global north.

AN ALTERNATIVE BIOGRAPHY OF CANCER: THE ROLE OF ENVIRONMENT AND THE IMPORTANCE OF LOCAL BIOLOGIES

In the foreword to this volume, Anastasia Karakasidou critiques Siddhartha Mukherjee's (2010) Pulitzer prize-winning book, *The Emperor of All Maladies: A Biography of Cancer* and argues for the importance of alternate perspectives if we are to construct a transnational, environmental history of cancer. Such a project is crucial, she maintains, in order to open up possibilities for understanding both the causes and appropriate responses to this disease globally (see also, Singer & Baer, 2011, pp. 226–230).

Karakasidou contends that cancer is something that occurs within our bodies but that interactions with our environments can determine how, when and even if the disease develops. By casting environmental theories aside, however, we are left with no choice but to internalize the biomedical explanation for cancer. It is time, she argues, to reexamine how we as organisms maintain our homeostasis within our environment in a more holistic manner.

This emphasis on homeostasis and the regulations of bodies with environments echoes Margaret Lock's initial formulation of her ideas about *local biologies*. In her 1993 book, Lock writes that her US informants frequently experienced hot flashes associated with menopause and many suffered extreme physiological symptoms because of them. Such reports were largely absent from Japanese women's discussions of this lifecycle phase. When Lock linked these symptom reports to established differences in the epidemiology of heart disease, osteoporosis and breast cancer between Japan and the West, she realized that more than cultural context was involved. Instead, she suggested that there were actual differences in women's bodies due to both culture and environment, perhaps as linked through diet. She then formulated the concept of local biologies to refer to the coproduction of biological and cultural contributions to embodied experience, which, in turn, shaped discourses about the body (Lock, 2001, p. 478).

As Brotherton and Nguyen (2013, p. 288) write, Lock's widely used concept "de-centers the modernist assumption of a universal material body, and postulates ceaseless interactions among bodies, environments (historical and local), and social/political variables." Therefore, if the development and experience of disease is linked biologically to variations in culture and environment, then cancer as a global category is likely comprised of many very different conditions with variant causes, developmental trajectories, symptomatic expressions and potentialities for treatment. Fouzieyha Tow-ghi's (2013) article on cervical cancer programs in India illustrates this view well. As she writes, it is well known biologically that the strains of HPV that cause cervical cancer vary geographically, but this knowledge remains unexamined in the global effort to develop, test and market HPV vaccines. Large pharmaceutical corporations are focused on a single strain HPV vac-cine as a key public health preventive strategy globally. Not only is a single strain vaccine likely to target the wrong variants of HPV in many areas, but overreliance on it ignores the reality that poor women in many parts of India lack access to basic screening through pap smears and to other health ser-vices that are more relevant to their needs. More importantly, a vaccination campaign to target all adolescent Indian girls would enrich multinational companies but bankrupt India's national health budget.

In an important recent article, Burke (2014) explores how the outsourc-ing of research and clinical trials conducted with "naïve" or untouched experimental populations often ignores the impacts of local biologies on the results. Yet findings from these trials may circle back to significantly impact health policy decisions in the global north. She analyzes the famous "Shang-hai Study," the first randomized controlled trial of breast self-exam (BSE), and how the policy recommendations it generated transformed the guide-lines for breast cancer screening and priorities for research in the United States. The popularity of BSE in the US took off in 1950 and continued with the rise of self-help and women's empowerment movements in the 60s and 70s (see Edwards, 2013). Yet even though the American Cancer Society heavily promoted BSE as a woman's responsibility to guard her own health and that of her family, many clinicians complained that BSE led to false posi-tive results and excess anxiety for female patients and called for research to demonstrate its efficacy.

The Shanghai study was conducted between 1988 and 1995. As Burke documents, scientists argued that it could not be undertaken in the United States because BSE practice there was so well entrenched. Therefore, instead of a treatment naïve population (Jain, 2013), researchers sought out a "screening naïve" population. The trial was designed to test the *teaching* of BSE in relation to breast cancer mortality; to assess the extent to which a health behavior, not a treatment, changed the number of deaths from the disease. The sites chosen were Shanghai Textile Industry Bureau factories because female workers resided on the sites in dormitories, received their medical care from the factories and had no mammographic screening avail-able. Women in the experimental groups were taught a three-step BSE tech-nique with reinforcement sessions whereas those in the control arms were not. Findings from the study unleashed a firestorm when reported back to the United States. The investigators concluded that BSE had no impact on breast cancer mortality and that a higher number of women who received BSE instruction reported false positives that required clinical investigation (Thomas et al., 2002).

Burke traces how the results of the Shanghai study traveled and were received among various stakeholders including researchers, breast cancer advocates, oncologists and breast cancer survivors in the United States, Canada, and Europe. Two important types of critiques began to emerge from these groups. The first, echoing Lock's notion of local biologies, questioned the assumption of the universal woman's body posited by biomedicine and argued that there might be important biological differences in the Chinese population related to genetic risk factors, tumor types and hormone receptivity as well as local variables of diet and environmental exposures that could limit the generalizability of the results to a much more biologically diverse US population with greater levels of social stratification. Secondly, Burke adapts the concept of local ecologies of care from Das and Das (2006) to discuss the impact of *local ecologies of screening* on the parameters of this study. The actual health behavior of BSE historically in the United States was regarded as essential to women's health and a part of women's activism and empowerment. It is not unreasonable to suppose that such a high level of commitment to and practice with this procedure might lead it to be performed differently in the United States than it was by a screening naïve population in China.

Despite these cogent and sometime virulent critiques, Burke reports that the American Cancer Society along with other influential breast cancer research and funding groups dropped recommendations for BSE as part of routine breast cancer screening in the United States. In so doing, she writes, the United States went from reliance on a low-level, low-cost technique under the control of women toward an exclusive reliance on more expensive screening procedures under the control of physicians, such as clinical exams and mammography, which as Mathews (2014) has demonstrated, are not equally available to all women. Moreover, once the screening recommendations shifted, research funding to evaluate the teaching or effectiveness of BSE was curtailed. Therefore, it has been virtually impossible within the United States to conduct further studies to verify or refute the findings from Shanghai. Burke concludes that the case of the Shanghai study illustrates the "influences of varying understandings of the biological and the local and their impact on what constitutes appropriate and valid evidence in breast cancer research" (p. 519). Her essay is also a reminder of the importance of Whyte and Gibbon's (2009) contention that the ways globalizing health practices become associated with public health, scientific research standards and ethics of care for underserved populations is of central importance for medical anthropology.

In her recent writing on the epigenetics of Alzheimer's disease, Lock (2013) proposes that the concept of *embedded bodies* may serve as a link between the epigenetics of the individual and the environments in which they live. She references the work of the anthropologist Niewöhner (2011) to define this concept as the idea that individual bodies are susceptible to changes in the social and material environment as inscribed by both evolutionary and transgenerational time (2013, p. 301). For example, some environmental epigeneticists suggest that the experience of social adversity in early life may profoundly affect health in later life. The implication is that groups unrelated biologically or by coresidence may still experience similar genetic and physiological changes based upon common social and historical influences. Lock argues that anthropologists need to embrace both the concepts of local biologies and embedded bodies to begin to explore biosocial differentiation, understood "as a product of individual lived experience in specific environmental, historical and sociopolitical contexts" (p. 303) in order to understand how these impact the experience of disease.

Lora-Wainwright's chapter in this volume undertakes such a project as she examines the ways that biomedical discourses of biology, risk and disease travel across national boundaries and intersect with local and traditional notions of the body as embedded in social and historical worlds in contemporary China. She draws upon ethnographic fieldwork and an extended case study of one family to argue that cancer in rural China presents a context through which family responsibilities are debated and past and current political economies are assessed. As people struggle to explain the presence of the disease, they emphasize different types of explanations depending on what is morally desirable at the time.

Lora-Wainwright focuses on a local condition known as *fighting for breath* and how it is understood by villagers. Although stomach and esophageal cancers are the most common in the region, notions about them have changed. In the recent past, she reports that these were classified and named in terms of their most obvious embodied effects including *vomiting illness* and *choking or spitting illness*. Now, however, the notion of the fight for breath encapsulates more than the physical to include the emotional and economic hardship presented by this often fatal disease, and it is variously attributed to suffering and hardship that occurred in the past during the Cultural Revolution as well as to present forms of suffering linked to industrialization and the use of farm chemicals, social changes and the ending of family lines, and the prevalence of bad habits such as smoking and drinking. As a result, ambiguity pervades cancer etiologies, imbuing them with both the potential to harm and to endow those who have the disease with moral characteristics. Lora-Wainwright concludes that examining the social, cultural and economic roots of etiologies and the ways in which their implications may change in the present both in radical and subtle ways provides insights into different types of social suffering and, as Lock would remind us, into variant biological experiences of disease.

THE POLITICS OF STRUGGLE AND ENGAGEMENT: PROBLEMATIZING NOTIONS OF BIOSOCIALITY AND GLOBAL BIOLOGICAL CITIZENSHIP

Lora-Wainwright's research shows that people's fundamental conceptions of cancer are shaped by history and by political motivations as realized in response to local, national and even global developments. But people do more than respond to structural forces, they use cancer as a way to think about and protest the conditions under which they live. In that sense, talk about cancer is often politicized and employed to make claims, struggle for rights, and protest labeling and stigma. As a group comes together around cancer-related issues, their collective as well as individual identifications may draw upon traditional frameworks such as gender, kinship, ethnicity and religion, or these may intersect with emerging forms of sociality rooted in emerging biomedical categories in novel ways.

Martha Balshem's 1993 book, *Cancer in the Community*, provides an example of the former. She documents struggles that play out along lines of social class and ethnicity in an inner-city Philadelphia neighborhood she calls Tannerstown, where white working-class community members of Polish descent often resisted the attempts of health educators and medical personnel—representatives of the professional, middle class—to attribute the cause of their cancers to poor lifestyle choices such as smoking and unhealthy diets. The residents felt they were being blamed and stigmatized, not so much for having cancer, as for being of an inferior social class and ethnicity. Balshem writes that "with regard to lifestyle and health, working-class people in particular are often judged as lacking" (p. 6). When health educators labeled the Polish diet as high fat and judged it negatively, community members reacted with anger. They correctly perceived that the medical establishment equated good health with the elimination of traditional lifestyles and beliefs in exchange for adherence to scientific pronouncements. Her informants responded by tempting health educators to eat tasty, Polish dishes at public meetings and by telling "defiant ancestor" stories about their relatives who had lived long and healthy lives despite smoking and drinking (1993, pp. 80–83). They also constructed an alternative explanatory narrative noting that their inner-city neighborhood, an official cancer hot spot, was surrounded by three chemical factories and suggested the life in a heavily polluted environment was more responsible for high cancer rates than personal lifestyle choices. Balshem points out that the maintenance of a rebellious consciousness based on ethnic and class identities was an attempt by the residents of Tannerstown to demonstrate the value of their lives and of their community, a way to claim the moral high ground (p. 87), echoing the concerns with demonstrating morality expressed by Lora-Wainwright's Chinese informants.

Around the time of Balshem's work, Paul Rabinow (1992, 1996) put forward the term *biosociality* to refer to aspects of biological nature, as revealed by science, and how these become the basis for new types of sociality. For example, emergent diagnostic technologies for genetic testing can create social difference and social groupings giving rise to new types of individual identities based upon shared biological statuses. Thus people diagnosed with specific diseases often form groups to exchange information, advocate for research and even to socialize. Similarly, therapeutic technologies, as Whyte (2009) points out, can form the basis for biosociality as in the case of support groups for people who have had mastectomies or transplants (p. 10).

Anthropologists have taken up the challenge to study emergent forms of biosociality and to explore how older categories of classification inform or exist in tension with new kinds of biological identities (e.g., Gibbon & Novas, 2007). In her chapter for this volume, Nancy Burke writes that ethnicity in particular remains under-theorized in this literature, particularly with regard to how it intersects with and influences (or is influenced by) immigrant status and medically underserved patient groups. She draws on ethnographic work with a Filipina community organization in the San Francisco area to show how its original purpose, to serve the needs of low-income immigrants and seniors of Filipino origin, shifted in response to material constraints. As Burke notes, many community groups compete against one another for scarce funding to continue their programs. When this particular group was asked to participate in a research study related to breast cancer and found an opportunity to apply for breast-cancer related funding, aspects of the mission and their activities had to change. Yet members and leaders struggled with changing from a more general ethnic affiliation to a narrower biosocial one. In the process, the women's conceptions of cancer and their roles related to health began to alter. Burke contends that the responsibility of knowing oneself biomedically in this biosocial paradigm is a new form of labor expected of everyone. Yet the group also resisted the biosocial. The leader continued to include survivors and nonsurvivors suffering from various types of cancer as well as from other health conditions such as diabetes. This leader emphasized the importance of Filipino identity and stated that segmenting members by type of disease was artificial. Burke concludes that thinking through biosociality in relation to ethnicity in cases such as this provides important insights into the very active and pervasive ways ethnicity shapes and informs support and care in the current moment.

Macdonald's description of the charity activities of breast cancer survivors in India provides a contrasting example. In an area where cancer is feared and stigmatized, women do not wish to admit to having the disease and have no interest in forming collective groups based on shared biosociality. Yet many still need information and someone to inspire hope. Macdonald shows how some volunteer survivors are developing novel forms for providing support based upon existing cultural traditions such as the aesthetics of vision as contextualized within the Hindu religion without creating groups organized around a biosocial category.

Alternatively, as Livingston's (2012) work documents in Botswana, where cancer is a low national priority and facilities and resources from the state are in short supply, people may not receive a diagnosis until they are close to death. In these extreme circumstances, there are no survivors who live long enough after treatment to form biosocial groups and there is no impetus for others to lobby the public sector for funding because little is available. Identifications based on kinship predominate as individual patients rely on their families to help them navigate the system to find diagnoses, secure drugs to relieve pain and confront death (see also Mulemi's chapter in this volume).

In a 1996 essay, Rabinow noted that older cultural categories have as much potential to be reinforced in relation to biosocial trajectories as novel modes of identity have of being created, but he does not specify what conditions might lead to one outcome versus another. Clearly, in areas where certain ethnic or class groups are discriminated against generally and live marginal lives in poverty, they may be reluctant to take on another stigmatizing identity rooted in illness, especially if they perceive they are being blamed for being victims. Moreover, as Roberts (2008) argues, the theory of biosociality implies the existence of a state that is stable and that can distribute desirable social welfare benefits (p. 93). If people have nothing to gain or lack the biocapital to organize, there may be little impetus for the formation of biosocial groupings. Gregg's (2003) work on cervical cancer in a favela slum in northeastern Brazil illustrates these observations. While the community has one of the highest rates of cervical cancer in the world, most women lack access to basic medical services. Because everyday existence under such extreme poverty is precarious, many women trade sex for favors from men to survive. Yet when they do contract cancer, health officials blame them for having led immoral lives. Gregg found, paradoxically, that while the women affected refused to let others know they had cancer for fear of negative gossip, they did not privately or publicly resist the stigmatizing discourse of health officials. Instead, they embraced these explanations and blamed themselves for having contracted the disease. In so doing, Gregg maintains that the women were able to emphasize continuity and mediate the disruption that cancer had on their lives (p. 78). Not surprisingly, in this community no biosocial groups existed and no one identified as a cancer victim or survivor. But the women did pursue treatment aggressively because they viewed the aftereffects of radiation, which made sexual activity difficult, as positive because it made them *pure* or *like virgins* again and therefore erased any potential biosocial stigma (79).

Aureliano's contribution to this volume documents the ambivalence that can occur for individuals caught between fears of stigma and biomedical prescriptions based on biosocial identifications. She studied two groups of breast cancer survivors from middle and working class families in a Brazilian city. She found that most women wanted to avoid stigma by returning to their chores as homemakers or to the work place immediately after surgery in order to preserve a sense of normality and keep others from finding out that they had cancer. In so doing, they emphasized the management and usefulness of their bodies as a way to normalize the experiences of everyday life after treatment (see also Manderson, 1999b for similar findings from Australia) and as a way to invert and challenge the dominant discourses in Brazil, which emphasized female sexuality as the core of identity. Their physicians, however, urged the women to rest and take it easy and instructed them to put their own health needs before those of their families. Aureliano shows that these survivors rejected a biosocial identification that they felt reduced them to a breast. Instead, they emphasized the importance of the whole person and viewed carrying on with their responsibilities at home and work as a sign of their strength. They also questioned the medical view that their needs should come before those of their families and placed greater priority on their identities as wives, mothers and daughters than as patients. Aureliano's example, like the case analyzed by Burke, demonstrates that family dynamics, material realities and the constraints imposed by government aid and private charity funding often affect the ways in which biosocial identities are established or attenuated, creating conflicts for individuals as they attempt to adjust their own self-identifications and images.

In addition, both the structure and ideology of a national health system can further influence the move toward or away from biosocial identifications. Sarradon-Eck's chapter in this volume examines the reasons why a psychosomatic model for the etiology of cancer predominates among middle- and upper-class French patients and many health professionals. The French have a system of universal access to health care and one of the best medical systems in the world. Yet this system does not promote patient involvement. Cancer patients in France, unlike those in other countries, do not organize for collective action and do not form social groupings based upon biosocial factors. Jeannine Coreil (2010) has proposed that the lack of cancer support groups in France may be related to a number of factors including an authoritarian, paternalistic medical system and a monopolistic national cancer organization *(La Ligue Contre le Cancer)*, an assumption of family responsibility for patient support, a socialist emphasis on sameness that undermines special programs for subpopulations such as cancer victims, an ethos of dependency on the state to meet health needs, and cancer patients' feelings of guilt and isolation that preclude activism. As a result, Sarradon-Eck contends that patients seek to avoid the attempts of health officials to blame them for poor lifestyle choices. By framing the etiological story of cancer around personal psychological traumas, patients are able to render the amorphous sense of social distress experienced in postmodern France intelligible and controllable.

Whereas theories of biosociality are premised upon the existence of a stable nation state (Roberts, 2008), many forces of communication and commerce are operating today at the supranational level. Rose and Novas (2004) refine Petryna's (2002) notion of *biological citizenship* to explore the connections made between biology and self-identity in these global spaces. They propose that in the global market place where new biomedical technologies and treatments are traded, people are increasingly made up not as citizens with rights and duties toward the nations in which they live but as biological consumers. Anthropologists have examined the ethical issues surrounding the outsourcing of clinical trials by pharmaceutical companies in the search for treatment-naïve populations in other parts of the world (Abadie, 2010; Fisher, 2006, 2009; Petryna, 2005, 2009).

Gibbon's chapter in this volume looks more specifically at the outsourcing of research as Western geneticists seek to collaborate with colleagues in Brazil to test for the distribution of genetic susceptibility to breast cancer in a wider segment of the population. In the Brazilian context, Gibbon reports that research becomes caught up with the constitution of clinical needs, rights and care. She conducted fieldwork in three urban locales and interviewed not only patients but providers and scientists as well. She found that genetic services were not part of the Brazilian public health system and hence operated in an interstitial space. Oncologists and scientists in Brazil were interested in figuring out the contribution of genetic risk to the rising rates of breast cancer in the country. They viewed collaboration with foreign institutions as a resource for finding these answers and for the development of better cancer prevention. Although free access to health care is defined as a basic right in the Brazilian constitution, in reality there are stark inequities within the system. As a result, many other people recruited for genetic testing viewed their participation as a way to access basic health services through identification as part of families predisposed to cancer. Thus for some, biosocial identifications emerged in an attempt to gain resources, but the impetus to define biological citizenship in this way was coming from the outside not from within these communities (see also, Rose & Novas, 2004).

These identifications, moreover, are beginning to transform the way that the question of prevention is unfolding in Brazilian cancer care. As Biehl and Petryna (2011) have documented, thousands of Brazilians from different social classes are now effectively suing the government for the right to health care resources as predicated on the constitutional commitment to access for all. Gibbon includes examples of patients without private insurance bringing letters from attorneys into clinics to demand genetic testing from the government as a *right* of public access. She notes that the phenomenon of patient litigants in the context of cancer genetics may put increasing pressure on the state to incorporate these tests as part of the public provision of health care. Hence the perception of the possibility of *damaged biology* (Petryna, 2002) is emerging as the basis for making citizenship claims under conditions of inequity and uncertainty.

Gibbon concludes by noting that participation in transnational and clinical trials research is embedded in complex structures of inequality and power that work to exploit as much as to aid the people involved. Her case study raises important questions about the multiple effects of global health partnerships explored elsewhere (see Beihl & Petryna, 2013; Crane, 2010, 2013; Janes & Corbett, 2009), such as who ultimately benefits from such relationships? Is the research relevant to addressing the needs of local researchers *and* participants? Does obtaining resources from research divert national governments from assuming responsibility for their share of basic care to meet human needs?

SUFFERING, THE MORALITY OF CARE AND SHIFTING DEFINITIONS OF PATIENTHOOD

Many of the authors in this collection engage experiences of cancer at the interstices of the body, community, and the various contexts in which suffering and care occur. In 2001, Frank argued that the inner sense of suffering is, to a certain extent, "unspeakable," and therefore our efforts to depict suffering in academic accounts of human experience are doomed to failure. Yet, as Hallowell (2006) eloquently contends, it can be argued that the meaning of suffering rests in public criteria, shared linguistic and nonlinguistic signs, what cannot be shared is irrelevant. Clearly, the experience of cancer is both personal and social. Because suffering extends beyond the biological experience of pain to encompass the anguish of lives disrupted, horizons cut short and intimate connections severed, anthropologists argue that it is vital to understand how patienthood and suffering are defined cross-culturally in order to situate and map the contexts in which suffering occurs and who it affects. Moreover, it is also vital to analyze the role of family and friends as caregivers and supports throughout the illness experience and during death because, as Livingston (2012) writes, caregiving "is at once deeply personal and deeply social, and it is a vital practical matter, crucial to patient well-being and survival" (p. 96).

Biomedicine as practiced in the global north privileges the individual patient as both sufferer and decision maker (Balshem, 1993, pg. 115). Yet analysts have pointed out that in many other parts of the world, family units are enmeshed in the dynamics of illness treatment and it can be difficult to determine the boundaries of patienthood. In her chapter, Bright writes about women diagnosed with breast cancer in India and the factors that influence their decisions to undergo treatment. She cites the work of scholars like Cohen (1998) to engage with previous anthropological research on the existence of a familial self in India, a self that is more relational than autonomous (Roland, 1987). Unlike Roland, who argues that the familial self develops from hierarchical relationships within the extended family, Bright argues for more specificity, showing that the relational self develops from and within local and transnational relationships necessary to enact and seek cancer care. For Indian women, a diagnosis of breast cancer is deeply upsetting and stigmatizing in the larger community. Bright shows that many women do not want to undergo treatment for fear that their illness will impinge upon the welfare of the family if they are unable to fulfill their household duties afterward or if treatment costs limit resources needed by others. Alternatively, Bright reports, when family members learn of a woman's problem, they are often the ones to insist upon treatment, making the decision on behalf of the patient, a decision she feels compelled to carry out because of these interdependent relationships. These relations of dependency and care extend across national boundaries when family members engaging in migrant labor in the Persian Gulf region send funds home to help relatives secure treatment. Alternatively, those who become ill while working abroad often return home to seek care because family is the unit to provide the assistance needed with decisions and recovery. Therefore, Bright concludes, relationships structure all forms of care in ways that blur the boundaries between things like home and hospital. Even when these spaces may seem to be at odds, such as when care is performed at home through an exchange based on kinship, whereas care in medical centers is purchased through the market, they do not operate in separate ontological or therapeutic worlds.

More importantly, she argues, crucial to care and how it is enacted is love. Women's narratives reveal love to be something more than an emotional impulse or show of solidarity. Bright proposes that what this love looks like is a complex scenario of mutual persuasion and regard, embedded in norms of kinship. Love is *like care*, but with a key distinction. Love is the place where individual and cultural aspects of relationships *meet* and make care tenable.

Anthropologists have recently turned their attention to how care and health are defined and understood by differently positioned individuals and political systems as well as the implications of such definitions. Brada (2011, p. 286) asks how "some places, people, and health inequalities fall under the purview of 'global health' while others do not?" and, subsequently, what effects follow from such a delineation? When both global and national governmental structures lay the care of cancer patients at the feet of families and communities, what are the implications of taking up this burden?

Benson Mulemi's chapter in this volume shows how caregiving is a necessity for family members in Kenya because the government has few facilities for cancer treatment and a shortage of trained doctors and medications. In rural areas, extended families and kin groups must work together to secure the necessities for a patient's survival. Families assist with navigating the different levels of referral in the health system, provide material support and physical care for the patient during the help-seeking process, and emotional support once the patient is admitted for cancer treatment. Because patients are usually diagnosed with late stage disease when little can be done for them medically, Mulemi finds that they are often sent home to rest or receive supportive care. At that point, family and kin assume total responsibility for the dying. In such situations of extreme need, these family groups work together to assist the patient rather than one individual being appointed and recognized as a caregiver with a limited role, and they see rendering assistance as part of the obligation of kinship rather than caring for cancer as a specialized task.

Although research on informal caregiving in the United States has increased over the last decade (Bee, Barnes & Luker, 2009; Harding, List, Epiphaniou & Jones, 2012; Osse, Vernooij-Dassen, Schade & Grol, 2006), few scholars have examined the dynamics of informal caregiving for those dying of cancer in other cultural contexts. Luxardo, in her chapter for this volume, turns the lens to look at this issue from the perspective of the caregivers themselves, to focus on what she calls, "the dark side of caregiving." She observed and interviewed caregivers of cancer patents in Argentina who were within six months of death and receiving palliative care or hospice care at home. She found that caregivers did not always choose their roles voluntarily. Because the Argentine medical system, a hybrid of public and private care in a middle-resource nation, lacked the facilities and resources to provide for the terminally ill, it was assumed they would die at home and that families would assume the burdens of care. Yet women, mainly wives or daughters, made up the majority of caregivers because culturally it was widely accepted that they would take on these roles as natural parts of their domestic duties. Many of the women, however, experienced great stress as they alone had to perform a variety of tasks for which they were largely unprepared. These included handling the physical needs of the patient as well as the administration of medications, managing the patient's emotional distress and handling the complex family dynamics that surrounded death. Not surprisingly, many felt resentment and frustration that remained often unvoiced but sometimes carried out in passive/aggressive strategies of patient neglect, and many experienced exhaustion because they also had to work or manage households while serving as caregivers. Others felt burdened to be there at the moment of death and to make sure it was a meaningful experience; yet for many patients, severe complications made hospitalization necessary. When patients died alone in the hospital, caregivers carried enormous guilt afterward. Luxardo concludes by arguing for a more nuanced and balanced view of the caregiver-patient relationship. Rather than being seen as sick and in need of counseling, caregivers should be viewed as unpaid laborers in dire need of practical support from the state. The stories recounted in Luxardo's work illustrate embedded practicalities and the value of listening to, and recording, people's "most pressing and ordinary concerns" (Biehl & Petryna, 2013).

Not only is the experience of suffering a social one, shared with intimates, the nature of how suffering is defined is also socially constructed. As Mulemi documents in this volume, rural Kenyans do not privilege cancer as producing more intense or more significant suffering than any of the other misfortunes experienced in daily life. Livingston (2012) writes that most families in Botswana have seen relatives die from HIV/AIDS and all manner of other accidental and infectious diseases. In these situations, where disease is widespread and adequate medical is lacking, pain is cited by 64% of terminally ill patients as their biggest problem (p. 264). Similarly, Murray, Grant & Kendall (2003) find that cancer patients in the Meru South district of Kenya have considerable unmet physical needs and that pain dominates their experiences of the disease. Governments in Kenya and Botswana do not prioritize pain relief and pain management is seen as a luxury; therefore, in many parts of rural Africa, patients want and need pain control but face the reality of a home death without either.

Alternatively, as Murray et al. (2003) note, African patients do not die alone. They are surrounded by kin and neighbors who help them with psychological and spiritual support that gives them emotional comfort in the hour of death. These findings parallel those of an earlier study by Bennett (1999) in rural northeast Thailand. There too, the terminally ill were sent home to die without access to pain medication. While patients were comforted by the proximity of kin, including senior relatives who slept in the house with them, Bennett notes that the taboo on talking about cancer and death often left relationship issues unresolved and patients and families lacked closure (p. 401).

Murray et al. (2003) document similar experiences among Scottish cancer patients but for different reasons. Scotland is a developed nation that provides free primary and secondary health care and a comprehensive social security system. Cancer patients can expect a hospital or hospice death with excellent medical care and access to sophisticated pain management. Yet many fear death and in the absence of family or others with whom to voice distress, they experience great but often unvoiced suffering. Lawton (2000) studied hospice patients in the United Kingdom and found that their greatest fear was "a drawn-out period of dependency, decline and social disengagement prior to death" (p. 171). She suggests that existential fears in the global north have shifted from being about death itself to being about the process of dying, and the professionalization of death care often leaves patients with no means of expressing these fears and little emotional or spiritual support.

Harris takes up these themes in her chapter for this volume. She explores how death and dying are talked about, managed and experienced in Scotland, noting that dying is hidden, and its meaning is privatized. The terminally ill often feel lonely and isolated, she writes, cut off from family and friends, and unable to talk about their fears of dying with anyone. Unlike the cancer nurses Livingston (2012, pp. 111–112) described in Botswana who expend great energy to create a warm, spiritual environment of the cancer ward, the goal of which is to humanize the patient, hospice workers in the United Kingdom are more emotionally distanced from the mental and emotional needs of patients. Reflecting on her personal experience caring for a family member with cancer and conducting research in a hospice setting, Harris recounts her own "profound deafness" when she simply did not hear the attempts of one informant to broach these topics. She notes that inadvertently she and others often foreclosed the possibilities for these conversations, causing hidden suffering for patients. Harris concludes that many in the postmodern world feel ill equipped to provide comfort and make sense of the incomprehensible in a secularized era so they simply do not hear the voices of those who wish to embark on new scripts.

Sarradon-Eck's chapter for this volume reflects a sense of hidden suffering among French cancer patients. High levels of uncertainty connected to the stresses of contemporary life contribute to their desire to pinpoint the causes of cancer and take actions to prevent recurrence. Many adopt a psychosomatic model, locating the etiology of cancer in psychological causes, including psychic traumas. Increasingly, these middle-class and affluent patients turn not to the French medical system but to alternative therapists such as the practitioners of the New German medicine or bio-decoding for help with uncovering the source of these traumas in order to prevent recurrence. Sarradon-Eck argues that the assertion that psychological causes are to blame for cancer enables patients to regain control over the management of the disease and over their day-to-day lives, enabling them to decrease uncertainty about prognosis and reduce anxiety and suffering.

Often suffering is the product of imagined losses, frequently social in nature. Cancer patients may imagine what their deaths will do to the people left behind or alternatively fear that they will die before having a chance to forge social relationships and continue family lines into the future. Hallowell's (2006) work on genetic risk and ovarian cancer illustrates the former. In interviews with women who tested positive for genetic risk for ovarian cancer in the United States, she sought to understand how they made decisions about whether or not to take action on risk and pursue annual screening or prophylactic surgery. She found that many had witnessed firsthand the deaths of other female relatives and could provide graphic accounts of the pain and suffering that illness and death had caused family members. To avoid inflicting a similar fate on their families, some women sought to be proactive. Others feared that death from cancer would terminate their social relationships and cause their spouses and children untold suffering into the future. These women too chose to be proactive in treatment so that their perceived familial obligations would not go unmet in the future. While many of them suffered the anguish of knowing they were at risk of a deadly disease, their decisions emphasized the imagined risk of social loss and emotional pain they projected onto close family members.

In her chapter for this volume, Karen Dyer reports that young adult cancer patients in Puerto Rico suffer when they discover, often after having undergone cancer treatment, that their future fertility is likely impaired. She documents the complex relationship between infertility due to cancer treatment, access to assisted reproductive technologies (ART), and cultural understandings of family and motherhood. As Dyer points out, children are highly valued in Puerto Rico. Yet few oncologists alert young cancer patients to the possibilities of freezing eggs or sperm in advance of treatment. She explores the reasons behind these silences on the part of professionals and proposes that both professional socialization and the complex history of dependency relations with the United States are involved. Most Puerto Rican specialists are trained professionally in the practice of oncology as it exists in the United States. As a result, providers prioritize treatment at all costs, with the preservation of life, not quality of life, as the ultimate goal. Therefore, oncologists in her study spent much more time discussing the side effects of hair loss and nausea than infertility. She explains that oncologists fear that if patients know about infertility risks, they might choose to delay or forego certain curative treatments.

Dyer also explores the history of sterilization of Puerto Rican women resulting from a eugenics logic that pervaded Western public health and development programs throughout the 20th century. Dyer postulates that this logic informs providers' assumptions that women who already have children do not need to have more, and thus do not need to learn about, or have access to, ART. In addition, access to ART services is limited and costly in Puerto Rico. Dyer finds that practitioners often make assumptions about the inability of patients to afford these options and thus omit discussions of them during consultations for treatment. Yet patients also interpret this lack of disclosure in the context of colonial history and fear that medical professionals are once again conspiring to keep down births or making judgments about who merits the opportunity to reproduce and who does not.

TRANSNATIONALISM, BIOMEDICAL TRAVEL AND DISCIPLINED BODIES

Dyer's work highlights how treatment protocols and expectations for care travel from US medical centers to Puerto Rican cancer clinics. Other contributors to this volume detail the movement of research protocols via international partnerships (Gibbon), the travel of biomedical discourses of biology, risk and disease across national boundaries (Bright, Lora-Wainwright, Sarradon), and the sometimes continuous and arduous travel of patients seeking appropriate care (Armin, Bright, Burke, Macdonald, Mulemi). In a globalizing world, ideas and practices spread rapidly, acting to erase the power and borders of nation states. On the other hand, as Gastaldo, Gooden and Massaquoi (2005) argue, the unprecedented movement of people across the globe is better defined as *transnationalism*, a process anchored in the experience of living between two or more countries. Therefore, they write, transnationalism is framed on territoriality and based on processes of cultural identity and difference, self and otherness, and the production of negotiated social spaces (2005, p. 1). Nowhere is this conjunction of global and transnational forces more apparent than in the arena of health care.

Much of the existing literature on transnational medical travel focuses on *medical tourism*, a phenomenon of the wealthy classes in the global north, sometimes referred to as "medical exiles" (Kangas, 2010), who seek more affordable health care in the global south (Ackerman, 2010; Aizura, 2010; Mazzaschi, 2011; Sobo, 2009). In some cases, such medical travel is a "pragmatic solution to limited insurance coverage and high prices" (Dalstrom, 2012, p. 163) sought by lower-income residents of high-resource nations. In their work among Mexican immigrants who return to Mexico for health care, Horton and Cole (2011) illustrate the ways in which such medical travel allows for class transformation. Medicaid dependents in the United

States, for example, become privileged users of the private health care system in Mexico, a system that they would have been unable to access previously as full-time residents of that country.

Increasingly, medical tourism is also practiced in the resource-poor nations of the global south, when the very wealthy are able to seek care for conditions such as cancer at state of the art facilities in the United States and Europe. Occasionally, these travels lead, as Moe, Pappas and Murray (2007) document for Jordan, to collaborative efforts to improve cancer facilities in the sending nation, but more often than not, the majority continue to lack access to adequate care for cancer in those countries (Whittaker, Manderson & Cartwright, 2010). People with the ability to travel, moreover, shop between and even within countries for the best services. Ellison (2014) chronicles the rise of *amenity wards* in the Tanzanian medical system, which once espoused heath care as a right of citizenship. In an effort to generate revenue from patients and integrate for-profit care into the system, these wards provide those with the financial means to purchase insurance access to higher quality care than is open to the rest of the population leading to increasing levels of biomedical stratification.

Nonetheless, as Livingston (2012) writes, people of all socioeconomic strata may attempt to cross boundaries for health care when it is a necessity. She documents the existence of an uneven regional landscape in health care in southern Africa that to a certain extent operates as a zero-sum game. In the past, patients with complicated cancers were sent to the Mpilo hospital in Zimbabwe for treatments unavailable in Botswana. By 2006, however, the economic collapse of Zimbabwe led to the ultimate failure of that health care system (p. 177). Practitioners fled, and faced with the lack of medications and services and long waits for care, those patients who could travel attempted to do so. The more recent recovery at Mpilo hospital, moreover, has been built on the privatization of services resulting in a further divide between those who can afford insurance and those who cannot.

In her chapter for this volume, Julie Armin investigates a different type of medical travel, one driven by necessity when transnational migrants are denied access to basic services in their new countries of residence. She conducted research with undocumented Mexican immigrants in the US state of Arizona where a number of recent laws have restricted the services open to them, broadened the powers of police to pursue illegal immigrants, and required federal health workers to report anyone who revealed that they were in the United States illegally. Those who failed to do so, moreover, were threatened with hefty fines.

Nonetheless, Armin documents how many local Arizona providers and charities spent years building cross-border relationships with the staff of a Mexican oncology clinic five hours distant and actively encouraged and assisted undocumented women without insurance or access to Medicaid funds to travel back to Mexico to receive affordable cancer treatment. The Mexican consulate in Arizona also assisted them with enrollment in the Mexican public health insurance program prior to their departures. However, the increasing militarization of the border in response to waves of anti-immigration fears has made travel for care dangerous, and many undocumented women fear that they may never be able to return to their families and jobs in the United States if they do travel back to Mexico. Armin's study examines the complicated strategies that these women and the administrators and providers of health services employ to find cancer care in contested social spaces.

A key element supporting transnational medical travel is the circulation of currency in the global market. In Kristin Bright's contribution, remittances are often sent from transnational workers in Dubai back to Kerala, India, to pay for cancer treatments for relatives. Yet currency is not the only factor of importance. As Gastaldo, Gooden and Massaquoi (2005) contend, trans-nationalism and decisions to travel are also rooted in processes of cultural identity and difference. For example, Bright documents the case of a young Indian woman working in Abu Dhabi when she was diagnosed with breast cancer. After consulting with family, she traveled back to Kerala for a second opinion and made the decision to leave her work in order to stay at home with family to receive her treatments. As Bright notes, in the Indian context, migration is often a financial necessity, but the importance of the relational self as constituted within the family is an emotionally salient factor in deci-sions about care. Similarly, in Armin's study, women's decisions about where to seek cancer care often hinged more on issues of family and belonging than on what would be most financially beneficial, in some cases opting to go without treatment altogether rather than to leave their homes behind.

Many of the world's peoples move across borders for reasons other than health; they may be seeking better economic opportunities, fleeing violence and political persecution, or involuntarily leaving war-torn areas. As these groups cross borders, they often become structurally vulnerable, stigma-tized and discriminated against for their status as outsiders. Inevitably large scale or ongoing relocations lead to debates within the receiving nations about whether or not transnational migrants deserve the rights and ben-efits accorded native citizens. In the early part of the 20th century in the United States, for example, waves of immigrants from Europe were met with fear and distrust by the residents of the large cities in which these groups settled. Facing increasing outbreaks of infectious diseases for which no cures could be found, Americans scapegoated immigrants as repositories of disease and stereotyped them as lazy, dirty, immoral and criminal. Veena Das (2001) points out that "threats of new diseases create anxieties that can be expressed through a political geography of blame not only in the popular discourse but also in the scientific discourse" (p. 9). Not surprisingly, the blame and stigma attached to immigrants for the spread of disease was part of the impetus behind both the early US public health and sanitation cam-paigns to clean up immigrant slums and the eugenics movement to restrict births among these supposedly inferior foreign populations.

The linkage of disease to fears about immigration resurfaced in the 1980s with the rise and spread of the AIDS epidemic and more recently with fears about immigrants transmitting Ebola into the United States and Europe. Yet there is also evidence that the fears associated with immigrants are shifting in the global north (Bloch & Schuster, 2002). The generalized sense of anxiety and uncertainty stemming from the global financial crisis and the unprecedented pace of technological change has focused public debate less on the threat of immigrants as the carriers of disease and more on immigrants as competitors for jobs and state benefits, including health and welfare services, intended for native born citizens.

Movements to disenfranchise immigrant groups often hinge on restriction and control; surveillance becomes the watchword and goal of the state. In his chapter, "Discipline and Punish, Panopticism," Foucault (1977) describes the measures taken by a 17th century European town to control the plague. Basic to surveillance was the institution of a system of permanent registration that recorded the name, sex, age, birth and death dates and any illnesses or irregularities associated with inhabitants thereby giving the magistrates total control over medical care. Foucalt writes, "the relation of each individual to his disease and to his death passes through the repositories of power, the registration they make of it, the decisions they take on it" (1977, p. 198). Foucault traces the emergence of new technologies of power throughout the 18th and 19th centuries in Europe as the state attempted to control unruly populations through the exercise of discipline. Discipline, for Foucault, is pervasive and indirect, produced in and through institutions of power (e.g. schools, hospitals, the military, government structures, etc.), and accepted as natural by its subjects, both individuals and families. It is a physics or an anatomy of power, a technology (1977, p. 201).

Armin's chapter expands upon these insights to show how documents function not only to structure immigrant Mexican women's access to health care but also to naturalize their place in the US social and economic hierarchy. Initially, the need to prove eligibility with immigration/citizenship documents functions to open or close the gates of access to basic health services. Once women are labeled *undocumented*, they must either return to Mexico for cancer treatments or attempt to find safe spaces in the system where charitable sources of care exist. Ironically, Armin notes that a federally funded program, Well Woman in Arizona, offers low- and no-cost mammography and Pap smears to women without health insurance and confirmation of citizenship status is not required for participation. However, if an abnormality is detected, these women must enroll in Medicaid to receive treatment, which is a program restricted to permanent legal residents. The only other local option, Armin reports, is an annual grant of $100,000 from a US foundation administered through a clinic to support the treatment of undocumented women with breast cancer. In this negotiated space, the medical record takes on enormous importance. To qualify for consideration, women must demonstrate that they have a diagnosis for this particular type of cancer. As a result, Armin writes, medical documents have symbolic importance as they have the potential to mobilize human and financial resources around these women. Medical records also serve to locate women both geographically (where the records are housed) and in terms of the socioeconomic hierarchy.

Yet Armin points out that other documents come into play once a diagnosis is made. In order to qualify for these charitable funds for treatment and other small forms of local assistance and in order to be deemed eligible for sliding scale fee at clinics, these women must surrender numerous financial documents along with a picture ID. However, not every patient is willing to share their information because they lack trust in the system. Staff members too have an ambivalent view of the process. They understand the trust issues, but are caught in a time of financial constraint related to the high costs of care. As Armin notes, despite its humanitarian mission, the clinic does play a role as an agent for the state's auditing practices. Moreover, the state and the clinic jointly create powerful documents—bills—that are actionable and that act to establish organizational legitimacy. In an in-depth examination of one patient's situation, Armin shows how medical bills project expectations for a patient's behavior toward the local health care system and, in turn, shape the patient's own perceptions about the possibilities for future treatments. Armin concludes by arguing that documents of various types act to naturalize a person's subject position. Exposed to economic exploitation and cultural insults (see also, Quesada, Hart & Bourgois, 2011), these women become located in a particular place in the social hierarchy, which affects how they see themselves and leads them to accept such positions as natural.

The strong disciplining nature of documents, however, does not necessarily, as Armin writes, foreclose the possibilities of protest. Yet rather than objecting to the need for documents at all, many of the vulnerable instead contest issues about what is included or left out of them, especially attributions that they fear will cast blame, stigmatize or cause them to be seen as morally culpable for this own misfortunes. In so doing, they often indirectly challenge the authority of those in positions of power.

Martha Balshem (1993) presents a clear example of this type of protest in her analysis of one working-class woman's dispute with her husband's physician about the information contained in his medical record in Tannerstown, Pennsylvania. After a prolonged illness, the husband traveled among hospitals seeking answers. Ultimately he was diagnosed with lung cancer and notations were made in the medical chart that he was alcoholic and had a 22-year history of cigarette smoking. His wife confronted the physician in charge about her fears that this erroneous information would be used by medical personnel to conclude that her husband's lifestyle had caused his illness. She wanted this information removed and details added about a previous accident suffered on his job in a chemical factory along with years spent living in a heavily polluted neighborhood. As Lora-Wainwright notes in her chapter on the ambiguity of blame in rural China, contending forms of morality are constantly produced through negotiations about cancer etiology. Eventually, the wife succeeded in getting a handwritten note added to the margins of the record indicating that her husband drank less than a case of beer a week. But neither the official diagnosis nor the indictment of lifestyle factors was removed. Balshem concludes that the wife's ultimate struggle concerned the exclusion of her own voice from her husband's medical record, which everyone saw as the authoritative text on his illness and death (1993, p. 107). The physician's response that the wife was "concerned about the wrong things" is, as Balshem notes, a veiled moral judgment. Patients and their families are viewed as morally culpable if they do not stay within behavioral boundaries proscribed by biomedical authorities because they view patient compliance as the only way of assuring a cure.

So although the power of medical dominance does not determine the wife's thoughts and feelings, the medical record itself continues to minimize or discount the social, cultural and environmental contexts of disease, and hence her attempts to exert control over the meaning of her husband's death go unfulfilled. Balshem concludes that the root problem in the clinic is not one of communication but one of power (p. 124). Protests over documents are often protests about authority and class and the subtle forms through which they come into play.

Concern about how documents can categorize and define a person following a cancer diagnosis emerges as an important theme in Aureliano's contribution to this volume. Her research on working-class women in Brazil with breast cancer showed their strong desires to return to a normal state after surgery by resuming household chores and paid work so that others would be unaware that they had cancer. Yet many of these women were responsible for the support of families whereas others who worked outside the home often had difficulties returning to paid employment due to the physical effects of surgery. In order to survive, they had to claim rights to pensions and social security support from the state. Much like the women in Armin's study, documents were required in order to secure pensions on the basis of disability. Taking such a rights-based approach enabled some women to experience financial independence for the first time in their lives. The process of doing so, however, established documentary evidence of their disabled status and identified them publicly as cancer victims, undercutting their attempts to reassert normality and changing the way that others viewed them. As a result, their identification as cancer survivors was situationally dependent and loaded with moral overtones.

CONCLUSION AND OUTLINE FOR THE VOLUME

The chapters in this volume demonstrate Manderson's (1999a) contention that anthropologists have much to contribute to the transnational study of cancer. These fine-grained ethnographic studies show that debates about cancer etiology in all parts of the world reflect the political and social tensions of the times as well as local, cultural conceptions about morally desirable behavior. It is not surprising, therefore, that in this contemporary moment in the global north, the predominant biomedical explanatory system encoded in scientific practice emphasizes cancer as the result of individual genetic predispositions activated by autonomous lifestyle choices. In an increasingly fragmented and uncertain era, such a metaphorical model provides the illusion of control and the future promise of personalized medical therapies that might one day cure this dreaded disease (see Gibbon's chapter in this volume). Although biomedicine has accomplished much using this paradigmatic framework, it has been blind to the repeated observation over many decades that environmental and chemical contaminants are equally responsible for the rapid rise of cancers the world over. Moreover, a model that holds the individual responsible for choosing health often leads professionals and others to blame and stigmatize the victims of cancer for their presumed morally deficient lifestyle choices. Indeed, as the chapters in this volume show, many of the world's people are uncomfortable with these moral implications, especially when socioeconomic realities limit their abilities to choose healthy lifestyles or escape from contaminated sources of food, water and air. In the absence of alternatives, they struggle to assimilate biomedical explanations to local understandings and to protest the perceived power imbalances manifested in clinical settings.

The biomedical framework also essentializes the nature and experience of cancer itself. The models we employ to understand the unknown are drawn from analogies with the known. In the United States, Canada and Europe, as Bell (2014) documents, breast cancer, thanks to the tireless work of advocates and the politics of research funding, has become the standard against which the experience of all other cancers is assessed. Yet cancers vary in etiology, symptomology and prognosis, and those in the global north who suffer from cervical, lung and other more stigmatized conditions have fewer options for therapy and less public and private support, especially when others blame them for contracting the disease. Alternatively, inhabitants of the global south are disproportionately affected by cancers related to infectious agents, such as those of the cervix, liver and stomach, and are more likely to suffer occupational and environmental exposures to contaminants leading to rising rates of lung and bladder cancers as well as leukemias and lymphomas. This differential distribution of cancers and their comorbidity with a variety of other infectious agents results in dramatically variant symptomatic manifestations and disease outcomes than those suffered by breast cancer patients in the global north.

In addition, researchers have documented the prevalence of one overarching narrative about the ideal patient and cancer survivor in the global north, also largely based upon public perceptions of breast cancer activists. The hero-survivor is one who complies completely with biomedical treatments and fights against the odds to survive while maintaining a cheerful attitude.

Eventually, this ideal survivor comes to view cancer as a transformative, not a disruptive and tragic life experience (Coreil, Wilke & Pintado, 2004). The goals framed by this type of explanatory framework, moreover, emphasize the push for constant surveillance and screening in order to promote early detection and increase the likelihood of survival from cancer. Yet, as the volume authors demonstrate, such emphases are often premature in areas of the world where people lack access to basic health services and there is an absence of personnel and facilities to provide cancer treatments. Where late stage diagnosis is the norm, survivorship is not a category, and patients instead need basic pain medications and more palliative care. Nonetheless, as Harris' essay reminds us, the definition of a good death is culturally specific. For many in the global north, pain relief and professional care are not enough when emotional and spiritual support are lacking.

A true transnational approach to the study of cancer helps correct both the ethnocentric nature of many biomedical assumptions encoded in international health initiatives and to illuminate the particular needs of local populations living within highly diverse political, social and economic systems. Koplan et al. (2009) argue for the adoption of the term, *global health* instead of *international health* as a way to acknowledge that the developed world does not have a monopoly on good ideas and better approaches to the prevention and treatment of common diseases, healthy environments, and more efficient food production and distribution (p. 1994). Moreover, such a terminology shift, they argue, recognizes the possibilities for real partnerships, the pooling of experience and knowledge, and a two-way flow between developed and developing countries to address health challenges such as cancer. The chapters in this volume are an important first step in efforts to construct a transnational approach to the study of cancer and its effects both globally and locally.

The chapters in this volume are organized under two general headings. The first group (by Lora-Wainwright, Sarradon-Eck, Gibbon, Armin, Burke, and Macdonald) is located in the part "Structural Matters: Technologies of Disease, Risk and Management." These chapters outline cultural shifts, transformations and transitions in meanings of cancer, risk, patienthood, survivorship and care within and interacting with varying social structures. The uneven availability of cancer treatment, technology and post-treatment support emerges across these chapters, as does the impact of differing political economies on possibilities for each. Of particular emphasis is a consideration of how inequality, pollution, sociopolitical ideologies and their ethical undercurrents, are linked to conceptions of bodily disorder and situated worldviews. Contributors attempt to illuminate the underlying processes by which certain types of authoritative and embodied knowledge and therapeutic management are legitimated or contested with reference to scientific developments, standards of clinical care and community aspirations. They also attend to organized collectivities and knowledge-practices, as when cancer is addressed by peer-support groups and forms of alliance between patients, health professionals and funding organizations with diverse agendas for sociopolitical action, crafted on discourses of empowerment, rights and control. In effect, the authors in this part provide theoretical elaboration on responses to cancer as a global health problem and begin to dissect and rethink the intentions and repercussions of paradigms related to patient autonomy, health disparities, charity and clinical need.

The second set of chapters (Bright, Mulemi, Aureliano, Luxardo, Dyer, and Harris), organized under the heading "Cancer and the Sociality of Care: Intimacy, Support and Collective Burden-Sharing" engage experiences of cancer at the interstices of the body, community and the various contexts in which disease management and care occurs. Contributors track the negotiations and challenges that emerge as cancer becomes an issue of collective burden-sharing, often against a backdrop of socioeconomic inequalities and health policies that fail to provide adequate care and support. Individuals experiencing the disease as well as those caring for patients come to various confrontations with the public scripts of cancer and possible challenges to established identities. Crucial to understanding identity practices is a consideration of how the symbolic and social representations of the body and appropriate role behaviors in specific cultural environments impact the illness experience. Cancer patients often struggle to escape being defined by the disease yet paradoxically, when they give voice to concerns about disfigurement and death, others may be unwilling to hear, engage with or support them. Across the contributions in this part, intimacy emerges in different ways, both as an aspect of relational experience and as an embodied process. Building on these insights, authors point to the complexity of interactions between the afflicted, local health systems and those providing care as these shape people's perceptions of risk, ideas about appropriate therapeutic actions and ways of dealing with the psychosocial aspects of the disease.

The volume concludes with an afterword written by Lenore Manderson, editor of *Medical Anthropology* and a researcher of distinction in the field of global cancer care. Her comments draw attention to some of the key issues facing us in the future as well as to new directions and challenges for anthropological research on the transnational nature of cancer and its care.

REFERENCES

Abadie, R. (2010). *The professional guinea pig: Big Pharma and the risky world of human subjects.* Durham, NC: Duke University Press Books.

Ackerman, S. L. (2010). Plastic paradise: Transforming bodies and selves in Costa Rica's cosmetic surgery tourism industry. *Medical anthropology, 29,* 403–423.

Adams, V., Burke, N. J., & Whitmarsh, I. (2014). Slow research: Thoughts for a movement in global health. *Medical Anthropology, 33,* 179–197.

Aizura, A. Z. (2010). Feminine transformations: Gender reassignment surgical tourism in Thailand. *Medical Anthropology, 29,* 424–443.

Balshem, M. L. (1993). *Cancer in the community: Class and medical authority.* Washington, DC: Smithsonian Institution Press.

Bee, P. E., Barnes, P., & Luker, K. A. (2009). A systematic review of informal caregivers' needs in providing home-based end-of-life care to people with cancer. *Journal of Clinical Nursing, 18*, 1379–1393.

Bell, K. (2014). The breast-cancer-ization of cancer survivorship: Implications for experiences of the disease. *Social Science & Medicine, 110*, 56–63.

Bennett, E. S. (1999). Soft truth: Ethics and cancer in northeast Thailand. *Anthropology & Medicine, 6*, 395–404.

Biehl, J., & Petryna, A. (2011). Bodies of rights and therapeutic markets. *Social Research: An International Quarterly, 78*, 359–386.

Biehl, J., & Petryna, A. (Eds.). (2013). *When people come first: Critical studies in global health*. Princeton, NJ: Princeton University Press.

Bloch, A., & Schuster, L. (2002). Asylum and welfare: Contemporary debates. *Critical Social Policy, 22*, 393–414.

Brada, B. (2011). Not here. Making the spaces and subjects of "global health" in Botswana. *Culture, Medicine and Psychiatry, 35*, 285–312.

Brotherton, P. S., & Nguyen, V. K. (2013). Revisiting local biology in the era of global health. *Medical Anthropology, 32*, 287–290.

Burhansstipanov, L., Gilbert, A., LaMarca, K., & Krebs, L. U. (2001). An innovative path to improving cancer care in Indian country. *Public Health Reports, 116*, 424–433.

Burke, N. J. (2014). Local biologies and ecologies of screening: Tracing the aftereffects of the "Shanghai Study". *Anthropological Quarterly, 87*, 497–524.

Burke, N. J., Villero, O., & Guerra, C. (2012). Passing through meanings of survivorship and support among Filipinas with breast cancer. *Qualitative Health Research, 22*, 189–198.

Cohen, L. (1998). *No aging in India: Alzheimer's, the bad family, and other modern things*. Berkeley, CA: University of California Press.

Comaroff, J., & Comaroff, J. L. (2012). Theory from the South: Or, how Euro-America is evolving toward Africa. *Anthropological Forum, 22*, 113–131.

Coreil, J. (2010). Overview: Social support, education and advocacy. Unpublished Manuscript prepared for Wenner Gren Conference on Metaphors of Cancer, New Orleans, LA: November.

Coreil, J., Wilke, J., & Pintado, I. (2004). Cultural models of illness and recovery in breast cancer support groups. *Qualitative Health Research, 14*, 905–923.

Crane, J. T. (2010). Unequal "Partners": AIDS, academia, and the rise of global health. *Behemoth, 3*, 78–97.

Crane, J. T. (2013). *Scrambling for Africa: AIDS, expertise, and the rise of American global health science*. Ithaca, NY: Cornell University Press.

Dalstrom, M. D. (2012). Winter Texans and the re-creation of the American medical experience in Mexico. *Medical Anthropology, 31*, 162–177.

Das, V. (2001). *Stigma, contagion, defect: Issues in the anthropology of public health*. Paper presented at Stigma and Global Health: Developing a Research Agenda conference, Bethesda, Maryland. Retrieved from http://www.stigmaconference.nih.gov/FinalDasPaper.htm

Das, V., & Das, R. K. (2006). Pharmaceuticals in urban ecologies: The register of the local. In A. Petryna, A. Lakoff & A. Kleinman (Eds.), *Global pharmaceuticals: Ethics, markets, practices* (pp. 171–206). Durham: Duke University Press.

Del Vecchio Good, M. J., Good, B. J., Schaffer, C., & Lind, S. E. (1990). American oncology and the discourse on hope. *Culture, Medicine and Psychiatry, 14*, 59–79.

Edwards, L. (2013). *In the kingdom of the Sick: A social history of chronic illness in America*. New York, NY: Walker & Co.

Ellison, J. (2014). First-class health: Amenity wards, health insurance, and normalizing health care inequalities in Tanzania. *Medical Anthropology Quarterly, 28*, 162–181.

Fisher, J. A. (2006). Coordinating "ethical" clinical trials: The role of research coordinators in the contract research industry. *Sociology of Health & Illness, 28,* 678–694.

Fisher, J. A. (2009). *Medical research for hire: The political economy of pharmaceutical clinical trials.* New Brunswick: NJ: Rutgers University Press.

Foucault, Michel. (1977). Discipline and punish, panopticism. In A. Sheridan (Ed.), *Discipline and punish: The birth of the prison* (pp. 195–228). New York, NY: Vintage Books.

Frank, A. W. (2001). Can we research suffering? *Qualitative Health Research, 11,* 353–362.

Garrison, K. (2007) The personal is rhetorical: War, protest and peace in breast cancer narratives. *Disability Studies Quarterly, 27,* 114–118.

Gastaldo, D., Gooden, A., & Massaquoi, N. (2005). Transnational health promotion: Social well-being across borders and immigrant women's subjectivities. *Wagadu, 2,* 1–16.

Geertz, Clifford. (2007). "To exist is to have confidence in one's way of being": Rituals as model systems. In N. H. Angela, E. L. Creager, & M. N. Wise (Eds.), *Science without laws: Model systems, cases, exemplary narratives,* (pp. 212–224). Durham, NC: Duke University Press.

Gibbon, S., & Novas, C. (Eds.). (2007). *Biosocialities, genetics and the social sciences: Making biologies and identities.* London: Routledge.

Gordon, D. R. (1990). Embodying illness, embodying cancer. *Culture, Medicine and Psychiatry, 14,* 275–297.

Gordon, D. R., & Paci, E. (1997). Disclosure practices and cultural narratives: Understanding concealment and silence around cancer in Tuscany, Italy. *Social Science & Medicine, 44,* 1433–1452.

Gregg, J. L. (2003). *Virtually virgins: Sexual strategies and cervical cancer in Recife, Brazil.* Palo Alto, CA: Stanford University Press.

Hallowell, N. (2006). Varieties of suffering: Living with the risk of ovarian cancer. *Health, Risk and Society, 8,* 9–26.

Harding, R., List, S., Epiphaniou, E. & Jones, H. (2012). How can informal caregivers in cancer and palliative care be supported? An updated systematic literature review of interventions and their effectiveness. *Palliative Medicine, 26,* 7–22.

Horton, S., & Cole, S. (2011). Medical returns: Seeking health care in Mexico. *Social Science & Medicine, 72,* 1846–1852.

Jain, S. L. (2013). *Malignant: How cancer becomes us.* Berkeley, CA: University of California Press.

Janes, C. R., & Corbett, K. K. (2009). Anthropology and global health. *Annual Review of Anthropology, 38,* 167–183.

Jemal, A., Center, M. M., DeSantis, C., & Ward, E. M. (2010). Global patterns of cancer incidence and mortality rates and trends. *Cancer Epidemiology Biomarkers & Prevention, 19,* 1893–1907.

Kangas, B. (2010). Traveling for medical care in a global world. *Medical Anthropology, 29,* 344–362.

Koplan, J. P., Bond, T. C., Merson, M. H., Reddy, K. S., Rodriguez, M. H., Sewankambo, N. K., & Wasserheit, J. N. (2009). Towards a common definition of global health. *The Lancet, 373,* 1993–1995.

Lakoff, G., and Johnson, M. (1980*). Metaphors we live by.* Chicago, IL: University of Chicago Press.

Lawton, J. (2000). *The dying process: Patients' experiences of palliative care.* London: Taylor & Francis.

Livingston, J. (2012). *Improvising medicine: An African oncology ward in an emerging cancer epidemic.* Durham, NC: Duke University Press.

Lock, M. (1993). *Encounters with aging: Mythologies of menopause in Japan and North America.* Berkeley, CA: University of California Press.

Lock, M. (2001). The tempering of medical anthropology: Troubling natural categories. *Medical Anthropology Quarterly, 15,* 478–492.

Lock, M. (2013). The epigenome and nature/nurture reunification: A challenge for anthropology. *Medical Anthropology, 32,* 291–308.

Manderson, L. (1999a). Editorial; New perspectives in the anthropology on cancer control, disease and palliative care. *Anthropology & Medicine, 6,* 317–321.

Manderson, L. (1999b). Gender, normality and the post-surgical body. *Anthropology & Medicine, 6,* 381–394.

Mathews, H. F. (2000). Negotiating cultural consensus in a breast cancer self-help group. *Medical Anthropology Quarterly, 14,* 394–413.

Mathews, H. F. (2014). Cultural broker or collaborator? Lessons learned from breast cancer survivor groups in eastern North Carolina. *Practicing Anthropology, 36,* 16–21.

Mathews, H.F., Lannin, D.R., & Mitchell, J.P. (1994). Coming to terms with advanced breast cancer: Black women's narratives from Eastern North Carolina. *Social Science & Medicine, 38,* 789–800.

Mazzaschi, A. (2011). Surgeon and safari: Producing valuable bodies in Johannesburg. *Signs, 36,* 303–312.

McMullin, J., & Weiner, D. (2008). Introduction: An anthropology of cancer. In J. McMullin & D. Weiner (Eds.), *Confronting cancer: Metaphors, advocacy and anthropology* (pp. 3–27). Santa Fe, NM: School for Advanced Research Press.

Moe, J.L., Pappas, G., & Murray, A. (2007). Transformational leadership, transnational culture and political competence in globalizing health care services: A case study of Jordan's King Hussein Cancer Center. *Globalization and Health, 3,* 11–23.

Mukherjee, S. (2010). *The emperor of all maladies: A biography of cancer.* New York, NY: Simon and Schuster.

Mulemi, B. A. (2008). Patients' perspectives on hospitalization: Experiences from a cancer ward in Kenya. *Anthropology & Medicine, 15,* 117–131.

Murray, S. A., Grant, E., Grant, A., & Kendall, M. (2003). Dying from cancer in developed and developing countries: Lessons from two qualitative interview studies of patients and their careers. *British Medical Journal, 326,* 1–5.

Niewöhner, J. (2011). Epigenetics: Embedded bodies and the molecularisation of biography and milieu. *BioSocieties, 6,* 279–298.

Osse, B.H., Vernooij-Dassen, M.J., Schadé, E., & Grol, R.P. (2006). Problems experienced by the informal caregivers of cancer patients and their needs for support. *Cancer Nursing, 29,* 378–388.

Petryna, A. (2002). *Life exposed: Biological citizens after Chernobyl.* Princeton, NJ: Princeton University Press.

Petryna, A. (2005). Ethical variability: Drug development and globalizing clinical trials. *American Ethnologist, 32,* 183–197.

Petryna, A. (2009). *When experiments travel: Clinical trials and the global search for human subjects.* Princeton, NJ: Princeton University Press.

Pigg, S.L. (2013). On sitting and doing: Ethnography as action in global health. *Social Science & Medicine, 99,* 127–134.

Quesada, J., Hart, L.K., & Bourgois, P. (2011). Structural vulnerability and health: Latino migrant laborers in the United States. *Medical Anthropology, 30,* 339–362.

Rabinow, P. (1992). Artificiality and enlightenment: From sociobiology to biosociality. In J. Crary & S. Swinter (Eds.), *Zone 6: Incorporations.* New York, NY: Zone Press.

Rabinow, P. (1996). Artificiality and enlightenment: From sociobiology to biosociality. In P. Rabinow (Ed.), *Essays on the anthropology of reason* (pp. 91–111). Princeton, NJ: Princeton University Press.

Roberts, E.F.S. (2008). Biology, sociality and reproductive modernity in Ecuadorian *in- vitro* fertilization: The particulars of place. In S. Gibbon, & C. Novas (Eds.),

Biosocialities, genetics and the social sciences: Making biologies and identities (pp. 79–97). London: Routledge.

Roland, A. (1987). The familial self, the individualized self, and the transcendent self: Psychoanalytic reflections on India and America. *Psychoanalytic Review, 74,* 237–254.

Rose, N., & Novas, C. (2004). Biological citizenship. In A. Ong & S. Collier (Eds.), *Global assemblages: Technology, politics and ethics as anthropological problems* (pp. 439–463). London: Blackwell Publishing.

Saillant, F. (1990). Discourse, knowledge and experience of cancer: A life story. *Culture, Medicine & Psychiatry, 14,* 81–104.

Singer, M., & Baer, H. (2011). *Introducing medical anthropology: A discipline in action.* New York, NY: AltaMira Press.

Sobo, E. J. (2009). Medical travel: What it means, why it matters. *Medical Anthropology, 28,* 326–335.

Sontag, S. (1979). *Illness as metaphor.* New York, NY: Farrar, Straus and Giroux.

Thomas, D. B., Gao, D. L., Ray, R. M., Wang, W. W., Allison, C. J., Chen, F. L., . . . & Self, S. G. (2002). Randomized trial of breast self-examination in Shanghai: Final results. *Journal of the National Cancer Institute, 94,* 1445–1457.

Towghi, F. (2013). The biopolitics of reproductive technologies beyond the clinic: Localizing HPV vaccines in India. *Medical Anthropology, 32,* 325–342.

Whittaker, A., Manderson, L., & Cartwright, E. (2010). Patients without borders: Understanding medical travel. *Medical Anthropology, 29,* 336–343.

Whyte, S. R. (2009). Health identities and subjectivities. *Medical Anthropology Quarterly, 23,* 6–15.

Whyte, S. R., & Gibbon, S. (2009). Special edition for anthropology and medicine: Biomedical technology and health inequities in the global north and south. *Anthropology & Medicine, 16,* 97–103.

Part I
Structural Matters
Technologies of Disease, Risk and Management

1 The Ambiguity of Blame and the Multiple Careers of Cancer Etiologies in Rural China[1]

Anna Lora-Wainwright

INTRODUCTION

On October 19, 2004, I followed Erjie to her natal village to celebrate her father's 62nd birthday. I had lived with her, her husband and their daughter since June in Baoma village, Langzhong county (Sichuan Province) to carry out fieldwork on experiences of health, illness and health care in rural China. The occasion was particularly poignant. Erjie's father, who I would learn to call Gandie (literally meaning dry father, a concept akin to Godfather), had been diagnosed with esophagus cancer some weeks earlier. However, as is often the case, his family had not informed him. During the half-hour walk to her hometown up and down the hill and past dozens of vegetable plots, Erjie argued at length that repressed anger caused Gandie's cancer. She was so adamant that her father would recover if he could just stop getting angry that I started to doubt he had been diagnosed with cancer at all. Around 50 people attended his birthday party, but Gandie was clearly not in the mood for celebration. He ate nothing, paced the courtyard dressed in his best traditional silk shirt, a dark blue jacket reminiscent of revolutionary times, and a hat. He looked unsettlingly tense and restless, and seemed to be in pain.

Over the coming months and the years that followed Gandie's death, his family put forward a range of shifting explanations for Gandie's illness as they struggled to make sense of it. In doing so, they also reinforced their memories of Gandie as a moral subject and reconfigured their relationships to him and to each other. This chapter illustrates that the ways in which cancer is explained and experienced are historically rooted but also inextricably related to attributions of blame and efforts to live morally. It suggests that attention to political economy and cultural analysis must be combined with close narratives of human experience. It does so by describing how causes of cancer may be linked to wider political economic contexts but also to the microtemporal shifts in how cancer is understood by the sufferer and his or her family in the course of illness and after death. Causes blamed for cancer change over time, but they are mapped onto overlapping rather than distinct moral and political economies and articulate ambivalence about both past and present. Cancer raises questions over individual culpability (e.g., the sufferer was predisposed to easily lose his temper, or drank heavily), but it also presents a context through which family responsibilities are debated and past and current political economies are assessed. Different elements are embraced as explanations for cancer when it is morally desirable. Many of these elements allow ambiguity over who or what is blamed and in doing so they become sites for negotiating social relations and values. Villagers' multifaceted and situationally contingent narratives about cancer causality serve as a prism to explore what is at stake in the contemporary reform era.

This chapter is based on almost two years of ethnographic fieldwork in Baoma village, including 15 months in 2004–2005 and regular yearly visits since then. During all visits, I lived with Erjie and her family. Serendipity brought me to focus on cancer. After Gandie was diagnosed with the illness, I spent much of my fieldwork with him and his family, gaining a firsthand experience of how they made sense of cancer and coped with it. This overwhelming focus on one extended family enabled a deeper understanding of how explanations for cancer are generationally, historically and socially situated. I complemented this focus with a study of other local families affected by cancer and numerous conversations with neighbors and relatives of cancer sufferers. Whereas in-depth engagement with a single case illustrates the microhistorical changes in cancer etiology, participant observation among several local families spanning almost a decade allows a broader analysis of the wider social, political and economic forces that affected local approaches to cancer causality and its treatment. The combination of these methodological strategies is intended to produce a more nuanced portrayal of cancer that combines macrolevel forces and intimate individual and family experiences.

POLITICAL ECONOMY, CULTURAL ANALYSIS AND EXPERIENCE: "FIGHTING FOR BREATH"

Critical medical anthropology has long advocated attention to the political and economic forces that affect the distribution of suffering and care (see Singer & Baer, 1995). The concept of "structural violence" for instance highlighted the dangers of resorting to culture to understand suffering (Farmer, 2003). In a classic piece, Nancy Scheper-Hughes and Margaret Lock (1987) portrayed medical anthropology as divided between political economic and post-structuralist analyses (a division much of subsequent literature has endeavored to overcome) and emphasized the need to study the subjective lived experience of illness. Tackling this challenge, the concept of "social suffering" (Kleinman, Das & Lock, 1997) allows a study of suffering as intersubjective without reducing it to cultural analysis or economic or historical determinism. The recent attention to "subjectivity" (Biehl, Good & Kleinman, 2007) is similarly an effort to combine a study of lived experience with one of micro- and macropolitics and inequalities as they impact on individual lives. With these conceptual frameworks in mind, I approach cancer in contemporary rural China as inseparable from poverty and inequality but also from the frenetic industrialization and development of recent years. The ways in which villagers make sense of cancer articulate deep ambivalence to their collective suffering and physical hardship in the past, but also to the new challenges and injustice of the present. At the same time, close attention to experience highlights the intersubjective dimensions of suffering for the cancer patient and his or her family and the ways in which it unfolds over time.

My attention to what I call *fighting for breath* is intended as a semiotic framework to encompass everyday efforts to make sense of cancer and treat it. As stomach and esophagus cancers—the most common types of cancer in Langzhong—have until recently been understood with reference to their most obvious embodied effects, respectively as "vomiting illness" (*huishi bing*) and "choking or spitting illness" (*gengshi bing*), the expression is particularly pertinent. It is intended to encapsulate the physical, emotional and economic hardship presented by this most often fatal disease. The fight for breath is both a physical and a social struggle to maintain integrity and to ensure family and neighborly support. It is not only about fighting for survival but also about the search for a moral existence in contemporary China. What kinds of moral claims are implied by attributing cancer to hardship, diet or anger? The post-Mao period has been frequently described as a fall "from heaven to earth" (Croll, 1994), as uncivic, individualistic and immoral (Liu, 2000; Yan, 2003). By contrast, I examine how contending forms of morality are constantly produced through negotiations about cancer etiology.

The fight against cancer, then, is deeply bound to efforts not only to maintain health but also to debate one's position within the family and the local community. Langzhong villagers experience daily life as an incessant struggle to make ends meet, made all the more poignant by comparisons with a past when living costs were lower and with urbanites who have fared much more favorably during market reforms. Cancer is experienced as an extreme embodiment of these routinized and recurrent forms of social suffering. It may variously be attributed to suffering and hardship in the past (starvation, food shortage, hard physical labor and humiliation during the Cultural Revolution) or in the present (consumerism requiring the use of farm chemicals or anxiety among men who failed to preserve the family line), as well as to bad temper or to socially valued habits such as smoking and drinking. The subtleties of their experiences and of what is at stake for sufferers and their families may only be conveyed through close ethnographic accounts of how they make sense of cancer and cope with it. The expression fighting for breath encapsulates these everyday struggles. This chapter starts by examining the historical roots of some of these etiologies and proceeds to portray the microtemporal and subjective ways in which etiologies change. Although these two dimensions are explored separately for analytical clarity, they are deeply interwoven. Together, they come to shape the variable and contested *multiple careers of cancer etiologies*, as they are molded by historical, ideological, social, cultural and experiential forces.

HISTORICALLY ROOTED VALUES: CANCER AND THE OVERLAPPING VALUES OF THE PAST AND THE PRESENT

Illness etiologies are deeply connected to the social, political and economic realities within which they are situated (see Martin, 1994). In *Illness as Metaphor*, Susan Sontag (1991) argued that the association of tuberculosis with low energy, consumption and wasting during the Victorian era "echo[ed] the attitudes of early capitalist accumulation," fears of not having enough energy, and the necessity of regulated consumption. By contrast, as "advanced capitalism requires expansion, speculation, the creation of new needs," cancer "evokes a different economic catastrophe: that of unregulated, abnormal, incoherent growth" (p. 64). Everett Zhang (2007) has made a related point in the Chinese context. He argued that the transition in moral codes from collectivism to economic reforms was embodied by the decline of spermatorrhea (*yijing*),[2] which was commonly diagnosed during Mao, and the increase in diagnoses of impotence in the present. For Zhang, this difference is due to different moral contexts: during Mao individual desire was unacceptable, and as a consequence people felt *yijing* to be a problem. By contrast, in the time of reform, individual desire is accepted. Consequently men are no longer preoccupied by *yijing* but by impotence, as they want to fulfill desires they finally have an opportunity to satisfy (as they have more money), but they are physically unable to do so.

Whereas these analyses are successful in highlighting the interplay between understandings of illness and broader social and economic change, they also run the risk of simplifying much more complex processes. With reference to sexuality, Sandra Hyde (2007) argued that there is no "linear progression from the ancient Confucian notion of the proper conjugal bed, through a Maoist code of containment, to emerge into sexual freedom and modernity. It is a story of ongoing and persistent conflicts among alternative regimes of power" (p. 191). Similarly, Judith Farquhar (2002) contended that the transformation from the ethics of serving the people to the reformist emphasis on consumerism occurred gradually and they both influence people's search for health. Likewise in Langzhong, villagers did not describe an individualist immoral present as opposed to a collectivist moral past nor, vice versa, did they categorically condemn the past and see the present as free and prosperous. A more complex relationship with both past and present was at play. The present was partly judged through the prism of the past, but villagers also constantly strived to recreate a moral universe to make sense of their present. This ambivalence about both collectivism and market economy was articulated in the ways in which villagers made sense of cancer.

Cancer etiology does not follow a chronological sequence that could be easily mapped onto political economic change. Rather, it reflects overlapping moral economies derived from experiences during collectivism and during reform. It is not a case of a new moral code eclipsing an outdated and irrelevant version but of a former moral economy coexisting with emergent ones. This, as we shall see, is further complicated by particular individual experiences and family contexts that influence explanations for cancer during illness and after death.

Stomach and esophagus cancers are also frequently referred to respectively as "vomiting illness" (*huishi bing*) and "choking or spitting illness" (*gengshi bing*). As a consequence, it is difficult to establish how locals explained the spitting and vomiting illnesses before cancer gained currency as an illness category. Whereas the former terms are rooted in folk explanations of disease, the latter is a quickly globalizing biomedical category that has come to largely overshadow and metabolize previous terminologies. Nevertheless, villagers' understanding of cancer causality draws simultaneously from biomedicine, Chinese medicine and folk explanations previously associated with the vomiting and spitting illness, such as hard work, poverty, food shortage and emotional distress. In practice, the divisions between these approaches to illness and healing are not neat in China's plural medical landscape. Sydney White (1993, 1999) has similarly shown that in rural Lijiang, common lay categories for understanding affliction—such as hot and cold or exposure to wind, damp or dryness—were remarkably consistent with the explanatory models of the medicine of systematic correspondence, also incorporating influences from biomedical discourses such as genetic heredity, germ theory and infectiousness (chapter 7, pp. 1340–1341). Villagers do not self-consciously choose between causalities rooted in Western or Chinese medicine because of predilections for one or other medical system, but rather approach them as part of an epistemological continuum that is shaped not only by official discourse and practitioners but also by sufferers themselves. As I will show, their accounts of cancer causality are rooted in historical contexts as well as in their shifting individual experience and family dynamics.

At present, villagers state that vomiting and spitting illnesses, common in the past, were due to poor diet and to the physical strain of working long hours on collective farms and infrastructural projects such as irrigation pools. These causalities have also become associated with stomach and esophagus cancer. That past suffering is blamed for a fatal illness in the present also articulates an implicit criticism of the past, a deep ambivalence toward poor diet and the need for physically demanding labor. During late reforms, villagers reflect on their historical experience and present the collective past as riddled by spitting and vomiting illnesses, illnesses of inability to consume. In doing so, they also portray the past as a time characterized by a ban on consumption, demonized as selfish. They critique its demands on productive bodies by attributing illness to poverty (lack of consumption) combined with the hardships of production (physically strenuous work for the collective). They see cancer in the present as partly caused by such suffering in the past. Esophagus and stomach cancer are experienced as an attack on the most vital requirements of village life: not only ability to eat but the related ability to work (see also Shao, 2006).

The correlation between cancer and limited ability to eat is embedded in past experiences of shortage and, conversely, it lends strength to the historically rooted equation between eating and health. This may be usefully understood as a form of habitus (Bourdieu, 1977, 1990), as the naturalization of living conditions characterized by food shortage whereby access to food in itself constitutes health. In this context, villagers regarded those who could eat particularly large amounts of food (for instance, two large bowls of staple food per meal) as unlikely to develop an illness, especially of the kind manifested as inability to eat, such as esophagus or stomach cancer. Even when the sufferer's ability to eat started to decline and thereby raised the doctor's suspicion, the sufferer and their families were still inclined to disprove this with reference to the person's track record as someone who is "good at eating" (*neng chi*). Conversely, when villagers' energy, appetite and ability to eat decreased, they were suspected of having developed cancer. Such suspicions were strongest in the cases of those seen to have had a particularly strenuous life. When a woman in her 60s (the wife of a barefoot vet) who was single-handedly farming all of her large family's allotment of land and caring for four grandchildren became weak and unable to eat in 2008, villagers reasoned that she probably had cancer. Even when suspicions may have been disproved by the diagnosis of heart disease, rumors that her family may simply be keeping the cancer diagnosis a secret persisted.

Gandie and those of the older generation who endured famines and food shortages acquired a "taste of necessity" (Bourdieu, 1984, p. 177), involving a diet of rice or noodles and salt-preserved vegetables. Salt-preserved and pickled vegetables are of particular interest because, as part of a wider trend of limited dietary variation, they are epidemiologically correlated with cancers of the stomach and esophagus (Chen et al., 2006). They constituted a central part of local diet in the past and still play an important role in the present, particularly between October and June, when fewer fresh vegetables are available. Villagers however were typically skeptical as to the harmfulness of preserved vegetables and largely refuted this biomedically rooted causality in the present. Their consumption then cannot simply be regarded as a form of poverty-related self-oppression.

The centrality of preserved vegetables to villagers' habitus as a widespread and long-standing practice partly explains why they are usually not considered carcinogenic in the present. Yet the processes and contexts by which cancer is or is not attributed to preserved vegetables are too complex to be elucidated with reference to habitus alone. The different positions of preserved vegetables in cancer etiology articulate perceptions of the moral economies of the past and present. That preserved vegetables are associated with cancer during times of shortage implies a judgment of such times as characterized by an immoral economy. This biomedically rooted explanation gains legitimacy to explain cancer incidence in the past not because of a belief in the primacy of science, but because of the values it embodies. During a time of relative prosperity such as the present, however, preserved vegetables have taken on different implications. The value of preserved vegetables, expressed in the denial of their carcinogenic potential in the present articulates a critique of the current market economy, which has made the widespread use of farm chemicals necessary. Indeed, farmers justify their consumption of preserved vegetables (on which few chemicals are used) as the healthy (and green) alternative to buying vegetables in the market without knowledge of what is used to farm them. Consumption of food with limited farm chemicals is also a way for villagers to reclaim agency in decreasing the likelihood of cancer and an effort to reconstitute a moral economy based on homegrown food free from chemicals. Conversely, the strong tendency to attribute cancer to farm chemicals suggests ambivalence towards present consumerism. The copresence of etiologies that attribute cancer to excessive production (physical hardship in the collectives) and deficient consumption in the past but also to excessive consumption of harmful substances such as farm chemicals in the present embodies overlapping moral economies.

The critical attitude to past shortages and suffering has not resulted in an unequivocal embrace of present prosperity. In its deprivation, the Mao period is recalled positively to critique present corruption and the lack of a welfare state to help with rising health care and schooling costs. Although there was little sign of a welfare state in rural China until 2005, comparisons to efforts in the 1960s and 1970s to provide health care, however basic, were cherished against a money-oriented present. In this context, rather than resign themselves to a failed morality and lack of state support, families recreate a moral universe by mobilizing resources to care for ill relatives. Even when the past political economy of food shortage and strenuous physical work in the collectives is blamed for cancer, the pride derived from having managed to provide for oneself and one's family also imbues such sacrifices with a moral connotation. The wife of a man who died of cancer in 2006 told me the following year that he had worked extremely hard in his youth to build the collective irrigation ditch and that this surely precipitated cancer later in life. Similarly, when Aunt Liu died of cancer in late 2007 villagers were adamant that her hardship—having had to shoulder all the family's farming alone as her husband was a teacher—must have contributed to her developing cancer. Both of them were seen to have acted for the wider good (of the collective and the family).

Macrolevel historical forces as described earlier powerfully shape cancer causality, but individual experiences and microtemporal shifts are equally important. Many local explanations for cancer draw on shared experiences such as food shortage, hard work and exposure to farm chemicals but not all are deemed to have suffered to the same extent. Some, friends and relatives argue, worked harder than others, endured more severe shortages and relied more heavily on farm chemicals. Explanations for cancer are not only historically shaped but also socially situated. Conversely, they position sufferers within their families and the wider social context. These etiologies then work in two ways: as unifying principles based on a common history and a common present but also as dividing principles, whereby suffering is unequally distributed. In this way, these elements serve to explain why particular individuals fall sick, but this does not entail that the individual himself is blamed for the onset of cancer. On the contrary, by being embedded in shared social and economic histories, these etiologies provide intersubjective ways of explaining cancer. They situate cancer causality between the individual and the social realm, making it the result of an individual sacrifice, but one that is socially recognized and valued.

Ambiguity pervades cancer etiologies, imbuing them at once with the potential to harm and at the same time endowing those who suffered the consequences with moral characteristics. Located as it is within a local moral world that both commends and condemns hard work, the ability to live on a limited diet and use of farm chemicals, cancer is experienced not as an individual pathology but as a form of social suffering (Kleinman,1995; Kleinman, Das & Lock, 1997). Combining an understanding of the complex historical forces that mold cancer causalities with the more subtle and microtemporal ways in which causalities change over the course of an individual's illness and after death allows a more nuanced understanding of social suffering. Conceptually and methodologically, it shows that both of these dimensions need to be part of the analysis and that they infuse each other in complex ways. In turn, this approach highlights the different facets and temporalities of social suffering and the various forms of subjectivity that they articulate.

MICROTEMPORAL SHIFTS, ETIOLOGIES AND MORALITY

Understanding how moral worlds are remade in the face of cancer requires "close attention not only to the content of narratives, but also to the processes of their formation within local communities" (Das & Kleinman, 2001, p. 5). Earlier, I have shown how this is the case for macrohistorical shifts. The same applies on a much more microtemporal scale: cancer narratives shift during illness and after death. Such changes are central to forming and contesting family relations, remembering the sufferer as a moral subject and reconstituting a moral universe in the face of loss. Close attention to specific case studies from the early stages of illness to well after the sufferer's death allows a better understanding of how cancer may be attributed to different causes throughout its development and why this may be so. It also addresses the balance between rooting attitudes to illness in political economic contexts and accounting for subjective experience beyond historical determinism.

It is widely accepted in medical anthropology that a serious illness is a moral event (see for example Good, 1994; Kleinman, 1980, 1986, 1995). Equally, experiences of cancer have been shown to be closely tied to discourses of blame and morality.[3] The question of how blame is attributed and to whom is highly disputed, and it is at the very core of negotiations about moral behavior. Cancer is often considered "the fault of someone who has taken part in 'unsafe' behavior: alcoholism, smoking, or working with chemicals" (Weiss, 1997, p. 457). Those affected however may not agree. Martha Balshem's (1991, 1993) research on cancer among working-class Philadelphians shows that the residents of the "cancer hot spot" refused to adopt changes in lifestyle advised by education programs. By attributing cancer to fate, they declined responsibility and avoided blame. In doing so, they also countered the hegemony of biomedicine and unequal power relations played out in clinical medical practice. In her study of cancer among Mexicans, Linda Hunt (1998) also suggested that cancer patients did not resort to biomedical notions to make sense of cancer. But where Balshem's informants did not accept individualized explanations for cancer, Hunt argues that sufferers and their families deny arbitrariness and seek to understand why specific individuals developed cancer by relating it to particular events in their lives.

Neither of these approaches fully applies in my case study. Building on Byron Good's (1994) understanding of illness narratives as unfinished, Veena and Ranendra Das (2006) stated, "People did not move through illness experiences with ready-made 'beliefs' about the causes of their illness" (p. 90). The same may be said of the ways in which Gandie's family made sense of his illness. Different etiologies were adopted at different times during illness and after death. When Gandie was first diagnosed with cancer in October 2004 but not informed of this diagnosis, his relatives confidently attributed his discomfort to repressed anger. This enabled them to hope that his illness could be cured, if only he learned to control his temper. At this time, they regarded Gandie's ability and fondness for smoking and drinking spirits as a sign of health rather than a cause of cancer. By the end of October 2004, Gandie had become aware of his cancer. As Erjie put it, "Of course he knows; when you can't eat like that, you know it's cancer—what else would it be?" Gandie's own realization that he had cancer through his decreased ability to eat—what Deborah Gordon (1990) called "embodied or unconscious knowing" (p. 276)—triggered a shift in the ways in which the family explained his illness. Above all, they ceased to reflect on what may have caused it and concentrated on the apparent evidence that Gandie was still in good health: he could after all still eat something and helped his wife doing some heavy farm work. Erjie explained, "That's normal; if he manages to eat he's fine, he has energy to work, and he doesn't want my mother to do it all alone" (November 3, 2004). It seemed that his family at this stage, however worried, was still hopeful. Their hopefulness was rooted in Gandie's strength and ability to eat. As these historically rooted parameters of well-being seemed to remain relatively unchallenged by cancer, his relatives told each other that he might well survive. The equivalence between eating and health rooted in experiences of shortage convinced them he was still healthy. Yet this measure of health was soon challenged.

Gandie's decreasing ability to eat presented a parameter through which he and his family measured his physical decline. When his ability to eat decreased further in late November and he became unable to work, his family gradually became convinced he was going to die. In particular, as death came to seem inevitable, they avoided tracing his illness to any etiology at all, commenting that "this is what this illness is like—you don't know why you get it, and you can't cure it" (a frequent statement). By December 2004, Gandie was unable to keep food down for any longer than a minute, and he would then spit it out. At this stage, he was still on various medications, including chemotherapy through intravenous drips. The family members could not explain what these medicines were, nor did they recognize the term "chemotherapy" (*hualiao*). They were, however, keen to emphasize that they cost them over 100 yuan per day.[4] Given that the local monthly income for a worker at that time was roughly 500 yuan and much less for farmers, this is a considerable sum. In their desperate attempts to cope with Gandie's decline, his family revised their definition of what constitutes eating to make sense of his condition and come to terms with it. No longer the hearty eater he had been, even swallowing a few grains of grapes now counted as "eating" for Gandie. Conversely, regarding his declining health as a consequence of inability to eat reinforced their sense of the centrality of eating to health. As Gandie became bedbound, he was also unable to continue with chemotherapy, which required him to go to the city's hospital. Some newspapers were cut and placed next to the bed to wipe his mouth and a bowl was put next to the bed for him to spit in. By this point, Erjie and I were visiting two or three times a week, but the room where he lay was mostly silent. Even asking him how he was had become too sensitive. By January 2005 his skin had turned much darker and hairier as a result of weight loss, his cheekbones and eyebrows were ever more pronounced, he spat blood, and he could hardly speak. He could no longer raise his head, so his wife put some paper next to his head for him to spit on. He was tearful in the morning and felt anxious and restless at night. Erjie reflected, "It's so painful this illness, it 'eats' all your flesh and only then it lets you die (*ba nide rou chiwanle cai youfa si*)." The idiom of eating here takes on a new form. As Gandie himself could no longer eat, cancer was now eating away at his body. His agony came to an end on February 6, 2005.

Attitudes to cancer during its course broadly reflect Sontag's (1991) sentiment that finding a meaning for cancer is "punitive" (p. 59). Indeed, having ascribed cancer to smoking or drinking would have implied that Gandie might be partly responsible for his illness. Likewise, attributing cancer to anger and anxiety would have resulted in attributing blame either to Gandie for his bad temper or to those who made him angry. And yet cancer sufferers and their families do not reject biomedical ideologies outright, nor do they do so for the strategic purpose of opposing hegemonic ideology, as Balshem (1993) would have it. Indeed, after the sufferer's death, searching for an explanation becomes acceptable and desirable. These explanations may rely on epidemiological knowledge, such as in the case of smoking or drinking, or survivors may search for morality by tracing cancer to traumatic events and the propensity to get angry. After Gandie's death, his family began to link his cancer to specific elements of his biography such as smoking, drinking and anger. As Linda Hunt (1998) put it, his relatives strived to compose a "unifying interpretation capable of giving the disease coherent meaning by relating it to other problematic events" within his biography (p. 310). In contrast to Sontag, for those left behind, finding an explanation for cancer helped them to cope with their loss and to remember their deceased relative as a moral subject.

In January 2005, less than a month before Gandie's death, Erjie's husband remarked with admiration that Gandie used to be very "fierce" at drinking and smoking (*xiong de hen*). This was seen as evidence of Gandie's excellent health rather than a possible cause of cancer. After his death however Erjie began to regard smoking and drinking alcohol as causes of cancer. She cautioned her neighbor, a notorious heavy drinker that "my father drank a lot, and he got cancer," implying a link between them. She similarly reflected "getting angry is not good for people, look at my father," once again linking cancer with anger. As Gandie's case shows, attitudes about illness and healing are never fixed: His family's views on the effects of his eating, drinking, smoking and temper were redefined in the course of illness and after death. Past experiences—for instance, of Gandie as a mighty drinker and a hearty eater—formed the background through which current experiences were understood. At the same time, new experiences (of Gandie's decreasing ability to eat) created new parameters. Different etiologies have different implications for who or what is blamed. Tracing changes in how his family understood cancer stage by stage highlights not only how illness itself develops but also how Gandie and his family attempted to rebuild their moral universe in the face of illness—to avoid blaming Gandie or other members of the family, while at other times actually blaming relatives' unacceptable behavior. Such shifts are also forms of family caregiving. They show both family relations and morality to be emergent and processual rather than firm and undisputed. Whether they avoid explanations or search for them, sufferers and their families produce a moral commentary not only on the sufferer's life but also on the past and present contexts more widely.

I have argued that historically rooted etiologies such as hard work and food shortage are situated between the individual and the social realm, making suffering at once individualized but also socially valued. A similar point may be made for other etiologies. Indeed, ambiguity as to whether cancer is the fault of an individual or of wider circumstances potentially works to reinforce the efficacy of a given etiology, allowing different interpretations of who is blamed as a consequence. Just as I explained above for hard work, in rural Langzhong, the relationship between health, smoking and drinking alcohol was perceived with ambivalence. Although locals admitted that excessive drinking and smoking were harmful, they also claimed that ability to drink and smoke was typical of healthy people. As the reasoning went, if one can engage in a harmful practice and still maintain health, it must mean that his body is "fierce" (*xiong*), as was noted of Gandie. Given that these activities are associated with strong males (by contrast, they are regarded as undesirable for women), they are part of how masculinity is defined, and as a consequence they are a habitual parameter of normality for men (Kohrman, 2007, 2008). Crucially, smoking and drinking alcohol are socially valued ways of fostering relationships (*guanxi*), which are the very texture of life and vital to providing support in times of need. As socially accepted and respected activities central to social life, smoking and drinking cannot be pathologized, nor can individuals who engaged in them be blamed for doing so.

Ambiguity also surrounded the link between negative emotions and cancer. This folk causality significantly overlaps with accounts rooted in Chinese medicine. A young village doctor who had studied both Western and Chinese medicine stated that the effect of smoking, drinking and consuming preserved vegetables on the development of cancer was proposed by Western medicine but not by Chinese medicine. According to the latter, he argued, cancer was due to pathogenic emotions. He combined Chinese and Western medical knowledge to explain that repressed anger and trapped qi (*ouqi*) cause infections (*fa yan*) that in turn lead to the development of cancer. Along similar lines, a *qigong* healer with whom Elisabeth Hsu trained during her fieldwork claimed that an accumulation of qi leads to the development of tangible lumps, some of them tumors (Hsu, 1999, pp. 83–85). When cancer is attributed to a tendency to become angry and anxious, this can amount to blaming victims for causing their illness (Farmer, 1992, p. 248). But anger and anxiety may also be seen to stem from wider conditions, difficult situations or family conflicts making the sufferer anxious and angered. In this scenario, blame for precipitating cancer is typically attributed to significant family members, very often women and younger generations who may have challenged existing mores. Attribution of blame for cancer may channel such tensions between siblings and their wives and reproduce unequal power relations.

Gandie's eldest daughter-in-law, Dasao, for instance repeatedly commented (May 2005, April 2006, July 2008) that Gandie's youngest daughter-in-law (Sansao) had behaved disrespectfully toward him and his wife, failed to care for them and that she "made him repress his anger to death" (*ba ta ouqi si le*). By attributing Gandie's cancer to Sansao, Dasao presented herself as a caring daughter-in-law and defined Sansao's behavior as so unacceptable that it could cause illness and death. In many other cases, men accused women of causing cancer (or risking to cause cancer) in other men: Erjie's husband accused his mother of threatening his father's health by irritating him and the former village teacher faulted three wives and a daughter of making their respective husbands and father ill by not caring for them or by divorcing. In these negotiations, failure to comply with established values such as the importance of marriage and caring for their husbands and parents-in-law is constituted as pathological. Yet women did not always consent to these accusations unquestioningly. They questioned the definition of acceptable behavior by using that very same etiology—repressed anger—to blame cancer on an individual's propensity to anger, thereby avoiding blame. In doing so, they partially challenged and subverted the underlying ideology that defined appropriate behavior for wives, daughters and daughters-in-law. Attributing cancer to negative emotions allows recognition of its social origins and articulates comments about social norms and values. Ambiguity over whether negative emotions are blamed on the sufferer or on significant others channels contrasting values and practices. In this way, cancer potentially lends itself to reinforcing the hegemony of China's still largely patriarchal society, but it also channels some potential for contestation and change.[5]

CONCLUDING THOUGHTS

Previous perspectives on social suffering have already highlighted its intersubjective nature and the need to avoid cultural and economic determinism (Kleinman, Das & Lock, 1997). This chapter addresses this challenge empirically by engaging with both the micro- and macrofacets of suffering. Methodologically, it tackles the conceptual challenge of linking these two levels of analysis by combining the focus on one extended family with participant observation in the wider community. It pays attention to the political and economic forces that affect experiences of suffering and its distribution, but it avoids an overly structural approach and historical determinism by simultaneously examining the complex intersubjective reasons why particular etiologies gain and lose relevance and legitimacy. Temporality and ideas surrounding moral behavior are central to these shifts: different moments in the course of illness and after death foster divergent attitudes to cancer. This in turn powerfully informs the sufferer's experience and the coping strategies of his or her immediate family. Examining the social, cultural and economic roots of etiologies and the ways in which their implications may change in the present both in radical and subtle ways provides insights into different layers of social suffering.

The ambiguity that pervades cancer etiologies serves as a key lens, which allowed analysis of the conceptual links between the microlevel of experience and the macrolevel of historical change. Hard work is valued as a marker of healthy and moral individuals, but also regarded as potentially harmful. Preserved vegetables are associated with suffering in the past, but in the present they embody a healthier alternative to marketization. Excessive drinking and smoking are seen to be harmful, but the ability to engage in these activities is also associated with health and with fostering relationships. Negative emotions may be branded as individual temper (therefore blaming suffering on individuals) but they may also be attributed to close relatives who seemingly failed to fulfill their familial duties. As these causalities allow multiple interpretations and channel potentially conflicting values and definitions of morality, they also embody diverse facets of social suffering. The globalizing medical discourse of cancer plays a role in sufferers' experiences but, like explanations drawn from Chinese medicine or from folk understandings of disease, it is only foregrounded when it is consonant with local values. Even when cancer may be attributed to drinking or smoking or to a poor diet, this does not result in blaming individuals for their suffering. Rather, unhealthy diet and lifestyle are understood as part and parcel of the wider social, cultural and economic context, making such suffering social rather than individual.

In its account of micro- and macrotemporal shifts in cancer etiologies, this chapter has portrayed suffering as a dynamic and multilayered process. Etiologies operate at several intersecting levels, ranging from the individual sufferer and their families to the local community and beyond it to their understanding of how broader social, political and economic forces may cause cancer. Some etiologies trace their origins to biomedicine, others to Chinese medicine and yet others to locals' embodied experiences. But all are equally suffused by sociocultural contexts and articulate social values and judgments about the sufferers, their relatives and society at large. Cancer in rural Langzhong may be understood as a form of social suffering to the extent that the ways in which is it explained draw on both individualized and social causes: Drinking and smoking are individual habits as much as they are a prerequisite for fostering relationships. Eating preserved vegetables is a family's choice of diet as much as it is rooted in historically molded taste and current attitudes toward market food. Situated as they are at the intersection between individual and social experience, these causalities play a crucial role in attempts by both sufferers and their families to rebuild morality.

By presenting an analysis of both micro- and macrotemporal shifts in cancer etiologies, this chapter also attempted to question the distinction between them and to show instead how they intersect. Acknowledging that locals regard cancer as a disease of production in its link with hard work but also as a disease of consumption (both excessive and deficient) does not amount to historical determinism, to somehow denying them agency or ignoring their subjective experiences of suffering. Here, these etiologies are explored as they are upheld by individual sufferers and their families alongside other causes of cancer. By highlighting that attempts to make sense of cancer enable particular relationships to the sufferer, this chapter balances attention to both large historical forces and how they permeate everyday life. The relative ambiguity allowed by many etiologies over where blame is placed in turn configures cancer as an illness with both individual and social facets. The experience of cancer is situated somewhere in this shifting balance.

NOTES

1. Some of the material and arguments in this chapter previously appeared in my book, *Fighting for breath: Living morally and dying of cancer in a Chinese village* (2013). I am grateful to the University of Hawai'i Press for allowing me to publish them here in a revised version. I am also immensely grateful to the book editors for their valuable comments.
2. Spermatorrhea is involuntary discharge of semen without orgasm.
3. For book-length accounts, see for instance Balshem (1993), Gregg (2003) and Sontag (1991).
4. On attitudes to the cost of treatment see Lora-Wainwright (2013, chapter 7).
5. These arguments are developed more fully and with reference to ethnographic examples in Lora-Wainwright (2013, chapters 4 and 6).

REFERENCES

Balshem, M. (1991). Cancer, control and causality: Talking about cancer in a working-class community. *American Ethnologist, 18,* 152–172.
Balshem, M. (1993). *Cancer in the community.* Washington, DC: Smithsonian Institution.
Biehl, J., Good, B., & Kleinman, A. (Eds.). (2007). *Subjectivity: Ethnographic investigations.* Berkeley: University of California Press.
Bourdieu, P. (1977). *Outline of a theory of practice.* Cambridge: Cambridge University Press.
Bourdieu, P. (1984). *Distinction. A social critique of the judgment of taste.* London: Routledge.
Bourdieu, P. (1990). *The logic of practice.* Cambridge: Polity Press.
Chen, J., Liu, B., Pan, W., Campbell, C., Peto, R., Boreham, J., Parpia, B., Cassano, P., & Chen, Z. (2006). *Mortality, biochemistry, diet and lifestyle in rural China.* Oxford: Oxford University Press.
Croll, E. (1994). *From heaven to earth: Images and experiences of development in China.* London: Routledge.
Das, V., & Das, R. K. (2006). Pharmaceuticals in urban ecologies: The register of the local. In A. Petryna, A. Lakoff & A. Kleinman (Eds.), *Global pharmaceuticals: Ethics, markets, practices* (pp. 171–205). Durham, NC: Duke University Press.
Das, V. & Kleinman, A. (2001). Introduction. In V. Das, A. Kleinman, M. Lock, M. Ramphele & P. Reynolds (Eds.), *Remaking a world: Violence, social suffering and recovery* (pp. 1–30). Berkeley: University of California Press.
Farmer, P. (1992). *AIDS and accusation: Haiti and the geography of blame.* Berkeley: University of California Press.
Farmer, P. (2003). *Pathologies of power: Health, human rights and the new war on the poor.* Berkeley: University of California Press.
Farquhar, J. (2002). *Appetites: Food and sex in post-socialist China.* Durham, NC: Duke University Press.
Good, B. (1994). *Medicine, rationality and experience.* Cambridge: Cambridge University Press.

Gordon, D. (1990). Embodying illness, embodying cancer. *Culture, Medicine, and Psychiatry, 14,* 275–297.

Gregg, J. (2003). *Virtually virgins: Sexual strategies and cervical cancer in Recife.* Stanford, CA: Stanford University Press.

Hsu, E. (1999). *The transmission of Chinese medicine.* Cambridge: Cambridge University Press.

Hunt, L. (1998). Moral reasoning and the meaning of cancer: Causal explanations of oncologists and patients in southern Mexico. *Medical Anthropology Quarterly, 12,* 298–318.

Hyde, S. (2007). *Eating spring rice: The cultural politics of AIDS in southwest China.* Berkeley: University of California Press.

Kleinman, A. (1980). *Patients and healers in the context of culture: An exploration of the borderland between anthropology, medicine, and psychiatry.* Berkeley: University of California Press.

Kleinman, A. (1986). *Social origins of distress and disease: Depression, neurasthenia and pain in modern China.* New Haven, CT: Yale University Press.

Kleinman, A. (1995). *Writing at the margin: Discourse between anthropology and medicine.* Berkeley: University of California Press.

Kleinman, A., Das, V., & Lock, M. (Eds.). (1997). *Social suffering.* Berkeley: University of California Press.

Kohrman, M. (2007). Depoliticizing tobacco's exceptionality: Male sociality, death, and memory-making among Chinese cigarette smokers. *China Journal, 58,* 85–109.

Kohrman, M. (2008). Smoking among doctors: Governmentality, embodiment, and the diversion of blame in contemporary China. *Medical Anthropology, 27,* 9–42.

Liu, X. (2000). *In one's own shadow: An ethnographic account of the condition of post-reform rural China.* Berkeley: University of California Press.

Lora-Wainwright, A. (2013). *Fighting for breath: Living morally and dying of cancer in a Chinese village.* Honolulu: University of Hawai'i Press.

Martin, E. (1994). *Flexible bodies: Tracking immunity in American culture from the days of polio to the age of AIDS.* Boston: Beacon Press.

Scheper-Hughes, N., & Lock, M. (1987). The mindful body: A prolegomenon to future work in medical anthropology. *Medical Anthropology Quarterly, 1,* 6–41.

Shao, J. (2006). Fluid labor and blood money: The economy of HIV/AIDS in rural central China. *Cultural Anthropology, 21,* 535–69.

Singer, M., & Baer, H. (1995). *Critical medical anthropology.* Amityville, NY: Baywood Publishing.

Sontag, S. (1991). *Illness as metaphor and AIDS and its metaphors.* London: Penguin (originally published, 1968).

White, D. (1993). *Medical discourses, Naxi identities and the State: Transformations in socialist China.* PhD Dissertation. Berkeley: University of California.

White, D. (1999). Deciphering "integrated Chinese and Western medicine" in the rural Li-jiang basin: State policy and local practice(s) in socialist China. *Social Science and Medicine, 49,* 1333–1347.

Weiss, M. (1997). Signifying the pandemics: Metaphors of AIDS, cancer, and heart disease. *Medical Anthropology Quarterly, 11,* 456–476.

Yan, Y. (2003). *Private life under socialism: Love, intimacy, and family change in a Chinese village, 1949–1999.* Stanford, CA: Stanford University Press.

Zhang, E. Y. (2007). The birth of nanke (men's medicine) in China: The making of the subject of desire. *American Ethnologist, 34,* 491–508.

2 The Psychogenesis of Cancer in France

Controlling Uncertainty by Searching for Causes[1]

Aline Sarradon-Eck

The exploration of suffering can illuminate how people interpret their lived experiences in relation to the social world. In contemporary French society, for example, the majority of people believe that mental and emotional processes, the experience of psychic traumas, and the stresses of modern life can cause cancer or impact the development of the disease. The results of the *Baromètre du cancer* survey conducted in 2010 on a cohort of 3,120 people over 15 years of age showed that most people in France believe that the following factors certainly or probably contribute to the occurrence of cancer: the "stress of modern life" (73.3% of the respondents), having been "perturbed by previous painful experiences" (60.9%), being "embittered by emotional or professional disappointments" (49%), or not managing to express one's emotions (38.9%) (Perretti-Watel, Amsellem & Beck, 2012). These figures had changed very little since the previous survey conducted on similar lines in 2005, in which it was observed that only 18.8% of the respondents did not agree that psychological problems are liable to influence the occurrence of cancer (Peretti-Watel, 2006).

This chapter will investigate why the psychosomatic model for the etiology of cancer is so widely adopted in French society by patients and by several health care providers (Bataille, 2003; Ménoret, 1999; Sarradon-Eck, 2009), outline the forms this cultural representation takes at present, and explore the effects of these beliefs on the individual's experience of cancer and uncertainty about recurrence. As complementary and alternative methods of treatment are becoming more available in France, many cancer patients are consulting practitioners such as "biodecoding" therapists, not to have their cancer cured, but to prevent the risk of recurrence (Cohen, Rossi, Sarrandon-Eck & Schmitz, 2010).[2] I hypothesize that people blame psychological factors for causing cancer because engaging in therapy enables them to regain a sense of control over the management of disease and of their daily lives and decreases uncertainty about prognosis, which may relieve anxiety and suffering for them.

Manderson (2011) points out that cancer is a unique disease in the level of fear it engenders and in the levels of uncertainty that surround determinations of risk and predictions of survival. In many ways talk about cancer is a way of talking about uncertainty and control. The context of suffering, however, is dynamic and multilayered. Just as people in contemporary French society are beset by social and economic uncertainties, they also have access to a medical system often said to be the best in the world. Yet this universal health care does not promote patient involvement. Cancer patients in France, unlike those in other countries, do not organize for collective action and do not form social groupings based upon biosocial factors (Rabinow, 1992). Jeannine Coreil (2010) has explained the lack of cancer support groups in France in terms of six factors: 1) an authoritarian, paternalistic medical system and a monopolistic national cancer organization *(La Ligue Contre le Cancer)*; 2) the belief in Mediterranean societies that support should be provided by the family; 3) the national ethos of "one country," that is "we are French," and diversity is therefore not an appropriate basis to develop special programs for specific subpopulations; 4) dependence on the State and the health insurance system to deal with all medical problems; 5) cancer patients' guilt and isolation prevent them from organizing collective movements of the kind existing for HIV patients; and 6) mainstream cancer populations are less ready to contest biomedical dogma than more marginal groups such as homosexuals and drug users. Because biomedicine does not admit the psychogenesis of cancer,[3] I hypothesize that sharing explanatory models of illness (Kleinman, 1980) focused on psychological and emotional causes for cancer is a form of *peerjectivity*. This neologism was first used by Dupagne (2009) to refer to the concept of peer-to-peer networks on the Internet. Peerjectivity means pooling the subjectivities to lend a form of expertise whose validity is based on sharing and recognition as widely as possible, but also on the balance of medical and scientific figures or media personalities (as artists or sportsmen). Peerjectivity is a sharing of micro-expertise and subjectivities (cultural representations, advice, opinions) in a virtual community of people—here, persons who are sharing cancer experiences because they (or their relatives) are sick. In this sense, peerjectivity is not only related to Internet users but can be extended to the users of all medias (press, books, television). Peerjectivity is being used here to illustrate how the widespread sharing of a psychosomatic model of cancer shapes the ways that individuals then make sense of suffering, take action to reassert personal control over risk and uncertainty and, as Herzlich (1969) showed in a past survey, express the conflicting nature of social relations. This peerjectivity does not take place in biosocial support groups for patients, but rather, emerges from ordinary conversations and encounters with the media (press, movies, television, internet) that convey testimonies of cancer patients who believe in a psychosomatic model for the etiology of cancer and who in turn create the "myth" of the psychogenesis of cancer (Darmon, 1993).

This article is based on data collected by the author in previous studies (Pellegrini et al., 2006; Sarradon-Eck, 2009) that investigated explanatory models of cancer among French cancer patients and examined how they managed the disease and its treatments (biomedical treatments, complementary and alternative treatments) and the relationships between patients and physicians and with the health-care system. I conducted 45 in-depth interviews with cancer patients (36 women, 9 men) with different disease status or recurrence in the south of France. Moreover, I conducted hospital ethnography at two French cancer centers (6 months each between 2006 and 2009) in the south of France (Marseille, Nice).

In this chapter, I follow the theoretical proposition of Dan Sperber (1982) who invites anthropologists to explain cultural representations by identifying the factors that define selection and sharing of some cultural representations in a social group, and by describing their transformations. In the first part, I describe contemporary reinterpretations of ancient beliefs and the meanings they carried. This analysis allows distinction of three forms that psychosomatic cultural representations of cancer take at present. The last part explores the cultural and social factors that could explain why the psychosomatic model of cancer persists in French society and how it shapes health identities and subjectivities (Whyte, 2009).

LAY PSYCHOSOMATIC INTERPRETATIONS

The narratives I have collected about how people who have undergone trial by cancer experienced the disease provide a good picture of how their imaginations respond to their bodies being subjected to the various aspects of this trial. By examining the causal factors mobilized and put into words by these patients, I propose to analyze not only the personal experience recounted, but also the syntax underlying the interactions between the patients' psyches and their afflicted bodies, reflecting the general culturally determined picture of how the experience of cancer becomes embodied.

Various ways of imagining pathogenic interactions between mind and body can be detected in these patients' narratives. The humoral theories that formed a bond of common knowledge between patients and doctors for more than 20 centuries (Rosenberg & Vogel, 1979)[4] seem to have left some persistent semantic traces such as the use of the verb "to secrete" (*secreting cancer*), whereas other semantic features shed light on these views of physiopathological disorder.

Thinking about Disease in Metaphorical Terms

Some people picture disease as if it were a language serving as a means of communication between body and mind, the social environment and the body. Physical lesions and organic deficits act like biological "words"[5] that make individuals aware of their ill-being, as expressed by a 48-year-old male patient undergoing treatment for cancer of the tongue, which he attributed to bottling up all the vexations that were "stuck in (his) throat."

Other respondents stated that traumatic personal events or their unbearable mode of life had *undermined* or *gnawed away* at them, depriving them of (*pumping away*) their energy. Here the semantic register focuses on the loss of *energy* and *stamina*. Either because the perturbed psychic processes take up too much energy, or because the speakers are exhausted by the modern way of life, they believe that their bodies are weakened and form a suitable breeding ground for cancer. Both weakness and strength are sometimes regarded as inherited characteristics (*that's just how one is made*), as suggested by the discourse of a female patient, who hinted at the strength that had enabled her to survive cancer and other diseases from which other members of her family had died. However, weakness is usually thought to be acquired as the result of traumatic personal events or depression, which have undermined the body. The concept of strength (*internal resources, the strength we possess*) is also used by some individuals in connection with the healing or remission of disease and the need to fight it and *not give in* to it, as if they regarded the body as a kind of battlefield.

Metaphors can also be used as a means of depicting the transmutation of social pressures into physical symptoms (Benoist & Cathebras, 1993). Thinking in terms of analogies sets up a system of correspondences between body and mind, which has been popularized by common psychoanalytical jargon. This system of correspondences is based on analogical and metaphorical associations between colorful French expressions and patients' diseases and symptoms, forming symbolic and semantic bridges between a patient's disease and the various events and experiences that have occurred during his or her lifetime.

Cancer as a Metonym for Social Experience

Many of the respondents interviewed perceived cancer as resulting from a chain of traumatic personal events (a separation, the death of a family member, legal proceedings, etc.). These people spoke about "being submerged" by a "series of painful events," as if their bodies had incorporated these unhappy experiences and transformed them into cancer. Anthropologists have frequently described disease as an event in a chain of misfortunes (Augé, 1984). People link together all the painful events they have undergone as if they formed a single causal chain and could all be interpreted in terms of the same etiological scheme, including those events concocted by believers in witchcraft, which have often been described (Favret-Saada, 1977; Zempléni, 1985). It has emerged from the surveys I have conducted, in line with Saillant (1988), that cancer is often taken to constitute the end of the painful chain, either because it is the end of the road (*the endpoint*) or because it causes a break in the cycle.

However, cancer is usually perceived as resulting from the internalization of deleterious social pressures. In the interviews I recorded, the respondents mostly spoke about the "pressures" from which they had suffered at work (heavy workloads, long hours, moral harassment, conflictual relationships) as well as in their personal relationships, and about family problems. The body was consistently perceived as a vessel that could only hold a certain number of pressures: "they go on accumulating, and one day everything explodes and you've got cancer." Whereas the use of metaphor makes it possible to think about physiopathological issues, attributing the occurrence of cancer or its onset to stress mainly constitutes a means of denouncing the conflicts and processes of domination encountered in the world of work. In this sense, cancer can be seen as an idiom of social suffering (Bourdieu, 1999). The verbal and symbolic violence to which people have been subjected in their social interactions is thought to be incorporated and inscribed in their bodies in the form of cancer. The disease thus becomes a metonym for an individual's personal physical and social experience.

In common usage, the word *stress* is generally taken to mean an emotional shock or a state of anxiety induced by social pressures and the economic or social problems that overwhelm people when they can no longer cope. The respondents in my surveys and those questioned by Manderson, Markovic and Quinn (2005) who explained that their cancers were due to stress tended to perceive their bodies like passive objects beyond their control, just as their whole lives had escaped their control because of the conditions under which they were living. Cancer, the uncontrollable development of cells in the body a metaphor for social disorder (Sontag, 1978), had therefore come to represent their loss of control over their own lives as well as the misery caused by social pressures and the degradation of family and occupational relationships (Manderson, Markovic & Quinn, 2005).

Mariella Pandolfi (1993) has spoken about the body as the locus where social communications occur and social norms are interiorized, as well as being where social malaise is transformed in the organs into suffering and disease. This *memorial body*, as Pandolfi has called it, is a place where individuals resist society and its constraints. However, it is not a passive body, because by telling the story of their disease, individuals are able to make a new start after all their failures and defeats: their etiological explanations are often a story of revolt about how their relationships with society and the world have been transformed. In their discourse about their disease, many respondents mentioned the changes they had made in their lives as the result of the disease. In many cases, cancer, via the workings of the psychic processes it triggered, "showed" what was wrong with their lives and subsequently brought about some salutary changes: feeling more detached from social constraints; adopting a way of life which left more scope for leisure activities, relaxation and spiritual enrichment; taking greater care of themselves (*thinking about myself, looking after myself, attending to my own needs*); changing their working patterns, or even making a change of occupation. These individuals made an effort to break away from the previous social constraints and became responsible for managing their own lives.

Beyond this phenomenological approach, psychological explanations for cancer can be seen as a way of making new identity claims: being a victim of the modern world damages people's roles and identities because of the "covert aggressions of working life" (Bourdieu, 1999, p. 629). Individuals in contemporary France often associate their experiences of cancer with the pressures of modern life and the structure of post-industrial labor. To transform one's identity to "a person with a disease" is a symbolic strategy employed at the individual level because French cancer activism does not advocate for recognition of social pressures as a factor in the disease process nor do patients have access to collective forms of social support as mentioned earlier. Lay explanations that blame illness on the modern lifestyle, moreover, are deep-rooted in French society and these have been a language used to express the conflicting relationships between individual and society, as Herzlich (1969) showed. The idea that contemporary society, and its institutions, is a source of social and psychological suffering is a generalized opinion in France (Ehrenberg, 2010). As Alain Ehrenberg (2010) wrote, discourses about "civilization and its malaise" can be summarized by the double assertion: the social link is weakened and, in return, the individual is overladen by new responsibilities and hardship (p.13), especially in today's world of work. This chapter explores the psychological results of experiencing cancer in a situation where patients have access to universal health care but not to collective support and activism. Their attempts to reassert control over the disease and the body often leads them to locate the link between cancer and labor in the mind rather than outside the body in the social and physical environment. Explanations for the cause of cancer then are often traced to psychological stresses or traumas that must be dealt with in order to prevent future recurrences of the disease.

CONTEMPORARY CULTURAL ETIOLOGICAL MODELS

In these respondents' narratives, the psychological factors responsible for cancer were rarely taken to be the sole etiological explanation. Other factors incriminated included collective risk factors (pollution, electromagnetic waves, medication, poor diet, etc.), individual behavioral risk factors (alcohol, smoking, overeating, etc.), and some people put forward more fatalistic explanations, blaming the occurrence of the disease on the hand of destiny (heredity, bad luck). Regardless of the other factors put forward, psychogenetic explanations for cancer dominated most narratives and were found to correspond to three models that have been widely adopted by present-day French society.

Cancer Attributed to Individuals' Inability to Express Their Emotions

In this model, cancer patients have a distinct personality with a "high strung" character, unexpressed emotions, emotional instability and psychological vulnerability, all of which lead to the development of the disease. People spoke about *giving themselves cancer*. They had *produced* their tumors, as the deleterious result of their psychological make-up. This cultural model, which has been described by Susan Sontag (1978), predominated in 1970–80 in North American society as well.[6] This interpretation was still present in the narratives I recorded, but it tended to be superseded by the other two cultural codes described next.

Cancer Regarded as the Scar Produced by a Traumatic Event

According to this interpretation, patients have suffered from a psychic trauma as the result of an untoward biographical event or unbearable social conditions. Their cancer is therefore regarded as a physical scar inflicted by this trauma, the bodily counterpart of a painful social experience. Patients, therefore, frequently attempt to pinpoint the biographical event that triggered their cancer, which is then raised to trauma status *a posteriori* because, as one of the respondents put it, "cancer is attributed only to people who have problems (family, occupational, or sentimental problems)." Apart from the need to find an explanation for the onset of the disease, this process of inquiry is driven by a more pragmatic urge to repair the damage: these people were often trying to repair their psychic lesions in order to prevent the risk of recurrence.

The "Psyche" Regarded as a Cancer Risk Factor

Many of the people interviewed seemed to be inordinately bent on identifying the risks to which they had been exposed, not only in order to explain the reasons for their cancer, but also to prevent its recurrence. This procedure resembles a kind of lay epidemiological investigation on the various possible real and imaginary risk factors involved, which is conducted by patients on similar lines to medical and public health research. However, lay epidemiological investigations tend to favor the risk factors that seem to be the most "acceptable" in the light of current social norms. They tend to neglect or minimize the behavioral factors for which present-day society might have held them responsible (poor dietary habits, smoking, lack of exercise, etc.) and to focus rather on risk factors such as heredity and painful biographical events, which free them of personal responsibility for their disease and lay no blame on their personal habits.

This "lay epidemiology" (Davidson, Davey Smith & Frankel, 1991), which places the emphasis on psychological cancer risk factors, is worth examining more closely because it leads people to develop certain kinds of risk prevention strategies: they often attempt to prevent the recurrence of cancer by seeking treatment for their psychological conflicts. For example, they may undergo conventional forms of therapy with a psychiatrist or a psychologist, group psychotherapy, or seek out alternative and complementary forms of care (physical methods of therapy, energy boosting treatment, relaxation, etc.) or treatment (such as *biodecoding*, in particular: see later in this chapter). They reconstruct or reorganize their lives by changing their lifestyles in order to reduce social pressures, seek spiritual fulfillment and invest more strongly in leisure activities. These preventive measures help to reduce the uncertainty about whether they have been cured for good. They are driven by pragmatic motives, which can be summarized in the phrase "to get rid of the disease, one must get rid of its causes."

How did the shift occur from cancer being attributed to repressed emotions to it being attributed to traumas or psychological risk factors? The explanation seems to be that this change was induced by various mutually reinforced social and cultural processes.

FROM THE REPRESSION OF EMOTIONS TO PSYCHOLOGICAL TRAUMA

In *Illness as Metaphor* (1978), Susan Sontag denounced interpretations of cancer that blame the victim and devalorize or even reject sick people and all those who do not pursue the moral goals of self-accomplishment. According to these interpretations, cancer is not so much a sign of transgressive behavior (as in the case of AIDS) as it is an indicator of the individual's many weaknesses and failures: the inability to express emotions and to symbolize experience; poor imaginative powers; and the lack of ability to form mental representations, articulate feelings and cope with stress.

During the 1970s, psychosomatic medicine became very popular in France, where the writings of Pierre Marty and his followers were well received by both general physicians and specialists. One might say that one of the social rules pertaining at that time was the need to keep a stiff upper lip and control one's emotions. The cultural revolution that broke out in the 1970s was all about denouncing these social norms, which were harmful to individuals, and challenging law and order, constraints and hierarchies. In proclaiming the right to spontaneity, authenticity, nonsubmission and informal forms of conviviality, this countercultural movement was promoting individuals' right to express both their positive emotions and their quandaries. Because cancer was thought by the proponents of psychosomatic medicine, in line with Georg Groddeck (1977), to result from repressed emotions, this interpretation was widely held during the 1970s, as shown by the success of Fritz Zorn's novel *Mars*, first published in 1976 (see Zorn, 1982).

As the sociologist Robert Castel (1981) has explained, the success of psychosomatic medicine reflected the "new psychological culture" that emerged in the 1960s. This phenomenon was characterized by "an increase in the consumption of psychology" by "normal" subjects and by "the promotion of working on oneself in a continuous fashion so as to produce an efficient and adaptable subject" (Rabinow, 1992, p. 242). This "psychologization of society" was accompanied by overemphasis on the psyche and psychological factors in all the spheres of social life. People were being encouraged to express themselves more freely, in keeping with the new social norm of narrativity.

Along with the "psychologization of society," trauma began to be recognized in the Western world as the result of several combined factors. This was the beginning of the cultural process that Fassin and Rechtman (2009, pp. 6–7) have called "the generalized traumatisation of existence." These authors claim that trauma is no longer a specialized psychiatric term, but has acquired a more general meaning, that of "the new language of events," the painful events and the accidents of life now being vaguely classified as traumas, which leave psychological traces and which implicitly carry the need to obey the latest imperative: to put these events into words.

Among the various unconventional therapeutic approaches focusing on the psychological causes of disease, there is one which subscribes in particular to the wave of interest in trauma. Its practitioners form an oddly assorted category of therapists known as "biodecoders." They contend that disease results from a psychological shock, mainly caused by conflictual relations inside the family, which triggers a biological conflict in a brain region commanding a specific organ or physiological function, damaging the corresponding tissues. This damage can be mended by *decoding* the psychological shock in order to identify and thus resolve the conflict. This decoding process is referred to as biological because the therapist starts with the damaged tissue, working back to the origin of the conflict, using a series of correspondences based on mental associations.[7] These new kinds of treatment (German New Medicine, Biodecoding, Total Biology, Psycho-bio-genealogy, Family constellations) emerged in Europe during the 1990s. They have spread since then to Canada and more recently to the United States via networks of practitioners and thanks to the publicity they have been given by the media (Sarradon-Eck & Caudullo, 2011).

In France, these new unconventional healing methods are becoming increasingly available and feature on many patients' therapeutic itineraries. It is difficult to determine exactly how many *biodecoders* exist because the occupational directories do not specify the fact that many manual therapists (such as osteopaths and Ayurvedic specialists), speech-oriented therapists (such as sophrologists and psychotherapists), physicians (homeopaths) and physiotherapists practice biodecoding. This approach is being used, however, for diagnostic purposes (to identify the "biological conflict") by many practitioners, who then treat their patients using other methods.[8] The large majority of cancer patients who consult biodecoders do not consult these therapists to have their cancer cured, but to prevent the risk of recurrence; biodecoding professes to offer them something that conventional oncology can not: the explanation of cancer and the suppression of *its* cause—one piece of the missing part of biomedicine (Cohen & Rossi, 2011).

In writing about rural Brittany, Badone (2008) argues that when cancer patients seek out alternative and complementary therapies, they are seeking alternative narrative frameworks within which to situate their experiences of illness. She reports that biomedicine in France often structures etiological explanations around metaphors of bodily disintegration and disruption that offer little hope for recovery, scant emotional support for patients and no meaningful etiologies for cancer. Alternative therapists, in contrast, provide a different way of explaining and conceptualizing cancer that offers support and hope to patients and makes their experiences of suffering comprehensible (Badone, 2008; Begot, 2010; Cohen et al., 2010; Schmittz, 2011).

... and the Psyche Itself as a Risk Factor

The field of epidemiology, with its predictive models and the practice of searching for risk factors, has contributed to promoting the idea that disease is a rationally explainable process. Disease is not just the fruit of chance, but results from the exposure of an individual to one or several risks (Berlivet, 2004). Talking about risk factors has gradually worked its way into social discourse about disease.

In addition, since 1970–1980, public health organizations in France have institutionalized the idea that individuals are responsible for promoting and maintaining their own health. Disease, especially cancer, is often taken to result from improper behavior (a poor diet and/or lifestyle) that is not in keeping with medical standards. Authors such as Katz (1997) and Zola (1981) have described public health recommendations as the latest form of "secular morality" based on similar principles of sin, punishment and redemption to those propounded by traditional Judeo-Christian morality. These authors have suggested that public health is now acting as a substitute for religion and the Law (Massé, 2003). The European Cancer Code, drawn up in November 1994 in Bonn by a group of cancer experts under the aegis of the European Commission, contains 10 measures and recommendations for preventing some forms of cancer. The public was informed about this Code in the European anti-cancer campaign conducted in 1995 and 1996. Due to the symbolic allusions associated with the number 10 (10 measures and recommendations) and the style in which these measures and recommendations are written, this Code implicitly mimics the 10 Commandments.[9]

The fact that people assimilated the notion of sins and faults because of the teachings of the Church during the Middle Ages and the Renaissance (Delumeau, 1983) has facilitated the induction of feelings of guilt as a means of social control in present-day Western societies. The current secular principle of self-management that has replaced the religious practice of self-reproach has resulted in the "micro-ethic" use of shame for social control purposes, which has been defined as "interiorised shame for not being healthy, energetic and productive, especially shame for not having done all one can to preserve one's health" (Lecourt, 1996, p. 115). Thus the assertion that psychic trauma or the stresses of everyday life cause cancer can be interpreted as a way of protesting against the attempts of the public heath establishment to blame individuals and their lifestyles for the occurrence and recurrence of the disease. Yet as Badone (2008) writes, the resistance of cancer patients "must be seen in the context of an ongoing dependence on and submission to biomedical authority" (p. 210).

CONCLUSION

Patients' interpretations of their disease can help them reconstruct their identities and reorganize their disrupted personal worlds by creating reference points and building symbolic bridges between events, thus making sense of the event of illness (Good, 1994; Kleinman, 1980). Patients' understandings of their illnesses depends on the types of illnesses in question and on the patients' cultural context, that is, on the whole universe of representations, norms, values and social relationships that make up their everyday lives. Biographical interviews may of course carry the risk of overestimating the narrative aspects of the causal attribution process. However, the idea that narrativity empowers patients by making them the subjects of their narration is particularly relevant in the field of cancer management, where the latest methods of supportive care (Gagnon & Marche, 2007) consist in asking patients to tell the stories of their own personal experiences of illness. Among the possible causes of cancer, psychological factors lend themselves best to narrative because they make it possible to form links between an individual's past, present and future. Patients tell their stories in a specially dedicated place with the approval of the caregivers and the institution. This approach focuses on persons rather than on their disease, by allowing the time required to let patients speak and by setting up conditions favoring closer exchanges between them and their caregivers.

Framing the etiological story of cancer around personal psychological traumas provides a narrative of illness that renders the unintelligible and amorphous sense of social distress experienced in postmodern France intelligible and controllable. Telling the etiological story about one's cancer and its possible psychological causes also makes patients feel that they are contributing to the management of their own treatment. The expertise deployed by patients who have determined the causes of their illnesses through a peerjective approach, when doctors have not expressed an opinion, confirms the rights of patients to produce a specific discourse about their bodies and their diseases (Herzlich & Pierret, 1987), thereby indirectly challenging the hegemony of biomedicine. In addition, focusing on the psychological factors possibly involved enables individuals to face up to the presumed causes of cancer, thus showing that they have the power to act. Blaming psychological causes, therefore, constitutes a means of regaining responsibility for the management of disease by taking control of one's life, because cancer is a metaphor for loss of control. In this way, adopting cultural representations in which cancer is blamed on psychological factors meets the current societal requirement that people should take control of their own lives (Massé, 2003), but at the same time enables them to escape from attributions of blame embedded in public health discourses that implicate bad lifestyle choices as the cause of cancer. At an individual level, the reassertion of control enables patients to participate more actively in their treatment by decreasing the uncertainty about their prognosis and in attempts to prevent recurrence by making lifestyle changes. Yet ultimately, the focus on the psychogenic causes of cancer is a symbolic acknowledgement by patients of the damages caused to them by life in the contemporary social world.

NOTES

1. The article is based on surveys funded by a grant from the Fondation de France and Institut National du Cancer (INCa). I would to thank Dr Jessica Blanc, who translated the original French version of this paper into English.
2. A minority of cancer patients consults to have their cancer cured, but the majority consults to reduce the side effects of the cancer treatments, to reinforce the body (*"le terrain"*) to fight the disease, to prevent the risk of recurrence and to regain control over the management of the disease (Cohen et al., 2010).
3. The documents published by organizations such as the World Health Organization, the French National Cancer Institute and the French Anti-Cancer League in which the known (and scientifically established) causes and risk factors are presented make no mention of psychological factors. Nor does the psychogenesis of cancer feature among the processes possibly responsible for cancer mentioned in the biomedical literature. This topic has been mainly addressed in the fields of health psychology and psychiatry, where the authors of many studies have attempted to prove or disprove the validity of the psychosomatic hypothesis about the etiology of cancer. However, none of the reviews of the literature in which it has been attempted to prove scientifically that there exist causal links between presumably distressing events and the development of cancer have led to the conclusion that psychic processes affect either the occurrence or the evolution of the disease (Garssen, 2004).
4. The Hipppocratic humoral theories, revisited by the physicians during the period of Enlightenment, attributed the origin of cancer to sadness, anger, worry and other emotions and mental disturbances (the term "stress" had not yet been coined) that trigger the production of melancholic humour "loaded with acid and a vicious carcinogenous yeast" (Darmon, 1993).
5. There is a play on words here because "words" in French (*"les mots"*) is homonymous with *"les maux"*, which means diseases, pains and evils: the teachings of Lacan have often been quoted in connection with this commonly used psychosomatic pun.
6. For lack of previous studies on French society, it is impossible to say whether there exist any differences between the North American and French representations of cancer, and whether the cultural models adopted during the last 30 years or so have changed in any way.
7. Breast cancer in a right-handed female patient is attributed, for example, to "a nest conflict" with a child, a childish husband, etc.
8. Homeopathy, for example. Some homeopaths practicing biological decoding methods prescribe a specific remedy for each type of shock: Muriaticum Acidum after the loss of the mother, Hura Brasiliensis after the loss of a child, Urtica Urens after the loss of the father, etc.

9. The first four measures are presented as follows, for example:
   1. Don't smoke. If you are a smoker, stop smoking as soon as possible and refrain from smoking in the presence of other people. If you are a non-smoker, do not give in to the temptation of cigarettes.
   2. If you drink beer, wine or alcohol regularly, reduce your rate of consumption.
   3. Increase your daily intake of fresh fruit and vegetables. Eat plenty of cereals with a high fiber content.
   4. Avoid being overweight, spend more time on physical activities and reduce your intake of fatty foods.

REFERENCES

Augé, M. (1984). Ordre biologique, ordre social : la maladie, forme élémentaire de l'événement. In M. Augé & C. Herzlich (Eds.), *Le sens du mal,* (pp. 35–91). Paris: Éditions des Archives contemporaines.

Badone, E. (2008). Illness, biomedicine, and alternative healing in Brittany, France. *Medical Anthropology, 27,* 190–218.

Bataille, P. (2003). *Un cancer et la vie. Les malades face à la maladie.* Paris: Balland.

Begot, A. C. (2010) *Médecines parallèles et cancer. Une étude sociologique.* Paris: L'Harmattan.

Benoist, J., & Cathebras, P. (1993). The body: From an immateriality to another. *Social Sciences and Medicine, 36,* 857–865.

Berlivet, L. (2004). Une biopolitique de l'éducation pour la santé. La fabrique des campagnes de prévention. In D. Fassin & D. Memmi (dir.), *Le gouvernement des corps* (pp. 37–75). Paris: Éditions de l'EHESS.

Bourdieu, P. (Ed.). (1999). *The weight of the world. Social suffering in contemporary society.* Stanford, CA: Stanford University Press.

Castel, R. (1981). *La gestion des risques. De l'antipsychiatrie à l'après-psychanalyse.* Paris: Les éditions de minuit.

Cohen, P., Rossi, I., Sarradon-Eck, A., & Schmitz, O. (2010). *Synthèses*—Rapport final pour l'Institut National du Cancer du programme *"Des systèmes pluriels de recours non conventionnels des personnes atteintes de cancer: une approche socio-anthropologique comparative (France, Belgique, Suisse)."* Retrieved from http://www.univrouen.fr/servlet/com.univ.utils.LectureFichierJoint?CODE=1338 363032014&LANGUE=0

Cohen, P., & Rossi, I. (2011). Le pluralisme thérapeutique en mouvement. *Anthropologie & Santé, 2,* Retrieved from http://anthropologiesante.revues.org/606

Coreil, J. (2010). Overview: social support, education and advocacy. Unpublished Manuscript prepared for Wenner Gren Conference on Metaphors of Cancer, New Orleans, LA: November 2010.

Darmon, P. (1993). *Les cellules folles. L'homme face au cancer de l'Antiquité à nos jours.* Paris: Plon.

Davidson, C., Davey Smith, G., & Frankel, S. (1991). Lay epidemiology and the prevention paradox: The implications of coronary candidacy for health education. *Sociology of Health and Illness, 13,* 1–19.

Delumeau, J. (1983). *Le péché et la peur en Occident. La culpabilisation en Occident XIIIe-XVIIIe siècle.* Paris: Fayard.

Dupagne, D. (2009). La « pairjectivité », une nouvelle approche scientifique? *Médicine, 5,* 29–33.

Ehrenberg, A. (2010). *La société du malaise.* Paris: Odile jacob.

Fassin, D., & Rechtman, R. (2009). *The empire of trauma: An inquiry into the condition of victimhood.* (R. Gomme, Trans.). Princeton, NJ: Princeton University Press. (Original work published 2007).

Favret-Saada, J. (1977). *Les mots, la mort, les sorts*. Paris: Gallimard.
Gagnon, E., & Marche, H. (2007). Communication, singularité, héroïsme. L'accompagnement et les gestions temporelles du cancer. In Rossi I (dir.) *Prévoir et prédire la maladie. De la divination au pronostic* (pp. 285–302). Paris: Aux Lieux d'être.
Garssen, B. (2004). Psychological factors and cancer development: Evidence after 30 years' research. *Clinical Psychology Review, 24*, 315–38.
Good, B. (1994). *Medicine, rationality and experience: An anthropological perspective*. Cambridge, MA: Cambridge University Press.
Groddeck, G. (1977). *The meaning of illness: Selected psychoanalytic writings*. (G. Mander, Trans.). Madison, CT: International Universities Press.
Herzlich, C. (1969). Santé et maladie, analyse d'une représentation sociale. Paris: Éditions de l'EHESS, Mouton.
Herzlich, C. and Pierret, J. (1987). *Illness and self in society*. (E. Forster, Trans.). Baltimore: Johns Hopkins University Press. (original work published 1984).
Julian-Reynier, C. (2010). Women's perceptions and experience of adjuvant tamoxifen therapy account for their adherence: Breast cancer patients' point of view, *Psycho-Oncology, 19*, 472–479.
Katz, S. (1997). Secular morality. In Brandt and Rozin (dir.), *Morality and Health* (pp. 297–330). New York, NY: Routledge.
Kleinman, A. (1980). *Patients and healers in the context of culture*. Berkeley, CA: University of California Press.
Lecourt, D. (1996). Le paradoxe moderne de l'éthique. *Le Magazine littéraire*, 112–115.
Manderson, L. (2011). Anthropologies of cancer and risk, uncertainty and disruption. In M. Singer & P. Erickson (Eds.), *A Companion to medical anthropology* (pp. 323–338). London: Wiley Blackwell.
Manderson, L., Markovic, M., & Quinn, M. (2005). "Like roulette": Australian women's explanations of gynecological cancers. *Social Science and Medicine, 61*, 323–332.
Massé, R. (2003). *Éthique et santé publique. Enjeux, valeurs et normativité*. Montréal: Les Presses de l'Université de Laval.
Ménoret, M. (1999). *Les temps du cancer*. Paris: CNRS Éditions.
Pandolfi, M. (1993). Le self, le corps, la "crise de la présence." *Anthropologie et Sociétés, 17*, 1–2, 57–77.
Pellegrini, I., Sarradon-Eck, A., Ben Soussan, P., Lacour, A. C., Largillier, R, Tallet, A. . . . Peretti-Watel, P. (2006). Ce que la population pense du cancer. Opinions, risques perçus et causes présumées. In P. Guibert, P. Peretti-Watel, F. Beck, & A. Gautier, (Eds.), *Baromètre du cancer* (pp. 31–52). Paris: Éditions INPES.
Perretti-Watel, P., Amsellem, N., & Beck, F. (2012). Ce que les français pensent du cancer. In F. Beck & A. Gautier (dir.), *Baromètre cancer 2010* (pp. 47–70), Paris: Éditions INPES.
Rabinow, P. (1992). Artificiality and enlightenment: From sociobiology to biosociality. In J. Carry & J.C.S. Kwinter (Eds.), *Incorporations* (pp. 234–252). New York, NY: Zone.
Rosenberg, C., & Vogel, M. J. (Eds.). (1979). *The therapeutic revolution*. Philadelphia, PA: University of Pennsylvania Press.
Saillant, F. (1988). *Cancer et culture. Produire le sens de la maladie*, Montréal: Editions Saint-Martin.
Sarradon-Eck, A. (2009). Le cancer comme inscription d'une rupture biographique dans le corps. In F. Cousson-Gélie, E. Langlois, & M. Barrault (dir.), *Faire Face au cancer. Image du corps, image de soi* (pp. 285–312). Boulogne-Billancourt: Tikinigan.

Sarradon-Eck, A., & Caudullo, C. (2011). Le décodage biologique. Diffusion d'une nouvelle médecine non-conventionnelle contre le cancer. *Anthropologie & Santé, 2,* Retrieved from http://anthropologiesante.revues.org/539.

Schmitz, O. (2011) Les points d'articulation entre homéopathie et oncologie conventionnelle. *Anthropologie & Santé, 2,* Retrieved from http://anthropologiesante. revues.org/701

Sontag, S. (1978). *Illness as metaphor.* New York: Farrar, Strauss & Giroux.

Sperber, D. (1982). Le savoir des anthropologues. Paris : Herman.

Whyte, S. (2009). Health identities and subjectivities. The ethnographic challenge. *Medical Anthropology Quarterly, 23,* 6–15.

Zempléni, A. (1985). La maladie et ses causes. Introductio", *L'ethnographie,* 96–97 (Causes et agents de la maladie chez les peuples sans écriture), 13–44.

Zola, I. (1981). Culte de la santé et méfaits de la medicalization. In Bozzini (dir.), *Médecine et société, les années 80.* Montréal: Éditions Saint Martin, 41–67.

Zorn, F. (1982). *Mars.* New York, NY: Knopf.

3 Anticipating Prevention
Constituting Clinical Need, Rights and Resources in Brazilian Cancer Genetics

Sahra Gibbon

The ubiquitous promise of personalized medicine associated with developments in genetic research, including the field known as breast cancer genetics, has long been grounded in an assumption that this knowledge will facilitate the movement towards individualized and targeted treatment based on knowing a person's genotype. Despite emerging possibilities for using knowledge of the two well-known inherited susceptibly genes, BRCA 1 and 2, in the treatment of sporadic cancers (see Bourrett, Keating & Cambrosio, 2014), this promise has been limited for the most part to the possibility of providing a personalized risk susceptibility estimate based on genetic testing to detect mutations on these genes. The normalization of the *anticipatory habitus* (Joseph, 2014) associated with predictive interventions related to new fields of clinical intervention such as breast cancer genetics is reflected in the growing incorporation of genetic testing for breast cancer as a standard of care across diverse fields of public and private health care, particularly in North America and Europe (see Gibbon et al., 2014). The announcement in 2013 by actress Angelina Jolie that she had undergone a prophylactic mastectomy following a positive result for a mutation on the BRCA genes provides a striking and very public example of this rationality in action, which as this chapter will illustrate, continues to have repercussions in many diverse cultural contexts, indirectly and directly informing the expansion of predictive interventions for cancer.[1]

The terrain on which genetics operates means that the promise of personalized medicine now coexists alongside an emerging field of public health genomics (Bauer, 2013; Brand, Brand, & in den Bäumen, 2008; Taussig & Gibbon, 2013). This is changing the boundaries of how and where genetic knowledge is being made relevant to health care as well as the parameters of what is described as a preventative approach to cancer. Genomic research is now directly tied to large-scale epidemiological studies for communicable as well as noncommunicable diseases. At the same time, newer and faster sequencing techniques and technologies, which enable thousands of mutations to be rapidly identified, are informing and propelling novel terrains of genetic and epigenetic research in relation to cancer and other diseases. Questions of human biological variation and population differences have also reemerged in recent years as central to, if problematic and evolving dimensions of, public health genomics. Some suggest that the turn to public health is about reenergizing a field of science that has failed to live up to expectations (Whitmarsh, 2013), helping to extend its importance and relevance (Lindee, 2013). However, as Karen Sue Taussig and I note elsewhere, also of significance is the "social action set in motion by researchers seeking to translate genomic knowledge and technologies into public health" (Taussig & Gibbon, 2013, p. 3).

Social science research has begun to examine the way that a range of high-end medical technologies are now being unevenly translated across diverse terrains of global health care delivery, such that these often coexist and are made available to patients against a backdrop of precarious public health care or a lack of basic health resources (Bharadwaj & Glasner, 2009; Biehl & Petryna, 2013). In such cases we see how hopes for and investments in medical technologies are being invigorated, even in arenas where there is a ubiquitous scarcity of other health care resources.

One striking example of the expanded terrain of specifically genomic health care is evident in the incorporation of some aspects of breast cancer genetics into public health in countries such as Cuba, as I have explored in previous research (Gibbon, 2009, 2013a). Nevertheless it is important to note the selective and partial nature of these developments, which often take place alongside a discomfort about and recognition of the difficulties associated with translating the potential of genomic interventions into health care, particularly in terms of the promise of personalized medicine. What has been described as the "absent presence" of predictive genetic interventions associated with an increased risk of breast cancer has also been noted by others in contexts such as India and Italy (Gordon, 2014; Macdonald 2014; see also Kampriani's work on Greece, 2009). In these domains, concerns about the lack of basic clinical care for those with breast cancer and/ or the irrelevancy of predictive interventions, in the light of often scarce resources, directly and indirectly informs diverse responses to and engagements with novel fields of health care intervention and technology. Despite these concerns, high-profile technologies such as breast cancer genetics have now become part of transnational fields of research carried out in relation to diverse and highly variable public health care provision (Gibbon et al., 2014). Such developments reflect and also fuel the extremely fluid relationship between research and care that has, as Hallowell and colleagues (2010) note, been a particular feature of cancer genetics.

Anthropologists who explore the now broad global terrain of clinical trial research have consistently demonstrated how participation in research is a process that can constitute subjectivity and citizenship in ways that both include and exclude (Biehl, 2007; Nguyen, 2010; Petryna, 2009; Rajan, 2005). Although inequities characterize these social relations, participation in clinical trial research can also become a strategy for obtaining medical care (Biehl, 2007; Fisher, 2009). In this way ancillary care has the potential to become an expression of the ethical variability (Petryna, 2009) of the global outsourcing of clinical trials. Marissa Mika (2013), exploring the social repercussions of global clinical trial research on the practice of oncology in Uganda, also points to the way that such research can become a resource for wider communities of health care professionals and practice.

This chapter examines how, in the context of Brazilian cancer genetics, research becomes caught up with constituting clinical need, rights and care. It explores the uneven and disjunctured ways that research on cancer genetics in Brazil is framed and reproduced as a resource. I show how patients and practitioners engage with and are constituted by predictive and risk-reducing interventions resulting in diverse forms of patient/professional activism. My goal is to shed light on the sociocultural dynamics and tensions by which prevention, public health and clinical need are being calibrated at the meeting points *and* interstices between global cancer genetic research, the limits of public health as well as its pursuit as a national imperative and the rising incidence of cancer in Brazil. In this way I illustrate how global research trajectories, propelled in part through an emphasis on genomics as a form of preventative public health, inform local clinical practice at the same time that inequities in the Brazilian health care system comprise and propel the pursuit of cancer genetics as both a right to health care and a resource for research.

The data discussed and presented here draw from 18 months of ethnographic research carried out in three urban locales in the southern region of Brazil, including periods of participant observation in cancer genetic clinics, interviews and questionnaires with patients and their families, and also interviews with medical practitioners and scientists in cancer genetic clinics linked to public and mixed private/public hospitals including cancer genetics specialists, oncologists, mastologists and biologists.[2]

ONCOGENÉTICA IN BRAZIL: BETWEEN UNMET NEED, RESEARCH AND PUBLIC HEALTH

The appearance of *oncogenética* or cancer genetics in Brazil is a recent development emerging in the last eight years partly in response to the high national incidence of cancer. Brazil has over 50,000 newly diagnosed cases of breast cancer each year, a rate that is comparable to the US population. According to the *Instituto Nacional de Câncer* (INCA, 2014) linked to the Brazilian Ministry of Health, based on data gathered from population registries, there are also regional differences in the incidence of cancer with the highest rates of breast cancer reported for the southern states of Brazil (see also Lee et al., 2012, p. e96). Whereas some northern states and cities are reported to have an incidence of breast cancer that is 10 times lower than some of these southern regions, the northeast and north have significantly higher rates of incidence and mortality from cervical cancer (Azevedo & Silva, 2010).

There have been recent efforts to address rising rates of breast cancer in Brazil, including legislation in 2009 by the Brazilian Ministry of Health to recommended mammography screening every 2 years for all women between 50 and 69 (and at 35 years of age for those with a family history). However, limited data suggest not only that the infrastructure for providing mammograms are starkly different between northern and southern regions, but overall national mammography screening rates remaining substantially lower than WHO recommendations to screen over 70% of the population, with doctors in Brazil reporting that 80% of breast cancer cases are identified and brought to their attention by patients (Lee et al., 2012; p. e96). Moreover a recent Brazilian study examining breast cancer outcomes across different regions in Brazil found that women who received public health care had more advanced disease, less access to modern health care and treatments, and lower survival than those treated at private institutions (Simon, et al., 2009).

These disparities in access to and provision of breast cancer services reflect the broader complexities of public health provision in Brazil. The constitutional right to health emerged in post-dictatorship Brazil, informed by the efforts of various social movements to democratize health care. Nevertheless, the changes that this brought about have been contradictory and uneven (Biehl, 2005; Edmonds, 2010; Sanabria, 2010). About 75% of the population has access to health care only through the public health care system or SUS (Sistema Único de Saúde), with the rest of the population making use of health plans and insurances.[3] At the same time, the availability and relative affordability of health insurance for the middle class has meant that many choose not to use public services, seeing them as offering substandard care, a process that Faveret and Oliveira (1990) describe as "excluding universalism." Nevertheless, there is, as Sanabria (2010) in her examination of hormones and public health in Brazil points out, a great deal of movement of doctors, patients and protocols between private and public health care domains.

Some of that movement is reflected in the context of cancer genetics in Brazil, which is nevertheless emerging mainly in the relatively wealthy southern regions of the country. With genetic services not currently covered by the public health care system, cancer genetics operates in something of an interstitial space between research and public health. That is, it is practiced at the meeting point and gaps between the research activities of individual Brazilian researchers or their teams involved in collaborations with other scientists in the United States, France and Portugal, and precarious and limited public health interventions including screening or monitoring interventions such as mammography.[4] In this way, Brazilian cancer genetic services, situated by those who work in the field in Brazil as a *preventative* approach in a context of scarcity and limited resources, is mobilized and enacted in part through globalized clinical and transnational research collaborations.

The first part of this chapter explores some of these dynamics from the perspective of health care practitioners and scientists. It shows how the *activism* of these individuals within cancer genetics must be understood and rendered explicit as it serves to constitute clinical need, situate and extend research priorities in relation to transnational research collaborations, and provide care as part of a neglected preventative approach in a context of limited resources. The second part of this chapter examines the experience of patients who participate in, and in some cases pursue the *right* to what is perceived as preventative health.[5]

ACTIVIST PRACTITIONERS: UNKNOWN RISK AND THE POLITICS OF PREVENTION

There has been growing attention to population difference in genetic research tied in part to the emergence of public health genomics. That is, as testing widens across a global terrain it reveals gaps in medical knowledge based on databases of known mutations in previously identified risk populations in national contexts such as the United States, Canada and Europe. This fuels and informs a focus on identifying variation on the *spectrum* of currently unknown mutations that might be implicated across different national contexts as part of the pursuit of public health genomics. For some this has been described as linked to an emerging trajectory associated with the pharmaceutical industry of niche marketing (Lee 2005). Others point to the tensions this has generated in the way that the so-called underserved needs of neglected groups and populations are being reformulated in terms of both a resource and right to research and care. As Rayna Rapp (2013) points out "multiple publics have become part of exquisitely stratified research populations that now serve as potential global resources and market beneficiaries" (p. 574).

As I have explored elsewhere, moves to expand cancer genetics in contexts such as Brazil are emerging alongside and in tension with transnational research agendas linked to population difference (Gibbon, 2013b; Mozersky & Gibbon, 2014). Within Brazil, an emphasis on the *unknown* contribution of genetic risk in understanding the rising rates of cancer in the country reveals the limits of international standardized risk models and fuels the pursuit and activism of practitioners caught up in Brazilian cancer genetics framed in terms of finding more appropriate local estimations of genetic risk for the Brazilian population. In practice, however, efforts to identify the particular genetic aspects of the Brazilian population that may be relevant in terms of genetic ancestry and establish the relevance (or irrelevance) of certain mutations linked to an increased risk of cancer can involve both the incorporation and simultaneous rejection of categories of race and ethnicity (Mozersky & Gibbon, 2014; see also Santos, Silva & Gibbon 2014).

Nevertheless, putting into practice Brazilian cancer genetics and constituting it as clinical need are closely tied not only to efforts by practitioners to attend to as yet unknown national parameters of population difference, but also to a moral economy that conceives of cancer genetics as prevention.

Such moves parallel broader shifts in the way that a focus on population difference, particularly in the field of BRCA genetics, has been constituted as a movement towards prevention.[6]

This was evident in the way one young trainee cancer genetic practitioner in Sao Paulo passionately described the necessity of cancer genetics in Brazil.

> Why do we need this? Because we see the importance when you interview a family that has multiple cases of cancer in the family and understand the desperation of those families when they ask, "what should I look for?" "What should I do?" "Who's going to help me get early screening for my daughter, for my sister?" Because of this, it's vital that Brazil has in its public health system, cancer genetic clinics to try and help these families, and to have in our Brazilian statistics understanding of the genetic diseases that we are transmitting to our families . . . the populations going to grow and develop and transmit these mutations, so we have to know how to deal with this in the long term.

Here we see how an emphasis on attending to underserved populations who do not have access to basic health services is entwined with the perceived need to understand and gain knowledge about Brazilian statistics related to genetic risk as part of an emerging preventative approach framed in terms of having access to early screening and care for those at risk in the family. Such sentiments were reflected in the comments of another practitioner who described cancer genetics in terms of "protection for the family," stating that such individuals could have "a higher risk of having a tumor." Likewise, she added "I really think that cancer genetics is prevention."

For many of those who worked in the cancer genetics field there was a great deal of frustration associated with trying to ensure those who had been identified as being at risk were offered appropriate *preventative* interventions. In the mixed private/public hospital where I worked in Sao Paulo, I frequently witnessed the convoluted tasks that nurses and geneticists engaged in trying to ensure all those potentially at risk in the family were able to obtain extra screening once a family member had been identified as carrying a mutation. When one person had a *convenio* or private health insurance that covered certain kinds of interventions such as extra screening but others in the family did not, doctors and nurses skillfully maneuvered between the limits of the public health system, research protocols, hospital provision and the rules and regulations of different health insurers to make every effort to ensure that as many family members as possible were able to obtain screening.

The logic of cancer genetics for health for many of these professionals was evident. They emphasized not only the moral economy of prevention in terms of care for the family but the cost–benefits of cancer genetics to identify those at risk compared with the cost of treating those who developed breast cancer. This was how one geneticist in Porto Alegre put it,

If you have a family who [has] every likelihood of carrying a BRCA1 and BRCA2 gene, it's much simpler to test and know who has the mutation and who doesn't, rather than to screen everyone. If you imagine that 50% have the mutation and 50% don't, for at least half of those you don't have to do anything and that's a saving. The problem is the issue of compromising. I'm seeing a family today that needs the test that I can offer but it's very expensive; *SUS* doesn't offer this. But what happens if I leave it there and not worry about this and pretend there isn't a problem? . . . I just can't for another ten years keep doing research to offer testing . . . with care being something peripheral that [is] just tacked on the side.

In this instance it is not only the logic of cancer genetics as public health and prevention that is articulated, but also a frustration engendered by attempting to manage a clinical service that is ultimately dependent on research funding. Nevertheless, it is important to note that the idea of creating cancer genetic services within public health as part of a preventative approach was not supported by all health professionals I met in Brazil. In one public health hospital where I discussed this possibility with those who worked in the broader field of mastology (a health care specialty focused on breast health), there was considerable doubt about the value of cancer genetics in a *SUS* hospital. One of the mastologists began our interview by pointing to the very same challenge that the Brazilian cancer geneticists had identified, the lack of knowledge relating to the relevance of current knowledge about genetic risk for the Brazilian population. As he said, "there isn't a study of the Brazilian population on wide scale as yet that says what size of the Brazilian population is affected whether its 5, 10 or 15% genetic risk—that data doesn't exist."

But he also by contrast drew stark attention to the costs associated with such interventions:

It [genetic testing] is just not very common here [referring to the public hospital where he worked] because this involves costs. A hospital like this that looks after essentially a socially insecure population doesn't provide this because of the costs involved in these kind of tests, if they were available and used more freely.

Relating this situation back to the lack of knowledge about cancer risk in Brazil he continued:

If you don't have the criteria, you start to waste money and here we don't have money to waste . . . perhaps there are other priorities that should be addressed and would help lessen the impact of a particular disease . . . we have to select where we are going to invest our money, resources and materials . . . so I think we still don't have a justification for having a big national program that would involve lots of human resources. The test isn't certain even, it just says whether you have a risk or chance of having it or not so perhaps sometimes we are creating problems that we can't resolve and for which we can't really offer a very good solution.

In this case, the moral framing of cancer genetics as prevention is contested and brought into question in relation to the unknown component of genetic risk in Brazil and the cost of such interventions in resource-poor contexts. For some medical professionals (in this case those working in a related specialty that in fact prides it itself on adopting a *holistic* approach to breast health and the treatment of breast cancer), cancer genetics sits outside the realm of public health care and prevention due to both cost, unknown relevance and the uncertainty that it intervenes upon and also generates. This points to the limits of practitioner activism highlighting greater variation and diversity in the affective framing of cancer genetics as prevention across diverse domains of breast cancer care within spheres of public health care provision in Brazil.

ACTIVIST PRACTITIONERS AND *ROAD TRIPS*: THE PURSUIT OF RESEARCH AND PREVENTION

Events that provided some informative ethnographic insight on how the *activism* of cancer genetic practitioners facilitated the productive conjunction between participating in global research agendas and pursuing cancer genetics as public health were what were described as *road trips* made by some of the researchers I met. These were often undertaken by teams of the local and international cancer genetic researchers and health professionals to the interior and rural parts of the southern states of the country, as they engaged in efforts to seek out and identify individuals and families affected by hereditary cancer syndromes.

I accompanied one group of health professionals to the interior of the state of Sao Paulo to meet with an extended family who had experienced many cases of cancer, and recount some of that event in the following excerpt from fieldnotes:

We arrived early one morning in a rural region at the family home of one young female patient in her mid-20s who had been treated some years earlier for cancer at the hospital in Sao Paulo. Sonja was a student in Sao Paulo but had a large family in the interior of the state, which she had returned to on an overnight bus to meet us early in the morning at her aunt's house. It was in this moment, noticing the slight anxiety of Sonja as she watched and greeted family members as they arrived, that it became clear how she had been a central figure in the gathering of her relatives to meet the cancer genetics team as aunts, uncles and young relatives arrived at the entrance to the house. Giving an impromptu talk to the families the practitioner described the visit in terms "a chance to participate in research" and "a way of preventing cancer in the future" and also a "an opportunity to see who is at risk so that they can be offered treatment in Sao Paulo." She added that it was not, of course, obligatory to participate in the research, which was totally voluntary. Later I was told by one member of the team that it was unlikely that many of the family had convenios or private health insurance and living in a rural part of the state were, as a result, without easy access to health care services such as routine basic health care screening. While not explicitly stating that being involved in the research was a means to secure routine preventative screening from the hospital in Sao Paulo it seemed from these remarks that, from the point of view of the health professionals involved, this was perceived as an indirect benefit of participating in research.

Sitting in the make-shift space for collecting blood samples for research, which had been set up in one of rooms alongside the nurse, it was obvious that many of the preoccupations of those who agreed to donate blood for research were related to more immediate health care problems rather than the future risk of cancer per se. One elderly relative had a lot of pain in her neck and she asked if she should see someone in the hospital in Sao Paulo. The response of the nurse in this instance was not to be concerned for the moment about these health problems as the first thing to do was to find out if they were carriers of the mutation that Sonja had, pointing out that if they also carried the same mutation then they would be able to have access to more investigations. It seemed then from what the nurse was saying that a preventative approach was therefore predicated on the necessity through research of identifying those at highest risk.

The steady flow of relatives willing to donate blood and participate in the research generated a good deal of energy and enthusiasm among the researchers. In the car on our return there was much excitement that they had been able to collect so many samples in one visit and discussion about whether this would enable to them to map further clusters of cancer in the region as they had already done with a number of other families. But there was also some discussion of the social context of the family and, given the lack of access to health care through private health insurance, the extent to which other family members might through research protocols be encompassed by the care provided under the aegis of the cancer genetic research protocols at the hospital. There was in fact heightened awareness that this was essentially precarious, predicated on continuous funding from international collaborations and the ongoing willingness of the hospital to include at risk family members, not just those with cancer, in the hospital's protocols for screening interventions.

The events such as the road trips say much about activism on the part of these professionals. I would argue that these are not entirely explainable in terms of a perspective that views them as examples of the exploitation of vulnerable communities simply for the purpose of research collaborations and publications. There are both moral and affective dimensions associated with practitioners' efforts to pursue cancer genetics as public health via collaborative transnational research. The seeking out families in this way was not then *only* about furthering research ends, or simply identifying those at most risk, but was also about facilitating access to basic health services in efforts to meet what these practitioners perceived as the neglected broader goals of a preventative approach to health care. Nevertheless, as the road trips make clear, the role of patients in facilitating and mobilizing cancer genetic research as prevention is also central. In the final part of the chapter I turn more directly to examine the experience and perception of patients engaged with cancer genetic research in Brazil.

A LONGING FOR CARE AND THE RIGHT TO HEALTH

Only a handful of the vast majority of patients I met while carrying out research in three urban centers was able to muster the $2–3,000 necessary to pay for a genetic test. Most had arrived in the cancer genetic clinics following referral by a family member who had been treated at the hospital for cancer and were for the most part *SUS* patients.[7] As a result, their own and their family members' eligibility for testing was, for the most part, tied to a specific study protocol. Many were waiting for test results but as part of a program of research were also in receipt of other basic screening and health monitoring services. For many of these individuals simply being within the parameters of the hospital's care through participation in research was perceived as prevention. As one middle-aged female cancer patient who had had breast cancer but was now part of a study protocol relating to research on the two BRCA genes put it, "this works as prevention . . . if there was more of this type of research perhaps persons wouldn't arrive with cancer as it was in my case." Referring to her children she added:

> My daughters will now have much more care, they will be examined much earlier, perhaps have preventative screening much earlier and perhaps not come having developed cancer—this is a procedure (*uma regra*) that would be useful for everyone.

For others, being involved in this type of program went beyond prevention to being actively part of the search for a cure. As the following comments from a female patient in Sao Paulo suggest, this perception resulted in an eagerness and willingness to be part of such study protocols, where being a *guinea pig*, far from being something negative, was actively sought out and valued. As she said:

> I think that the future cure for cancer is in genetic research. Look take my cancer cells and make a vaccine! I think this will happen. I think

that genetics isn't just about prevention but a question of cure as well. Whenever they have this kind of research at the hospital I always say yes, I would really like to be a guinea pig in the cure for cancer.

Although these sentiments were shared by a number of patients, the majority of those I met felt a sense of relief that by participating in the research provided by the hospital they had access to regular screening and specialist health care. As we saw in the case of the road trip described previously, patients recruited into research perceived this as a means of accessing basic health care. This was also the case for Maria, a cleaner in her 40s who worked in Porto Alegre, as she talked about what it meant to her (and the difficulties she had also experienced) in her efforts to be under the aegis of the specialist hospitals' cancer genetic services:

When you manage to get a consultation with the doctor you're relieved but to arrive here you have to go through tremendous bureaucracy, queue for hours. In other hospitals you have to wait nearly one year to do a mammogram or 8 months for meeting with the doctor—the problem is getting in here [referring to the hospital associated with the cancer genetic research]. Once you arrive here everything's a blessing (*tudo e a abencoada*)—the problem is in getting here. [Now] I feel protected, I have screening and if I have a problem I know that I can have chemotherapy or surgery . . . I don't have the words to describe how grateful I am to you for all that you are doing here.[8]

The ways patients describe their experiences of participation in research reveal then a particular scale of investments that constitute an expanded space of possibilities for cancer genetics in Brazil. For these individuals this includes hopes for prevention or cure and participation in research becomes a strategic means of accessing often precarious or hard-to-get basic care and resources.

In an examination of the newly emerging field of public health genomics in Barbados, Ian Whitmarsh (2013) suggests that as genetic diagnosis, monitoring and surveillance are increasingly conceived as forms of preventative public health and a social good, there is an ethical imperative for individuals to fashion and discipline themselves into what he describes as new subjects of "biomedical compliance." Although some elements of these forms of subjectivity may be apparent in the narratives recounted in this paper there is, as Biehl and Petryna (2013, pp. 14–15) point out, a need to guard against a "uniform and unilateral diagnosis" to examine the "granular ways" in which supposedly neoliberal principles, tied in this instance to proactive patienthood required by genetic screening interventions, become "part and parcel of public health landscapes and social relations in resource poor contexts." As Petryna (2013) has noted elsewhere, there are often novel possibilities for the crafting of rights and responsibilities in such contexts that must be attended to and accounted for.

One very powerful illustration of this is evident in an emerging phenomenon in Brazil that is transforming the parameters and pathways by which patients are accessing health care services, linked to a process described as the judicialization of health and the phenomenon of patient litigants. In conclusion, I show how this is becoming evident within and developing as a direct consequence of the interstitial space in which Brazilian cancer genetics operates. Such phenomenon serve to further illuminate the diverse vectors through which an anticipatory habitus embedded in the preventative promise of cancer genetics is becoming part of new and novel claims and rights to health in Brazil.

As noted in recent studies by Joao Biehl and Adriana Petryna (2011, 2013), thousands of Brazilian patients across different social and economic classes are effectively suing the government for the right to health care resources such as medications, but also now other treatments, examinations and tests, predicated on a constitutional commitment in Brazil to provide health care for all. Patients litigants, who appear to comprise a broad section of social classes, are not simply "waiting for the high cost of medicine technologies to trickle down" but are instead "using public assistance and the levers of a responsive jury to gain full access now" (Biehl & Petryna, 2011, p. 363). Whereas the first such successful cases of judicialization have occurred in the context of participation in clinical trial research for medication related to mainly rare genetic conditions, increasingly patients are pursuing and successfully obtaining the right to health care resources outside these parameters by accessing mostly free legal services. As I illustrate next, this now includes the right to have a predictive genetic test for breast cancer.

In October 2013, I returned to Brazil as part of a research visit to the southern part of the country. Within minutes of meeting friends and colleagues working in one of the cancer genetic clinics there were numerous comments about Angelina Jolie's announcement made six months previously. From what they said it was clear that this had generated a lot of polemical discussion in the Brazilian media, as well as significantly raising the profile of cancer genetics in the country. "Thank goodness for Angelina Jolie," said one genetic practitioner casually as she talked to me of how the numbers at the cancer genetic clinic in a mixed public/private hospital in Sao Paulo had grown exponentially since the highly public statement by the actress and the ensuing media focus. While also pointing out she had as a result been approached by numerous television, radio and media outlets to comment on the announcement, she told me how referrals to the clinic and interest from publics had increased threefold in the ensuing six months. In another public hospital in Rio, it was notable while sitting in on a couple of consultations with practitioners whom I had gone to meet that Jolie's name was mentioned again, this time in the process of explaining the risk of having a BRCA mutation to a patient. The nurse genetic counselor used reference to Jolie's announcement as a way it seemed of almost normalizing the procedures that she was offering the patient; in this case, the possibility of having a genetic test linked to a particular research protocol. But it was at another public hospital in Porto Alegre where another dimension of these developments came to light.

The genetic practitioner there told me how in the last few months at least one or two of the 30 or so new patients without private health insurance seen each week had come armed with letters from lawyers saying that they were going to "*entra na justicia*" (go to the courts) to demand the government pay for them to have a genetic test, saying that they have a "right" (*um direto*) to the test that Angelina Jolie had. Although not totally supportive of judicialization as the best means by which patients should have access to health care (or equally that the action of celebrities should have this effect rather than reasoned science and research), the doctor I met acknowledged that the phenomenon of patient litigants in the context of cancer genetics was changing the health care landscape in which they were working. Moreover, she thought this was likely to put increasing pressure on the state to incorporate cancer genetics as part of the public provision of health care, a goal that was much sought after by many of those who worked in this emerging field of cancer care in Brazil.

The full consequences of the expansion of judicialization processes to include procedures such as predictive genetic testing is still unfolding in Brazil with cases being examined at federal and state level in what is normally a fairly drawn out process that can take many years. Nevertheless, the very fact that this phenomenon is happening now in Brazil further illustrates the complexities of the interstitial spaces in which Brazilian cancer genetics is coming into being and the way that an anticipatory habitus is becoming bound to a discourse of rights, not in this case to access treatment, but to pursue genetic testing as part of what is seen as preventative approach.

CONCLUSION

In this chapter I have explored the tensions and dynamics surrounding the way one domain of high-technology medicine associated with a transforming terrain of public health genomics is being mobilized and constituted as a social good, linked in part to a discourse of cancer prevention. In Brazil this is emerging in the not-easily-disaggregated meeting points between transnational research and precarious public health care provision in efforts to address and ameliorate the effects of rapidly rising cancer incidence and mortality. As Whitmarsh (2013) points out, while the pursuit of genetic research in resource-poor settings might be seen simply as an effort to simply "join in on cutting edge biomedicine," it also informs and transforms what counts as public health.

In Brazilian cancer genetics, patients participate in research in hopes of accessing basic health care services and what is perceived as the right to pursue prevention. At the same time, the activism of health professionals is central to collaborations in transnational research on the unknown genetic risks of breast cancer for the Brazilian population and to addressing underserved health care needs as part of a neglected preventative approach to health care. Yet this moral and affective framing of cancer genetics as prevention is not shared by all of those who work in related fields of health care, pointing to the limits of such activism and to differing perceptions about how public health and prevention should be pursued. Nonetheless, the anticipatory habitus constituted by fields of knowledge such as breast cancer genetics in Brazil seems to have found new expression in the wake of the activities of one global celebrity, which in conjunction with an expanding arena of judicialization in Brazil may potentially inform public health in as yet unknown ways.

Transnational research, and particularly clinical trials research, is embedded in complex structures of inequality and power that can work to exploit. At the same time, the particular institutional configuration of research and clinical intervention outlined in this chapter related to cancer genetic research in Brazil is also the context through which patients seek and often obtain basic health care in pursuit of prevention. It is similarly a nexus through which national research initiatives are nurtured and developed, previously nonexisting clinical specialties and professional identities are forged, and the means through which collective demands for wider public health care provision can be made to foreground an ethic of prevention.

As others have noted, the boundary between research and clinical care is often thin in the context of genetic research where research participation is often regarded as having diagnostic consequences or therapeutic benefits (Hallowell et al., 2010). This is particularly so in the context of cancer genetics where many hybrid activities take place given its inherently translational dimensions (Hallowell, 2009). Highlighting how the moral framing of research and clinical care are often closely and complexly entwined, Wadman and Hoeyer (2014) point out that it is important to not see this necessarily as a dilemma or obstacle but as a way to understand how both can thrive on coexistence and the way that knowledge, work ethics and emotions emerge in tandem (p. 7; see also Timmermans, 2010). While the enmeshed boundaries between research and care in transnational research generate different questions and challenges, given inequities and disparities in resources, it is important to see how and in what ways for different groups and individuals in specific local contexts research is constituted as a resource and resourcefully acted upon.

As the changing techniques, including the rapidly diminishing price of genomic screening for diseases such as cancer, are unevenly incorporated across and within developed and also increasingly emerging and developing country contexts, it will be important to monitor in comparative cultural arenas the ways that clinical need, prevention and rights to health become part of diverse efforts to shape and reshape the making of public health genomics.

NOTES

1. This development has generated much discussion across a range of public and social media and there is increasing evidence that the so-called "Angelina Jolie effect" has led to a marked increase in enquiries and referrals to cancer genetic clinics in the UK and elsewhere (Joseph, 2014; Retassie, 2013).
2. This work was funded by the Wellcome Trust (grant WT084128MA) as part of a project titled "Admixture, Ancestry and Breast Cancer in Brazil: An Ethnographic Investigation of Population Genetics, Disease Risk and Identity." Research included participant observation in cancer genetic clinics over a period of 18 months in three different urban centers of Brazil, interviews with patients and family members attending cancer genetic clinics (over 100 in total), and interviews with practitioners and scientists working within or alongside cancer genetic specialists (over 40 in total). Participating patients were attending cancer genetic clinics and were either undergoing, had received, or were awaiting the result of a genetic test on BRCA1 or BRCA 2 or R337h (a mutation thought to have a high frequency in the southern part of Brazil). Whereas the majority were women there were a number of men also recruited in the study, all were over 18.
3. See "Brazil's March towards Universal Coverage" in Bulletin of WHO, Volume 88, pp. 641–716.
4. In 2012 private insurance companies in Brazil agreed to pay for genetic testing for those with insurance schemes or *convenios*. During the time of most of my research however this was not the case, although a number of patients were advised to approach their health insurance provider by cancer geneticists in the hope of being able to secure a test.
5. The activism of health care practitioners is also an aspect that I've explored in the context of research on cancer genetics in Cuba (Gibbon 2013a).
6. This is evident in the growing calls in Canada and Israel for programs of population-wide screening of all Ashkenazi Jewish women and increasing interest in targeted screening interventions for certain populations, such as African American women with breast cancer diagnosed at a young age, with family history or with triple negative tumors (see for instance Churpek et al., 2013 and also Joseph, 2014).
7. Approximately 15% of the over 100 families and individuals who were interviewed had *convenios* or private health insurance and under 5% privately paid for genetic testing.
8. This patient quote also appears in Gibbon (2013b).

REFERENCES

Azevedo & Silva, G. (2010). Cervical cancer mortality trends in Brazil 1981–2006. *Cauderno da Saude Publica, 26,* 2399–2407.
Bauer, S. (2013). Modeling population health: Reflections on performativity of epidemiological techniques in the age of genomics. In K. S. Taussig & S. Gibbon (Eds.), Public health genomics. Anthropological interventions in the quest for molecular medicine. *Medical Anthropology Quarterly. Special Issue: Public Health Genomics, 27,* 510–530.
Bharadwaj, A., & Glasner, P. (2009). *Local cells, global science: The proliferation of stem cell technologies in India.* New York, NY: Routledge.
Biehl, J. (2005). *Vita: Life in a zone of social abandonment.* Berkeley, CA: University of California Press.

Biehl, J. (2007) *Will to live. AIDS therapies and the politics of survival.* Princeton, NJ: Princeton University Press.
Biehl, J., & Petryna, A. (2011). Bodies of rights and therapeutic markets. *Social Research: An International Quarterly, 78,* 359–386.
Biehl, J., & Petryna, A. (2013). Critical global health. *When people come first: Critical studies in global health.* Princeton, NJ: Princeton University Press.
Bourret, P., Keating, P., & Cambrosio, A. (2014). From BRCA to BRCAness: Tales of translational research. In S. Gibbon, G. Joseph, E. Kampriani, J. Mozersky, A. zun Nieden, & S. Palfner (Eds.), *Breast cancer gene research and medical practices: Transnational perspectives in the time of BRCA* (pp.175–193). ESRC Genomics Network Genetics and Society Book Series. London: Routledge.
Brand, A., Brand, H., & in den Bäumen, T. S. (2008). The impact of genetics and genomics on public health. *European Journal of Human Genetics, 16,* 5–13.
Churpek, J. E., Walsh, T., Zheng, Y., Casadei, S., Thornton, A.M., Lee, M.K., . . . Olopade, O. I. (2013). Inherited mutations in breast cancer genes in African American breast cancer patients revealed by targeted genomic capture and next generation sequencing. *Journal of Clinical Oncology, 31,* (suppl; abstra CRA1501).
Edmonds, A. (2010). *Pretty modern: Beauty, sex and plastic surgery in Brazil.* Durham, NC: Duke University Press.
Faveret, F., & Oliveira, P. J. (1990). A universalização excludente: reflexões sobre as tendências do sistema de saúde. *Planejamento e Políticas Públicas, 3,* 139–162.
Fisher, J. (2009). *Research for hire: The political economy of pharmaceutical clinical trial.* New Brunswick: Rutgers University Press.
Gibbon, S. (2009). Genomics as public health? Community genetics and the challenge of personalised medicine in Cuba. *Anthropology and Medicine, 16,* 131–146.
Gibbon, S. (2013a). Science, sentiment and the state. Community genetics and the pursuit of public health in Cuba. *Medical Anthropology Quarterly. Special Issue: Public Health Genomics, 27,* 531–549.
Gibbon, S. (2013b). Ancestry, temporality, and potentiality: Engaging cancer genetics in southern Brazil. *Current Anthropology Special Issue on Potentiality and Humanness: Revisiting the Anthropological Object in Contemporary Biomedicine, 54,* S107–S117.
Gibbon, S., Galen, J., Kampriani, E., Mozersky, J., zur Nieden, A., & Palfner, S. (Eds.). (2014). *Breast cancer gene research and medical practices: Transnational perspectives in the time of BRCA. ESRC Genomics Network Genetics and Society Book Series.* London: Routledge.
Gordon, D. (2014). It takes a particular world to produce and enact BRCA testing: The US had it, Italy had another. In S. Gibbon, G. Joseph, E. Kampriani, J. Mozersky, A. zun Nieden, & S. Palfner (Eds.), *Breast cancer gene research and medical practices: Transnational perspectives in the time of BRCA* (pp. 109–126). London and New York: Routledge.
Hallowell, N., Parry, S., Looke, S., Crawford, G., Lucassen, A., & Parker, M. (2010). Lay and professional understandings of research and clinical activities in cancer genetics and their implications for informed consent. *American Journal of Bioethics Primary Research, 1,* 25–34.
Hallowell, N., Cooke, S., Grawford, G., Parker, M. & Lucassen, A. (2009). Distinguishing research from clinical care in cancer genetics: Theoretical justifications and practical strategies. *Social Science and Medicine, 68,* 2010–2017.
INCA (Instituto Nacional de Cancer). (2014). *Estimativa. Incidencia de Cancer no Brasil.* Retrieved from http://www.inca.gov.br/estimativa/2014/index.asp.
Joseph, G. (2014). Genetics to the People: BRCA as public health and the dissemination of cancer risk knowledge. In S. Gibbon, G. Joseph, E. Kampriani, J. Mozersky, A. zun Nieden, & S. Palfner (Eds.), *Breast cancer gene research and medical*

practices: Transnational perspectives in the time of BRCA (pp. 57–72). *ESRC Genomics Network Genetics and Society Book Series.* London: Routledge.

Kampriani. E. (2009). Between religious philanthropy and individualized medicine: situating inherited breast cancer in Greece. Biomedical technology and health inequities in the global north and south. *Anthropology and Medicine Special Issue, 16,* 165–78.

Lee, B.L., Liedke, P.E.R., Barrios, C.H., Simon, S.D., Finkelstein, D.M., Goss, P.E. (2012). Breast cancer in Brazil: Present status and future goals. *The Lancet, 13,* e95- e102.

Lee, S.S.J. (2005). Racializing drug design: Implications of pharmacogenomics for health disparities. *American Journal of Public Health, 95,* 2133–2138.

Lindee, S. (2013). Commentary: A return to origins. Public Health Genomics. Anthropological Interventions in the Quest for Molecular Medicine. *Medical Anthropology Quarterly. Special Issue: Public Health Genomics, 27,* 570–572.

Macdonald, A. (2014). Situating breast cancer risk in urban India: Gender, temporality and social change. In S. Gibbon, G. Joseph, E. Kampriani, J. Mozersky, A. zun Nieden, & S. Palfner (Eds.), *Breast cancer gene research and medical practices: Transnational perspectives in the time of BRCA* (pp. 83–94). *ESRC Genomics Network Genetics and Society Book Series.* London: Routledge.

Mika, M. (2013). Research is our resource: Political oncology in Uganda. Paper presented at *AAA Panel Global Cancer: Institutions, Challenges and Stakes,* November 20–23, Chicago, IL.

Mozersky, J., & Gibbon, S. (2014). Mapping Jewish identities: Migratory histories and the transnational framing of the "Ashkenazi BRCA mutations" in the UK and Brazil. In S. Gibbon, G. Joseph, E. Kampriani, J. Mozersky, A. zun Nieden, & S. Palfner (Eds.), *Breast cancer gene research and medical practices: Transnational perspectives in the time of BRCA* (pp. 35–66). *ESRC Genomics Network Genetics and Society Book Series.* London: Routledge.

Nguyen, V-K. (2010). *The republic of therapy: Triage and sovereignty in West Africa's time of AIDS.* Durham: Duke University Press.

Petryna, A. (2013). The right of recovery. *Current Anthropology. Special Issue on Potentiality and Humanness: Revisiting the Anthropological Object in Contemporary Biomedicine, 54,* S67–S76.

Petryna, A. (2009). *When experiments travel: Clinical trials and the search for human subjects.* Princeton, NJ: Princeton University Press.

Rajan, K.S. (2005). Subjects of speculation: Emergent life sciences and market logics in the United States and India. *American Anthropologist, 107,* 19–30.

Rapp, R. (2013). Commentary: Thinking through public health genomics. Public health genomics. Anthropological interventions in the quest for molecular medicine. *Medical Anthropology Quarterly. Special Issue: Public Health Genomics, 27,* 573–576.

Retassie, R. (2013). The Jolie effect: Breast cancer gene testing increases, but so do surgery requests. *Bionews, 725,* Retrieved from http://www.bionews.org.uk/page_ 349931.asp.

Sanabria, E. (2010). From sub- to super-citizenship: Sex hormones and the body politic in Brazil. *Ethnos, Journal of Anthropology, 75,* 377–401.

Santos, R.V., Silva, G. & Gibbon, S. (2014). Pharmacogenomics, human genetic diversity and the incorporation and rejection of color/race in Brazil. *Journal of Biosocieties.* doi: 10.1057/biosoc.2014.21

Simon, S. D., Bines, J., Barrios, C., Nunes, J., Gomes, E., Pacheco, F., . . . Vasconcellos, C. (2009). Clinical characteristics and outcome of treatment of Brazilian women with breast cancer treated at public and private institutions—the AMAZONE project of the Brazilian breast cancer study group (GBECAM). *San Antonio Breast Cancer Symposium, 69,* San Antonoio, TX, Abstract.

Taussig, K. S. & Gibbon, S. (2013). Introduction. Public health genomics. Anthropo-logical interventions in the quest for molecular medicine. *Medical Anthropology Quarterly. Special Issue: Public Health Genomics, 27,* 471–488.

Timmermans, S. (2010). Reconciling research with medical care in RCTs. In C. Will & T. Moreira (Eds.), *Medical Proofs, Social Experiments: Clinical Trials in Shifting Contexts* (pp. 17–31). Farnham, UK and Burlington, VT: Ashgate.

Wadman, S., & Hoeyer, K. (2014). Beyond the therapeutic misconception: Research, care and moral friction. *Biosocieties, 9,* 3–23.

Whitmarsh, I. (2013). The ascetic subject of compliance: The turn to chronic disease in global health. In J. Biehl & A. Petryna (Eds.), *When people come first: Critical studies in global health* (pp. 302–325). Princeton, NJ: Princeton University Press.

4 Managing Borders, Bodies and Cancer
Documents and the Creation of Subjects[1]

Julie S. Armin

> Unauthorized entry, the most common form of illegal immigration [to the United States] since the 1920s, remains vexing for both state and society. Undocumented immigrants are at once **welcome and unwelcome**: they are woven into the economic fabric of the nation, but as labor that is cheap and disposable.
>
> —Mae M. Ngai, Impossible Subjects: Illegal Aliens
> and the Making of Modern America
> (2004, p. 2; author's emphasis)

This chapter examines access to cancer care among a structurally vulnerable population by noting how documents work to naturalize the place of unauthorized immigrants in the social and economic hierarchy in the United States. Documents structure access to health care. They foreclose some avenues for agency while opening up others, and they do the work of the state in disciplining *illegal* immigrant bodies. Drawing upon anthropological research into health care's role in producing the limited social inclusion of immigrants (e.g., Fassin & d'Halluin, 2005; Horton, 2004; Ticktin, 2006), I examine how undocumented women's structural vulnerability is reproduced by networks of health care providers who construct and circulate financial and medical documents. In doing so, I look to four general types of documents, discussing how they shape access to health care among the women in my study: 1) immigration/citizenship documents, which determine eligibility for public insurance; 2) medical records, which provide opportunities for health care access without political recognition; 3) financial documents, including bills and financial statements, which discipline subjects in a context of perceived scarcity; and 4) insurance documents, which provide uncertain stability and protection against debt. I examine how these various documents reflect and reinforce the social marginalization of unauthorized women, while also producing limited opportunities for action.

The fieldwork reported in this chapter was conducted from June 2010 until December 2011, with some additional interviews and participant observation taking place in summer and fall of 2012 in a major city in southern Arizona. In this study, I focused on women living with breast cancer who were either uninsured or eligible for the publicly funded insurance program called Medicaid. I employed ethnographic methods, including in-depth interviews, focus groups, and participant observation. I interacted with health care providers at three primary field sites: 1) a large academic cancer center, which I call Desert Cancer Center; 2) a federally qualified health center, which I call Saguaro Clinic; and 3) a small clinic staffed by a combination of volunteer and paid clinical professionals, which I call Mercy Clinic. Although I interviewed staff at all three locations (n = 33), most of my patient participants (n = 7)—both uninsured and Medicaid-eligible—were recruited through Mercy Clinic.

I employed a longitudinal qualitative research design and conducted one in-depth, in-person interview every three months with each woman living with cancer over the course of nine months. This approach facilitated insight into the ways in which thoughts, constraints, opportunities and challenges changed over time. During my visits with women, I collected information about the practical support they received at home, their medical bills, the financial support received from friends, family or charitable institutions (including health care providers). I also interviewed family members living in the home (n = 4). I rounded out my knowledge about the cancer care context by attending community events, such as Race for the Cure, by taking part in professional training and patient education events, and traveling to a major clinical breast cancer conference.[2] In the following, I focus on the detailed case of one of my participants to illustrate the complex role documents play in shaping the illness experiences of all participants.

This research uses the concept of structural vulnerability (Quesada, Hart, & Bourgois, 2011) as an analytic for understanding the health effects of unauthorized immigrants' position in a social hierarchy that takes as *natural* immigrants' social construction as "an embodied geography of disobedience to the law (a criminal)–in effect, a disobedient body"(Sandoval, 2008, p. 582). As Mae M. Ngai (2004) argues in her history of the making of "illegal aliens" in the United States, immigration policy in the early part of the 20th century reinforced racial and national hierarchies that privileged the entry of certain groups of immigrants, while blocking the entry of others. Furthermore, she writes, "Immigration restriction produced the illegal alien as a new legal and political subject, whose inclusion within the nation was simultaneously a social reality and a legal impossibility–a subject barred from citizenship and without rights" (p. 4). Illegality, in this case, shapes individual and community health and well-being, putting individuals and populations at-risk for poor mental and physical health.

AMBIGUOUS SUBJECTS: UNAUTHORIZED IMMIGRANTS AND HEALTH

At last estimate, 11.2 million people (3.7% of the total population) live in the United States with unauthorized status, and most of these individuals are originally from Mexico (Passel & Cohn, 2011). Arizona is among the states with the largest number of unauthorized immigrants, yet this population is only 6% (400,000) of Arizona's total population of more than 6.5 million people (Passel & Cohn, 2011). In Arizona, the large Mexican and Mexican-American population (Brown & Lopez, 2013) reflects the history of the state as once part of Mexico.

The historical relationships between the United States, Mexico and Central America that produce immigration flows are often overlooked when policy makers propose solutions to unauthorized immigration. As Linda Green (2011) points out, unauthorized immigration is produced through a complex web of multinational institutional relationships influencing the accumulation of capital. Therefore, solutions to the "problem" of immigration "leave the vast reach of neoliberal market fundamentalism and state measures to support it untouched and unaccountable" (Green, 2011, p. 368). One of the women in my study acknowledged that in her country (Honduras) she would be dead from breast cancer, so she was grateful to reside in the United States, a place that has advanced treatment technology. Her comment evokes a history of inequality in the Americas and particularly, the political, capital and military disenfranchisement of Honduras and other Central American countries by US interests (Foster, 2000).

Despite the great diversity of immigrant populations, current biomedical research on undocumented US residents often lumps them with their broader immigrant groups, such as Latinos (e.g., Betancourt, Carrillo, Green, & Maina, 2004). There are, however, notable studies that examine undocumented immigrants' access to or use of general health care (Chavez, 2012; Maldonado, Rodriguez, Torres, Flores, & Lovato, 2013; Ortega et al., 2007; Vargas Bustamante et al., 2012), much of which points to their underutilization of services due to a variety of factors, such as lack of health insurance and fear of deportation (Montealegre & Selwyn, 2012). Some health researchers have noted that immigration policy environments may shape health outcomes. For example, Iten, Jacobs, Lahiff and Fernández (2014) found that undocumented Mexicans receiving diabetes treatment at clinics in two *sanctuary* cities, where immigration status was not collected or discussed in the clinic, showed similar clinical outcomes to documented Mexican-born immigrants and US-born Mexican-Americans.

Because undocumented immigrants are barred from receiving public benefits in the United States, they may receive care through charity or safety net clinics. Anthropologists have examined how humanitarian and charity approaches to immigrant health care reproduce inequality (Castañeda, Carrion, Kline & Tyson, 2010) and how state processes of immigrant inclusion and exclusion are enacted in the clinic (Horton, 2004). Documents have figured prominently in anthropologists' understanding of these processes. For example, Fassin and d'Halluin's study of refugees in France (2005), described the use of medical records to transform refugee bodies into *political resources* for asylum. Miriam Ticktin's (2006) study of undocumented immigrants in France found that people attained political recognition as a result of a French law that confers legal residence permits for medical treatment that cannot be received in the immigrants' home countries. Ticktin (2006) critiques this form of humanitarianism for its limited concept of humanity "put into play by a politics of compassion that emphasizes benevolence over justice, standards of charity over those of obligation" (p. 42).

IMMIGRATION POLICY, A MILITARIZED BORDER AND OPPORTUNITIES FOR HEALTH CARE

Shortly before I began research in Arizona, the state had passed a number of anti-immigrant laws. SB1070, which garnered national and international attention for its assertive enforcement of federal immigration law, required law enforcement personnel to obtain proof of lawful presence in the United States, if they *reasonably suspected* that someone was an unauthorized resident. In the fall, prior to passage of SB1070, the Arizona legislature passed HB2008, which required workers who administer federal health and economic security programs in the state to report anyone who disclosed that they were an unauthorized resident. To neglect this responsibility put one at risk of being charged a hefty fine. These laws, particularly HB2008, had a chilling effect on people's willingness to interact with representatives of the state, including medical clinics that administered federal benefits programs.[3] Because of these developments in Arizona, I was uncertain that women would want to talk to me about their experiences with breast cancer.

Moreover, certain assumptions structured my initial expectations about the research. I had heard that many undocumented Mexican nationals diagnosed with cancer in the area traveled across the heavily militarized border for cancer care.[4] Although I did visit an oncology center in a Mexican border state, I did not do so with any of the women in my study. In fact, the women in my study were able to remain in Arizona for care due to their relatively *privileged* disease type, breast cancer, which is illustrated in the experience of one of my key informants, Ynez Flores, whom I met through a clinical contact.

In my initial conversation with Ynez, I could see that she was troubled by her diagnosis and the uncertainty of accessing treatment as she sought information from anyone offering guidance. As we settled in her small living room, *telenovela* playing on the television and the Virgin of Guadalupe on the wall observing us, Ynez explained that she had been diagnosed with breast cancer about a month before. She was distraught and confused, with feelings similar to those of many other women facing a cancer diagnosis, but her concern seemed to be amplified by her uncertainty about how she would pay for her treatment. Ynez did not have health insurance. She had canceled her policy when her insurer began probing her about the cancer diagnosis, and she could not qualify for Medicaid due to her undocumented status in the United States. She described feeling adrift without a sense of her next steps:

> They had me going from one [clinic] to another, just to check me, and they told me it was very bad because I have very aggressive cancer. They have told me to get medical attention, but no one has said they will be able to treat me. . . . I see that there is a lot of information [about cancer] on television, and many programs but, like they all say, you have to have insurance, be a citizen or [documented/authorized] resident of the US. Even US citizens have trouble getting help for serious illnesses like this. I think I don't have any other option but to go back to Mexico and be treated there. That way I will not be wasting my time here. Here, no one can assure me of anything.

As the conversation progressed, it became clear that Ynez was working to find cancer treatment in the United States so that she would not need to leave her home and family for months, or even years, in order to access care in Mexico.

Ynez's last resort for treatment, traveling to Mexico, her natal home, is an option offered to many Mexican nationals by their US-based providers. With the border less than an hour away by car and the closest Mexican oncology center five hours away, providers described this as an acceptable solution when cancer care is not locally available. There are networks of clinicians who have spent years building cross-border relationships so that patients can, ostensibly seamlessly, access care in Mexico after a cancer diagnosis in Arizona. Many of these clinicians and health professionals work in trusted safety net clinics that see socially and economically marginalized patients and are run by charitable organizations or receive federal funds for operation. And, although these cross-border networks are functional, they ignore the potential risks of leaving the United States, such as the inability to return or arrest.[5]

Nurse practitioner Katherine O'Rourke coordinates the breast cancer program at Mercy Clinic, one of the sites where I recruited patients and collected data. Sitting in her small beige office at the clinic, she explained to me that she encourages many Mexican national women who do not have insurance to go to Mexico for cancer care, where their treatment can be subsidized by the Mexican government depending on income. A social worker in Hermosillo, Sonora, arranges lodging during treatment and the clinic ensures the patient has her medical records in-hand before travel. However, Katherine acknowledged that many women refuse to go because they do not want to risk being separated from their families. "They are willing to live with an untreated cancer," she lamented, especially after the passage of SB1070, which prompted women to ask her, "What if I can't get back?" While emphasizing the deep commitment she has to her patients and her ambivalence about encouraging women to leave the United States for care, Katherine explained the difficulty in making charity funds stretch to meet the costs of expensive cancer treatment.

TRANSNATIONAL MANAGEMENT OF THE UNAUTHORIZED
IMMIGRANT WITH CANCER: CULTIVATING PERSONAL
RESPONSIBILITY AMONG DISOBEDIENT BODIES

In my conversations with providers, the subject of patients' US residency documentation rarely came up unless I mentioned it, possibly due to the social and geographic organization of health care in this particular context. Those who did mention it unprompted were frequently the charity providers like Katherine who took on the responsibility for helping undocumented people get the health care they required. Katherine and other providers in my field site described cultivating and maintaining institutional relationships with oncology centers in Mexico to facilitate treatment, if travel is necessary. Unlike the protocols of Arizona hospitals that repatriated hospitalized patients against their will (Sontag, 2008), these relationships offered an "opportunity" to patients who could not afford the cost of care in the United States. Recognizing the transborder possibilities for health care, the local Mexican Consulate in Arizona sponsors a program called *Ventanilla de Salud*,[6] which not only provides health education and connections to health care, but also provides applications for *Seguro Popular*, a Mexican program that offers health care services to its beneficiaries.

Official US immigration documents are critically important if an authorized immigrant needs medical treatment, does not have insurance and cannot afford to pay for treatment out-of-pocket, because they can enable her to sign up for public insurance, Medicaid.[7] Yet, as Wong-Kim, Chilton, Goh and Gines (2009) note, the current federal health care safety net policies in the United States acknowledge the need for health care among undocumented people only in emergency situations.[8] Supplementing emergency Medicaid are local programs shaped by local needs, resources and politics. These local programs are often dictated by what Anahi Viladrich describes as *frames* for thinking about undocumented people's health. As Viladrich (2012) argues, many of these frames serve to highlight "worthy" immigrant groups, such as the elderly or children, at the expense of others. Certain diseases, such as breast cancer, also garner significant federal and local funding and provide an opportunity for the uninsured and undocumented to gain access.

A federally funded initiative, Well Woman HealthCheck Program in Arizona, offers low- and no-cost mammography and Pap smears to women without health insurance. As a result of significant public and political pressure in the late 1990s, most women diagnosed with breast cancer through Well Woman are enrolled in Medicaid for treatment. Health education outreach workers in southern Arizona, often called *promotoras*, enroll eligible women in Well Woman. Importantly, confirmation of citizenship status is not required for Well Woman enrollment; however, citizens or women with certain legal resident status who are diagnosed with breast cancer through Well Woman receive all the benefits of the US public insurance program, Medicaid, which in Arizona is called the Arizona Health Care Cost Containment System (AHCCCS, pronounced "access"). Women without documented status may be screened for and diagnosed with cancer but they are ineligible for treatment support through Medicaid. A community health professional, recognizing the contradiction in this policy, commented that it does not seem fair to screen people for cancer if you are not going to treat them.

Filling in where public benefits leave off, a US-based foundation provides more than $100,000 per year for breast cancer treatment of un- and under-insured women in Southern Arizona. Although this seems like a large sum, providers at Mercy Clinic, where the grant is administered, reported that the grant ran out of funds every year and that women often needed to wait until the next funding cycle to learn if their breast cancer treatment could be covered. Moreover, because these funds must be allocated to a number of patients, there is no guarantee that one's entire treatment will be covered. An example of the limitations of this funding is the deprioritization of therapies only indirectly related to treatment of the primary cancer. One woman in my study was unable to receive help from the fund when she discovered that her eyelashes, which she had lost during chemotherapy, re-grew *into* her eye, an irritating side effect of treatment.

Ynez considered returning to Veracruz, Mexico, her home state, or to Sonora, Mexico, for treatment. In discussing the difficult decision to leave the United States for care, she said, "If I leave, it will be a big change. I have lived here for many years; I'd be leaving everything to go there. I have family [in Mexico] and everything but, I've lived my life somewhere else." She was reticent to leave her family—including a partner and son—in Arizona while she received treatment. Instead, she mused that she might leave Arizona to seek care in another US state where she also has family. Initially, she was concerned that she might be wasting her time staying in Arizona, where she was given the option to travel to Mexico and little hope of staying in residence for treatment. "Here no one can assure me of anything," she explained.

When she tried to seek out information about the costs of specific cancer therapies, Ynez described receiving oblique and vague responses, such as "It's very expensive." Yet she continued to hunt for available funds, explaining that she called many charities and clinics to find help, and emphasizing the *possibility* of finding a donation: "The clinic where I go [Mercy Clinic], they also operate with donations, and they haven't had any [recently] and they don't let you know if they receive funds. They could have donations today or not . . . or have some in a week—they don't have a date—you have to be on the lookout."

In the end, Ynez was informed that she had received charity funds and she initiated the most expensive aspects of cancer treatment (surgery and chemotherapy) five months after she was diagnosed. Indeed, the uninsured and undocumented women in my study remained in Arizona to receive cancer care, paid for with charity funds for uninsured breast cancer patients. Whereas there are many other cancers that do not attract charity funds for treatment, breast cancer's socially *privileged* position enabled

Mexican-national women to receive treatment while remaining in their adopted home, with the support of husbands, partners and family members and without the risk and cost of border-crossing.

MEDICAL RECORDS: HEALTH CARE WITHOUT POLITICAL RECOGNITION

Medical records have practical and symbolic meaning, in that they mobilize individual knowledge and collective resources. Several women developed an increasing awareness of the importance of understanding one's documented diagnosis to make sure you get the best care possible. One woman lamented the time lost when she and her family *ignored* her breast cancer diagnosis, so that when the cancer was finally treated, her lump had grown significantly. Another woman, who was dealing with a recurrence when she and I met, reflected on her lack of knowledge about her first diagnosis *and* her current diagnosis, explaining that the support group meetings at Mercy Clinic were helping her understand the need to press her doctor for details. As they moved through treatment, women conveyed an interest and concern for the biomedical details of their records, as communicated to them through their providers. In this way, medical records played a part in the *biomedicalization* (Clarke, Shim, Mamo, Fosket & Fishman, 2003) of women, as they began to understand their bodies in new ways.

Furthermore, medical documents have symbolic importance, as they have the potential to mobilize human and financial resources around women, whether in Arizona or in Mexico. As women moved through the illness experience, those who were nearing the end of their (acute) treatment phase articulated their trust in the network of people and institutions that had mobilized around them as a result of their documented diagnosis. One woman in particular explicitly noted the importance of staying in southern Arizona for the rest of her life because "I have my medical records here." In this way, while medical records are a reminder of illness, they represent a history of access to care and the possibility for future access, as well.

In addition to the official medical record, which is housed in the medical facility where treatment takes place, participants in my research often displayed medical documents that they received during their visits. In my last meeting with her, Ynez began presenting her lab reports, unprompted, in describing the chemotherapy she received. Referring to treatment documents from her oncologist, she articulated an understanding of her body and personal agency as it pertained to her health:

> These are the three treatments I am receiving at the hospital. The chemo every Wednesday and these are the results of the blood test that day. [The blood test] is done before the chemo, and then I see how I'm doing, if I have no infection, how my body is reacting to the medicine. The

nurse gives me a copy so I can compare, if I'm too low on something I have to go to the doctor right away.

Using the documents to frame a narrative that reflects a new understanding of her body, she invoked the data contained therein to describe, with certainty, her cancer treatment in the recent past and her anticipated treatment in the near future.

The medical documents seemed to put an end to her uncertainty, although they did little to fix Ynez's ambiguous statuses as a patient and as an unauthorized presence in the United States. Ynez once waited to find out if she would receive charity funds or to learn the cost of treatment to see if she and her family might be able to cobble together a way to pay for treatment. Her description of chemotherapy and blood draws using her medical documents appeared to illuminate what Javier Auyero (2012) refers to as subjugation through the uncertainty and arbitrariness of waiting. Although the documents seem to ameliorate this state on one hand, they cannot address Ynez's status as undocumented and uninsured, which coproduces her tenuous access to medical care and limited social belonging.

As other anthropologists have noted (Kaufman, 2005), medical records may structure one's illness experience, especially as diagnoses and procedures relate to health care financing. While these records give Ynez a new understanding of her body and its needs, the presence of a medical paper trail also connects Ynez and other women to a network of health care providers who have provided care in the past and who may provide care in the future. This network is strong yet limited: it links medically marginalized patients like Ynez to health care institutions, but its provision of treatment is limited by the availability of charity funding and patients' ability to pay for care out-of-pocket.

FINANCIAL DOCUMENTS: MANAGING DISOBEDIENT IMMIGRANT BODIES IN A CONTEXT OF PERCEIVED SCARCITY

At Mercy Clinic and other safety net clinics, the staff routinely request financial documents from their patients in order to determine sliding-scale pay rates, to apply for Medicaid funds and to submit requests for County Medical Access (CMA), a countywide health care discount program in which citizenship status is irrelevant. Like many large and small clinics, there are a number of eligibility staff who request documents and process paperwork for patients. In order to qualify for Mercy's sliding scale, a patient needs a picture ID, proof of income (e.g., paystubs or a letter from her employer) and an address. If she does not have any income, she completes a third-party payer form, in which someone else takes responsibility for her expenses. CMA has similar guidelines but requires an additional step if a person is self-employed: Women who are self-employed or in a semi-formal work environment where they are paid under-the-table must request their employer sign and notarize their employment information.

When I conducted this research, Mercy was undergoing a massive economic shift as it struggled under state budget cuts that reduced funds to help pay for care for the uninsured. Staff tried to leverage any state funds available to help pay for patients' care both at their own clinic and for specialist care outside the community clinic. When a new patient arrived to register for the clinic, the eligibility staff person determined if she qualified for Arizona's public insurance program, AHCCCS, and then the patient had to complete an application or lose the sliding scale available at the clinic. For undocumented people who could not qualify for AHCCCS, but who had serious medical issues such as cancer, CMA was a cost-effective way for the clinic to help them. Therefore, in the service of its own survival, Mercy Clinic put bureaucratic processes in place to ensure that needed financial documentation was elicited from patients.

However, not every undocumented patient was willing to share this information. Margo, one of the nurses from Mercy, shared her struggle with patients who would not submit their financial documents to the clinic. "It's frustrating when you can see both sides of the situation," she said, emphasizing that she could sympathize with the patient who was suffering but also understood the financial constraints of the clinic. "There's a balance you have to strike," she explained. "You want to help but you also want patients to do as much as possible for themselves." It was therefore expected that patients would turn over their financial documents and information to the clinic. Clinic personnel acknowledged that a great deal of trust is involved this kind of disclosure, but they also commented that the clinic has built a reputation as a safe space and trusted source of health care in the community for many years. Margo's expression of sympathy and exasperation not only illustrated her frustration at the patient's lack of trust in the clinic, but also revealed the tension between the clinic's moral inclination to provide health care to everyone in need and the financial constraints of high-cost care.

On the other hand, in its role as an agent for the state's auditing practices, the clinic participated in the construction of the profiles of undocumented and uninsured patients. Michael Power (1997) argues, "the idea of audit shapes public conceptions of the problems for which it is the solution; it is constitutive of a certain regulatory or control style which reflects deeply held commitments to checking and trust" (p. 7). The problem clearly emerges when people without citizenship documentation need expensive care in an environment of scarce resources. Through the practice of auditing, requiring patients to submit legal and financial documents, the problem is rendered manageable for a state and local health care system trying to minimize costs. These practices, as Dorothy Smith (1990) suggests, make "the world bureaucratically and professionally actionable," "clean" and "uncluttered" (p. 104). Yet, at the same time, through the selective production of evidence by patients and staff, a narrative develops about the patient that shapes her subsequent experiences with the health care system.

One powerful way in which the state and local health providers act jointly to shape patient experience through auditing is in the creation of bills for services. These are actionable and, as Power (1997) contends, establish organizational legitimacy. Ynez was qualified for CMA when she was diagnosed with breast cancer. It helped pay for the hormone injections that her doctor recommended to try to shrink the tumor while she waited for chemotherapy. Despite her participation in the discount program, she owed the hospital quite a bit of money for her visits to the doctor and for placing a catheter in anticipation of chemotherapy. Ynez received bills that contained the total amount charged for the medical services minus the CMA discount, so that she could see what she would pay without the discount. She explained that, without the CMA discount, she owed more than $4000 to the doctor. The CMA discount reduced the bill, but she was still required to pay a portion of this total immediately or she would forfeit the discount and pay 100% of the cost. Ynez seemed concerned and confused about what the bills told her. In her words:

> They sent me a bill charging for the doctor services, and another for the place and tools used and for the anesthesiologist. I would say [they are charging me for] the catheter, otherwise [am I] being charged double? One [bill] came for $1,800 and the other . . . in total it was four thousand and something. But I had already covered $279 and now I have the doctor's [bill] of $3,800. The CMA covers [part of the cost] if I pay first. Then they [will] pay. They say that is how it works. I have to pay over a thousand dollars right now.

She explained that CMA would cover the other 80% of her costs, if she paid $1000 first. This $1000 must be paid in a lump sum of money she and her family did not have. She described her discussion with the hospital:

> I asked them to let me make payments because I am not working and I have no money. I am willing to pay but they said there are no payment plans. I have to pay the total amount. If you do not pay then you will be sent to the credit bureau and then you have to pay in-full because it will not be covered. . . . I told my husband that we have to get that money anyway [because there will be other expenses] . . . I still haven't started treatment and they are charging me all that—imagine when I start treatment! I do not want to have debts pending. I don't know if the CMA will cover me [in the future]. I was told an amount for the radiation. They said I would have to pay about $13,000 because the treatment was for five weeks, daily.

Ynez's current bills helped form her perspective on future treatment, as she anticipates future debt and faces uncertainty about whether CMA will pay a portion of her cost. Returning to Power's insight about the audit process maintaining organizational legitimacy, we can see here that Ynez's medical bills shape her behavior toward the local health care system (including the CMA program and the hospital that bills her), in which Ynez is expected to maintain financial responsibility for her health. The bills, therefore, discipline an inherently "disobedient" unauthorized immigrant body (Sandoval, 2008). By reorienting Ynez's responsibility toward the health care system, the billing hospital and the CMA program do the work of the state by disciplining her body while they care for it.

INSURANCE DOCUMENTS: ORIENTING RESPONSIBILITY WHILE PROVIDING UNCERTAIN PROTECTION AGAINST DEBT

Two undocumented women in this study reported having health insurance in the past, yet their narratives reflect the uncertainty of health insurance coverage experienced by many Americans.[9] Insurance often comes and goes with job changes, unemployment and company policy changes. One woman, who had been insured through her husband's job in the past, explained that he had been irregularly employed for a year. She discussed how she felt when she was diagnosed with cancer while uninsured: "I felt bad that my husband had no work, we had no insurance, we had no money . . . What was I supposed to do? . . . I've always been afraid of having any debts here [in the United States]. Everything is so expensive. I [wonder] how I will pay."

Ynez had health insurance when she was diagnosed with breast cancer. Yet when I first met her, Ynez had just stopped paying for her policy. She and her family were convinced that the policy was not comprehensive enough to pay for her cancer care. She explained that when she was diagnosed with breast cancer, she was asked to sign a letter authorizing the company to access her medical records. She complained about the company's frequent calls to investigate the details of her medical care: "They said, we need to investigate the type of cancer. I understand that you need chemotherapy, but we must investigate. He [the insurance company representative] made me feel like a liar. I told them wherever you call and ask about me, they will tell you. . . . There are records. You can ask the doctors. I am not lying." The company had been scrutinizing her medical records for a month without word whether they would cover her treatment.

Ynez lamented, "The economy is really bad and people have insurance with low coverage. When you need help with a serious illness like mine, which is very expensive, then they tell you, 'you don't have enough coverage,' but at the time that they sell you the package they tell you they will." Ynez's concern about her insurance coverage for cancer treatment was not unfounded, as there has been a trend in private and public insurance programs toward reducing benefits while increasing the premiums and deductibles paid by their members (Shields, McGinn-Shapiro & Fronstin, 2008). Importantly, her disinterest in pursuing her rights as a consumer must be viewed in light of her socially and economically marginalized position, in which she is granted limited social inclusion and highly circumscribed economic opportunities. In the United States, where most private insurance coverage is job-based, many unauthorized immigrants work in low-wage, contingent jobs that do not provide health insurance benefits, such as the kitchen position in which Ynez worked. Furthermore, their ability to bear the costs of individual plans may be hampered by a low median household income (Passel & Cohn, 2009).

DOCUMENTS, STRUCTURAL VULNERABILITY, AND THE MANAGEMENT OF INCLUSION AND EXCLUSION

As Ynez negotiated limited belonging in the United States and her desire (and need) for cancer treatment, she weighed the possibilities available to her. She could remain in Arizona and await the availability of charity funds, which were uncertain and limited, or she could continue to pay her health insurance premium, and hope that the company would not refuse to cover her treatments. Alternatively, she could travel to Mexico for treatment, facing the risk of being away from her family and home for months or even years if she were unable to cross the border and return to Arizona. Finally, she could begin treatment with help from family and friends, managing bills as they arose and accepting increasing levels of debt. Ynez wanted to receive treatment in Arizona in order to remain in her home with her family, yet her ability to do so was defined by agents of the state, which acts to make certain bodies illegal.

In Ynez's story, it is possible to see how immigration policy enforcement extends beyond the official entities such as the Border Patrol or US Immigration and Customs Enforcement (ICE). In the state of Arizona, recent legislation enlisted school principals, welfare program caseworkers and police officers in the management of unauthorized immigrants' inclusion and exclusion. Less directly, health care workers employ bureaucratic paperwork to determine inclusion in the social body as they seek out non-state resources to treat undocumented women with cancer. Ynez's ability to remain at home in Arizona for treatment depended upon the medical records that documented details about her cancer diagnosis. Because funds were available only for women with breast cancer, the diagnosis, along with other measures of eligibility, such as lack of insurance and income verification, became the basis for her inclusion in the treatment group.

Critiques of medical humanitarianism (Ticktin, 2006) highlight the power of medical experts who are designated to determine eligibility for care based on sentiment, in lieu of political rights. Mercy Clinic staff operating within this framework of humanitarianism tried to negotiate individual idiosyncrasies and arbitrary determinations of worthiness by implementing a committee for allocating charitable funds to breast cancer patients. In the past, allocation was done on a person-by-person basis and only one staff member was responsible. Josie, a member of the new allocation committee, argued that making determinations as a group ensured that the responsibility did not fall to one person. Also, it made it possible to strategize the distribution of funds more effectively. The new committee tries to manage the funds so that they help more people. When Josie and I spoke, she told me the group was planning to discuss whether it was better to help just one woman or to help seven people. This determination would then guide their allocation policies in the future. For instance, she explained, one of their patients received $29,000 for treatment previously and now was back with a recurrence; how should they allocate funds for her? An examination of women's medical records and bills guide the actions of the committee.

The committee is charged with an unenviable task: to facilitate potentially life-saving care for some women, but not for others. In rationalizing the allocation of charity funds, Josie and her colleagues engage in *fair* distribution, maintaining a transparent and collective decision-making structure based on data from patients' medical and financial documentation. The contradictions inherent in this well-meaning committee's work did not seem lost on Josie, who appeared uneasily resigned to do the best she could to help women with whom she and other clinic staff had a personal relationship. Wishing they could help everyone who needed it, Josie and her colleagues instead acted as brokers, negotiating these personal relationships and broader state processes that socially and politically exclude unauthorized immigrants from the *right* to certain social programs.

CONCLUSION

In understanding the role documents play in (re)producing structural vulnerability and in writing the course of medical treatment, it is important to consider how they serve to naturalize one's position in a social and economic hierarchy. Ynez and other unauthorized immigrants with cancer are, as Quesada, Hart & Bourgois (2011, p. 340) put it, "subjected to economic exploitation and cultural insult" which leads to the social acceptance of such a position as natural. Yet there may still be protest along with acceptance of their positionality. Ynez commented that the US health care system offers great treatments. "But," she conceded, "it's best for the people who . . . were born here. But for those of us who come here to work . . . [trails off] Even if we have a lot of years here and worked hard paying our taxes." She then quickly reassured me that everyone has been helpful since her diagnosis, confirming that the oncologist gives her all the information she needs and the social worker looks out for her. Ynez's ambiguous social position emerged again in her final thoughts about what she planned to do if she were not able to find help in Arizona:

> I hope I will still have time to go somewhere else where I can be treated. These are hard decisions that one has to make, but you have to make them. My life is at play; I should not let any more time pass and make a decision quickly. That is it; I hope I can find an open door. I don't care if I have to work all my life to pay [for treatment]. I know my family is going to help me with that, to pay. But since [my providers] don't tell us an amount, or anything . . . They just say it is very expensive, but not how much . . . [trailing off] I have other options, to go to Mexico.

Ynez clearly articulates the tension between disciplining state processes and the possibilities available to her as a health care consumer who is severely constrained due to her social and economic position in the United States.

The illness experiences of unauthorized immigrants with cancer are influenced by an overarching structural vulnerability due to their undocumented status. Documents such as financial records, medical bills, medical records and insurance policies mitigate and reinforce inequalities, which place unauthorized immigrants within "diverse networks of power relationships and effects" (Quesada et al., 2011, p. 341) that shape vulnerability. Furthermore, the clinic and hospital and its staff are constrained by multiple state and institutional requirements for legitimization. However, as Mercy staff are implicated in the reproduction of inequality, they also challenge it. They use financial documents to slot uninsured (and potentially undocumented) patients into sliding scale or discount health care. They acknowledge patients' undocumented status and try to find ways to side-step conventional processes of state-funded cancer care for the uninsured. In doing so, they are also aware of the clinic's vulnerability. Josie noted that the clinic fields many calls from people who are opposed to unauthorized immigrants receiving care there. "But what can you do?" she asked, rhetorically. She quietly accepts the clinic's risk, which expands the field of vulnerability from the individual undocumented body to the collective body.

NOTES

1. I humbly acknowledge the women living with breast cancer who generously shared their stories and opened their homes to me. I also offer thanks to the health care providers who took the time to speak with me. These providers do their best to care for underserved people living with cancer by deftly negotiating an environment of scarce medical resources. I appreciate the work of my research assistant, Azucena Sanchez, who helped me conduct interviews and contributed much to my analysis. Finally, I would like to thank the editors for their insightful feedback on previous drafts of this chapter.
2. This research was approved by the Institutional Review Board at the University of Arizona. Because the study involved immigrants who might not have

legal status in the United States, I asked for the consent of participants verbally and I used pseudonyms in transcriptions. Furthermore, I secured a Certificate of Confidentiality from the National Cancer Institute, which protects my data against deposition. Because this work engages substantially with national and local health policies and organizations, I use the actual name of the programs (e.g., Medicaid), when their programs are publicly known.

3. Meanwhile the US-Mexico border continued its military build-up of personnel and technologies for managing the flows of people and goods. The Department of Homeland Security trumpets its doubling of "boots on the ground" since 2001 and its use of unmanned aircraft to patrol the Southwest border (US Department of Homeland Security, 2013). Arizona's border has its own additional perils, in that crossers have to make their way under the hot, unrelenting sun and waterless landscape of the Sonoran desert. Despite this risk, southeast Arizona contains the most traveled corridor for migrants along the entire US-Mexico border. The University of Arizona's Binational Migration Institute (Martinez et al, 2013) estimates that approximately 163 migrants a year perish in the Arizona desert.

4. Research reveals that Mexican-national migrants may return to Mexico—and often their state of origin—for the care of particular illnesses, including cancer (González-Block & de la Sierra-de la Vega, 2011).

5. News stories have detailed the Border Patrol practice of arresting unauthorized immigrants as they leave the US (Robbins, 2014).

6. For more information about this program, see http://ventanillas.org/index.php/es/.

7. Immigrants who have been admitted to the United States as permanent residents must live in the country for five years before they are eligible for Medicaid or other public means-tested services.

8. In her history of undocumented immigrants' access to health care in the United States, Beatrix Hoffman (2006) points out that two notable cases in the state of Arizona in the early 1970s effectively challenged laws that excluded nonresidents or noncitizens from emergency health care. As a result of these two cases, undocumented people cannot be turned away from hospitals in the event of an emergency. Treatment for cancer is often not deemed an emergency until it is well advanced and affecting bodily function.

9. Many Americans move in and out of both public and private insurance schemes as a result of shifting job status (Holahan, Garrett & Institute, 2009), income (Hill & Lutzky, 2003; Sommers & Rosenbaum, 2011), program fragmentation or administrative barriers (Lopez, 2005; Price, Boswell, Lessard & Wood, 2006; Sommers, 2005), and the cost of individual policies (Sered & Fernandopulle, 2005).

REFERENCES

Auyero, J. (2012). *Patients of the state: The politics of waiting in Argentina*. Durham, NC: Duke University Press.

Betancourt, J. R., Carrillo, J. E., Green, A. R., & Maina, A. (2004). Barriers to health promotion and disease prevention in the latino population. *Clinical Cornerstone, 6*, 16–29.

Brown, A., & Lopez, M. H. (2013). Mapping the latino population, by state, county and city. Washington, DC: Pew Research Center.

Castañeda, H., Carrion, I. V., Kline, N., & Tyson, D. M. (2010). False hope: Effects of social class and health policy on oral health inequalities for migrant farmworker families. *Social Science & Medicine, 71*, 2028–2037.

Chavez, L. R. (2012). Undocumented immigrants and their use of medical services in Orange County, California. *Social Science & Medicine, 74*, 887–893.

Clarke, A. E., Shim, J. K., Mamo, L., Fosket, J. R., & Fishman, J. R. (2003). Biomedicalization: Technoscientific transformations of health, illness, and U.S. biomedicine. *American Sociological Review, 68*, 161–194.

Fassin, D., & d'Halluin, E. (2005). The truth from the body: Medical certificates as ultimate evidence for asylum seekers. *American Anthropologist, 107*, 597–608.

Foster, L. V. (2000). *A brief history of Central America*. New York, NY: Facts on File, Inc.

González-Block, M. A., & de la Sierra-de la Vega, L. A. (2011). Hospital utilization by Mexican migrants returning to Mexico due to health needs. *BMC Public Health, 11*. Retrieved from http://www.biomedcentral.com/1471-2458/11/241

Green, L. (2011). The nobodies: Neoliberalism, violence, and migration. *Medical Anthropology, 30*, 366–385.

Hill, I., & Lutzky, A. W. (2003). Is there a hole in the bucket? Understanding SCHIP retention. Washington DC: The Urban Institute. Retrieved from http://www.urban.org/UploadedPDF/310792_OP-67.pdf.

Hoffman, B. (2006). Sympathy and exclusion. In Keith Wailoo, Julie Livingston & Peter Guarnaccia (Eds.), *A death retold: Jesica Santillan, the bungled transplant, and paradoxes of medical citizenship* (pp. 237–254). Chapel Hill, NC: The University of North Carolina Press.

Holahan, J., Garrett, A. B., & The Urban Institute. (2009). Rising unemployment, medicaid and the uninsured. Washington, DC: Kaiser Commission on Medicaid and the Uninsured. Retrieved from http://kff.org/other/issue-brief/rising-unemployment-medicaid-and-the-uninsured/

Horton, S. (2004). Different subjects: The health care system's participation in the differential construction of the cultural citizenship of Cuban refugees and Mexican immigrants. *Medical Anthropology Quarterly, 18*, 472–489.

Iten, A. E., Jacobs, E. A., Lahiff, M., & Fernández, A. (2014). Undocumented immigration status and diabetes care among Mexican immigrants in two immigration "sanctuary" areas. *Journal of Immigrant and Minority Health, 16*, 1–10.

Kaufman, S. R. (2005). . . . *And a time to die: How American hospitals shape the end of life*. Chicago, IL: University of Chicago Press.

Lopez, L. (2005). De facto disentitlement in an information economy: Enrollment issues in Medicaid managed care. *Medical Anthropology Quarterly, 19*, 26–46.

Maldonado, C. Z., Rodriguez, R. M., Torres, J. R., Flores, Y. S., & Lovato, L. M. (2013). Fear of discovery among Latino immigrants presenting to the emergency department. *Academic Emergency Medicine Journal, 20*, 155–161.

Martinez, D. E., Reineke, R. C., Rubio-Goldsmith, R., Anderson, B. E., Hess, G. L., Parks, B. O. (2013). A continued humanitarian crisis at the border: Undocumented border crosser deaths recorded by the Pima County Office of the Medical Examiner, 1990–2012. The University of Arizona Binational Migration Institute. Retrieved from http://bmi.arizona.edu/sites/default/files/border_deaths_final_web.pdf.

Montealegre, J. R., & Selwyn, B. J. (2012). Healthcare coverage and use among undocumented Central American immigrant women in Houston, Texas. *Journal of Immigrant and Minority Health, 16*, 204–210.

Ngai, M. M. (2004). *Impossible subjects: Illegal aliens and the making of modern america*. Princeton and Oxford: Princeton University Press.

Ortega, A. N., Fang, H., Perez, V. H., Rizzo, J. A., Carter-Pokras, O., Wallace, S. P., & Gelberg, L. (2007). Health care access, use of services, and experiences among undocumented Mexicans and other Latinos. *Archives of internal medicine, 167*, 2354–2360.

Passel, J. S., & Cohn, D. V. (2009). A portrait of unauthorized immigrants in the United States. Washington, DC: Pew Research Center. Retrieved from http://

www.pewhispanic.org/2009/04/14/a-portrait-of-unauthorized-immigrants-in-the-united-states/

Passel, J. S., & Cohn, D. V. (2011). Unauthorized immigrant population: National and state trends, 2010. Washington DC: Pew Research Center. Retrieved from http://www.pewhispanic.org/2011/02/01/unauthorized-immigrant-population-brnational-and-state-trends-2010/

Power, M. (1997). *The audit society: Rituals of verification.* New York, NY: Oxford University Press.

Price, J., Boswell, J., Lessard, M., & Wood, K. (2006). Why parents disenroll children from public health insurance: The case of southeastern North Carolina. *Journal of Applied Social Science, 23,* 92–106.

Quesada, J., Hart, L., & Bourgois, P. (2011). Structural vulnerability and health: Latino migrant laborers in the United States. *Medical Anthropology: Cross Cultural Studies in Health and Illness, 30,* 339–362.

Robbins, T. (2014, April 23, 2014). The curious practice of bringing immigrants back—to deport them, *National Public Radio.* Retrieved from http://www.npr.org/2014/04/23/306238506/the-curious-practice-of-bringing-immigrants-back-to-deport-them

Sandoval, T. S. (2008). Disobedient bodies. *American Behavioral Scientist, 52,* 580–597.

Sered, S. S., & Fernandopulle, R. J. (2005). *Uninsured in America: Life and death in the land of opportunity.* Berkeley, CA: University of California Press.

Shields, A. E., McGinn-Shapiro, M., & Fronstin, P. (2008). Trends in private insurance, Medicaid/state children's health insurance program, and the healthcare safety net: Implications for vulnerable populations and health disparities. *NYAS Annals of the New York Academy of Sciences, 1136,* 137–148.

Smith, D. E. (1990). *The conceptual practices of power: A feminist sociology of knowledge.* Boston, MA: Northeastern University Press.

Sommers, B. D. (2005). The impact of program structure on children's disenrollment from Medicaid and SCHIP. *Health Affairs, 24,* 1611–1618.

Sommers, B. D., & Rosenbaum, S. (2011). Issues in health reform: How changes in eligibility may move millions back and forth between Medicaid and insurance exchanges. *Health Affairs, 30,* 228–236.

Sontag, D. (2008). Immigrants deported, by U.S. Hospitals, *New York Times,* August 3, 2008. Retrieved from http://www.nytimes.com/2008/08/03/world/americas/03iht-03deport.14962642.html

Ticktin, M. (2006). Where ethics and politics meet: The violence of humanitarianism in France. *American Ethnologist, 33,* 33–49.

US Department of Homeland Security. (2013). Border security results. Retrieved from http://www.dhs.gov/border-security-results.

Vargas Bustamante, A., Fang, H., Garza, J., Carter-Pokras, O., Wallace, S .P., Rizzo, J. A., & Ortega, A. N. (2012). Variations in healthcare access and utilization among Mexican immigrants: The role of documentation status. *Journal of Immigrant and Minor Health, 14,* 146–155.

Viladrich, A. (2012). Beyond welfare reform: Reframing undocumented immigrants' entitlement to health care in the United States, a critical review. *Social Science & Medicine, 74,* 822–829.

Wong-Kim, E., Chilton, J. A., Goh, S. S., & Gines, V. (2009). Breast health issues of undocumented women in California and Texas. *Journal of Cancer Education, 24,* S64–67.

5   Filipina, Survivor or Both?

Negotiating Biosociality and Ethnicity in the Context of Scarcity[1]

Nancy J. Burke

Celestina smiled and waved me in after my soft knock on the exam room door. She was back for her monthly check up at the breast clinic, where she was being seen for her Stage II breast cancer. She told me she had heard from her daughter in the Philippines, who was taking care of Celestina's youngest son. Her daughter had called to confirm that she had received the money Celestina sent to pay for his care and for her granddaughter's college tuition. She smiled tiredly, pleased that they were okay. She told me that her arm was hurting, likely due to the lifting she had to do in her job as a caregiver for an elderly man. She had found the job through friends when she came to San Francisco the prior year. Celestina's story is a little different than many of the other Filipina breast cancer patients I have interviewed and visited in the public hospital breast clinic over the four years of this study. She was not diagnosed after arrival; rather she came to San Francisco knowing she had breast cancer and that she would have to work here while receiving treatment. She felt she had no choice. She had tried to get access to cancer treatment through a clinical trial conducted by an international pharmaceutical company in Manila once diagnosed there, but was found to be ineligible. There was no way she could pay the fees associated with treatment in Manila, and her son's increasing mental health issues were taxing the family's already tight budgets. Moving to the United States, where she could get treatment through the safety-net system and find work to support her family seemed the best option available to her.

I met Celestina while conducting an ethnographic study of breast cancer support for Filipina immigrants living in San Francisco, California. As part of this study, my colleague Ofelia Villero and I participated in and observed over sixty cancer support group meetings (Filipina only and mixed ethnicity groups). We conducted participant observation in church events, the safety-net hospital clinic where most women received their diagnosis and committed to a treatment plan, and community-based organization meetings and events between 2007 and 2011. We interviewed 51 women, ranging in age from 40 to 78 who had been in the United States for anywhere from 5 to 50 years. In addition we interviewed 15 family members.

Women in our study accessed a variety of community services, from financial support through the Breast Cancer Emergency Fund to the breast cancer survivor support group at a local Filipino community based organization. I was particularly interested in understanding when and how women came to the Filipina support group, what happened once they became a part of it, as well as why and how some women decided not to access this form of support. One reason I was interested in these processes was to get a sense of what new forms of sociality, or potentially biosociality, were emerging in the context of the rising numbers of Filipina breast cancer survivors in the United States. I was also interested in the ways that Filipino ethnicity intersected with biosociality among women with breast cancer.

The concept of biosociality was introduced in Paul Rabinow's 1992 essay "Artificiality and Enlightenment: From Sociobiology to Biosociality" (Rabinow, 2008). Using the Human Genome Project, at that time in its initial stages, as a site for the study of the *practices of life*, or the ways in which the natural becomes artificial and is remade as technique (Franklin, 1995), Rabinow's essay suggested that the *social* as *a whole* or *domain of study* be dissolved and replaced by biosociality. In positing biosociality as a reforming of sociality by remaking nature-as-culture, Rabinow employed Michel Foucault's notion that scientific knowledge is a key force reshaping life, labor and language (Franklin, 1995; Rabinow, 2008). Specifically, he conceptualized life as language that is subject to the scientific labor of decoding (e.g., decoding the Human Genome) in order to change it. Sara Franklin (1995), reflecting on Rabinow's work, argued that such an understanding "cannot be seen as separate from the intensification of power-as-knowledge through such practices, inevitably implying concomitant changes in cultural practice, from self-making to capital accumulation practices" (p. 177).

Anthropologists and other social scientists have used the concept of biosociality to understand the emergence of biologically defined patient affinity groups and the ways these groups become engaged in science. Much of this literature chronicles the ways patients and lay persons help raise funds for biomedical research, facilitate collection of blood and tissue samples, collect and share experiences with and data about a disease, influence legislation about biomedical research, etc. (Epstein, 2009a, 2009b; Gibbon, 2007; Gibbon & Novas, 2007a, 2007b; Rapp, 2003; Reiter, 1999; Rose & Novas, 2008). Novas (2007) furthers Rabinow's original exploration of the concept and the ways it has been taken up in the social sciences by arguing for the need to push beyond the patient group to understand, instead, how biosociality introduces new ways of thinking through and understanding the natural. Rabinow's introduction of the concept, he states, is an attempt "to get us beyond starting with preconceived notions of what persons, nature, genetic advocacy groups, culture, firms, or the self are, and to inquire into how persons, nature, genetic advocacy groups, culture, firms or the self are made up through a range of practices" (pp. 137–8).

Missing from much exploration of biosociality is how it intersects with and influences (or is influenced by) ethnicity and ethnic identity, particularly in immigrant and medically underserved patient groups. In the following, I draw attention to the ways in which labor, such as Celestina's work as a caregiver and the work community-based breast cancer support programs engage in to remain afloat, and the need for capital accumulation in the context of economic scarcity interact with self- and group-identity practices to create a particular kind of biosociality among immigrant women with breast cancer. In order to do so, it is necessary to first map the structures that have contributed to understandings of *populations* and *disparities* within US-medical research as these inform the financing available to community-based organizations offering breast cancer support. Next, I trace the emergence of a Filipina breast cancer support program in the mid-2000s at a time of economic retraction and increased recognition and funding of health disparities on a national level in the United States. I highlight structural, interorganizational and interpersonal factors that impact the forms and practices *support* and *care* take within this community-based organization. My aim is to explore the intersections of biosociality and ethnicity within a community-based organization and among a group of Filipina breast cancer survivors as they interface with funders and negotiate funding policies and expectations—a particular context in which life, language and labor are reconfigured.

THE EMERGENCE OF *DISPARITIES POPULATIONS*

M'Charek (2005), followed by Montoya (2007) and Marks (2008), has argued that populations are neither natural nor essential, but rather are coproduced through a complex overlapping whereby sociohistorical and biological processes are grafted onto one another. In the United States, various government initiatives over the last two decades—including the establishment of an Office of Research on Minority Health in 1990, a federal mandate (the NIH Revitalization Act) to include minorities in clinical research in 1993, a National Center of Minority Health and Health Disparities in 2000, and a National Institute of Minority Health and Health Disparities in 2010—have informed the establishment of a disparities infrastructure that has led to the legal definition of *disparities populations*.

> A population is a health disparity population if there is a significant disparity in the overall rate of disease incidence, prevalence, morbidity, mortality or survival rates in the population as compared to the health status of the general population.
>
> (Minority Health and Health Disparities Research and Education Act United States Public Law 106–525, 2000, p. 2498; National Cancer Institute, 2010)

Steven Epstein (2004, 2009b) has explored the processes underlying these legislative and institutional changes in depth, highlighting the inferred but unstated role of race or ethnicity in the definition of disparities populations. Utilizing registry surveillance data that report higher rates of morbidity and mortality for major chronic diseases including cancer, this definition helped to characterize certain population groups, such as Latinos and African Americans as disparity populations when compared with other subpopulations. For example, the 2014 American Cancer Society *Cancer Facts and Figures* reports that African American men and women have the highest cancer mortality rates of any racial and ethnic group. Asian and Pacific Islander men and women are reported to have the lowest cancer death rates, which are about half the rates of African American men and women, respectively. Survival rates among African American men and women are more than 10% lower than among Whites for 9 out of 11 major cancer sites, including breast and colon cancer. Contributing factors include the lower likelihood of African Americans receiving a cancer diagnosis at an early stage, when treatment is more successful, and receiving appropriate cancer treatment. Unequal access to medical care, differences in tumor characteristics unrelated to early detection and differences in the prevalence of comorbidities (other health conditions) have been identified as other contributing factors (American Cancer Society, 2014).

While Asian Americans in general experience less cancer than either White, Hispanic or African American women, recent work to disaggregate cancer statistics among Asians in the United States has revealed important differences in incidence and mortality. Filipinas, for example, are more likely to be diagnosed with cancer than women of other Asian groups, and die from the disease at the highest rates among Asians in California (Cockburn & Deapen, 2004; Gomez et al., 2010; McCracken et al., 2007). Breast cancer is the most commonly diagnosed type of cancer for Filipinas and the leading cause of cancer death (Gomez et al., 2010). Annual percentage increases in breast cancer incidence between 1988 and 2004 have been reported as high as 4% per year among US-born Filipinas (Gomez et al., 2012; Gomez et al., 2010).

With attention to persistent and increasing disparities in cancer outcomes such as these (Byers, 2010; Smith, Smith, Hurria, Hortobagyi & Buchholz, 2009), many US-based cancer foundations began prioritizing funding community-based organizations that work directly with such *disparities populations*. Filipina immigrants in the San Francisco Bay Area constitute one such population due to comparatively high breast cancer incidence rates and disproportionately high mortality. The Filipino Community Group serves as an example of one such community-based organization, originally designed to serve the needs of poor immigrant Filipino seniors and veterans, that received funding through a community-based, disparities-focused grant mechanism of a national breast cancer foundation.

IDENTITY AND BIOLOGICAL SUBJECTIVITY WITHIN
A CANCER SUPPORT GROUP

Fieldnote: March 12, 2008

*The graduation ceremony of the Filipina breast cancer support group was
well attended, with over 30 women and two men in the audience. Everyone
was seated in rows in the hall outside the office, the white plastic chairs
smashed in close together, and there was lively chatter in Tagalog, Ilocano
and Visayan echoing from the walls while music played loudly from
the karaoke machine. Food was spread out on several tables. Many of the
women had contributed a dish and the director had made her signature
ginisang munggo (mung bean dish). After eating and talking for a while, the
director, Lenny, walked from her seat beside me to the front of the room
and welcomed everyone, speaking through the microphone, which had an
eerie reverb echo effect. She said those who had attended all 12 meetings of
the support group would receive certificates, but first, she wanted participants to get up and talk about their experience as cancer survivors. Several
women spoke, at her invitation. The first said she was taking Arimidex,
later someone mentioned Procrit. Marisol, when she spoke, talked about her
negative experience as part of a clinical trial for Femara, and another talked
of her positive experience with the same drug. It was amazing to note how
their self-representations had changed since the beginning of the group three
years ago. They were identifying as survivors now, and seemed to have fallen
into that set narrative I have noted in other support groups (name, diagnosis
experience, treatment description, relying on God and prayer).*

This fieldnote excerpt and others that follow come from events held in
the offices of one of our primary partners in this study, the Filipina Community Group. We partnered with several organizations in the course of this
work, largely due to changes in the original partnering organization. I was
approached by the director of the first organization (which I will call "The
Center") in 2005 to help develop a research study based on their support
program to help answer the question of what was working in the group
and what was not (they had adopted a standard support group model in
collaboration with the university cancer center in 2004 and attendance was
sporadic at best), and to help bring funds into the agency.

Due to a scandal involving Medicaid fraud and misuse of funds, The
Center's director left the organization and was replaced with one who had
little knowledge of, or interest in, the breast cancer support group at just
about the time our research was funded. Under his direction, and due to the
medical leave of the support group facilitator, the Center's support group
disbanded. At this time the city was undergoing an economic downturn and
city contracts, upon which many community-based organizations relied,
had become scarce. In response to the technology bust and the housing
market crash, many city agencies were undergoing cuts, centralization and

efficiency became retrenchment strategies, and the public health department underwent a reassessment of the meaning of *direct services* in order to streamline spending. The result was a divestment in social and psychosocial resources that did not show a direct or immediate impact. Consequently, community-based organizations that had previously held discrete city contracts were placed in competition with each other for a reduced number of such contracts. In addition, the failing economy affected the availability of philanthropic support, which exacerbated an already dire situation as community-based organizations providing breast cancer support resources worked to distinguish their programs from each other in terms of population served, resources provided and linkage to care. It was a moment in which the dependency of such organizations on donors became clear, and in which the capacity of each to refashion itself to meet funders' criteria became paramount.

Lenny, the Filipino Community Group Director, had started working with our research team as The Center's group began to decline. Like the community-based organizations with which we worked, a funding agency was supporting our research. This agency had expectations of a certain number of interviews and observations to be completed, as described in our grant application. Lenny had agreed to help us recruit women to interview. At about this time, Lenny realized that many of the women who had attended The Center's breast cancer group also attended events at the Filipino Community Group. Once she learned that The Center's group had disbanded and there were breast cancer survivors coming to her programs, she decided to officially start a breast cancer support group. The Filipino Community Group received funding for this group from a the local chapter of a national breast cancer foundation that had begun funding community-based organizations serving medically underserved breast cancer patients in the 1990s. The rationale behind the foundation's funding initiative was that the people who know how to provide culturally appropriate support to breast cancer patients of different ethnicities are the community-based organizations already serving these subpopulations. Those closest to the ground, according to this logic, just needed support to continue the work they were already doing. By providing grants to these agencies, the National Breast Cancer Foundation was able to meet its goal of addressing breast cancer disparities. The Filipino Community Group also received funds from the local safety-net hospital foundation, which had a strong interest in facilitating and supporting ethnic-specific support programs. The hospital foundation had been instrumental in starting several such programs for Chinese and Latina patients.

In the course of our study and our work with the Filipino Community Group, we observed how the group negotiated the expectations of other community-based organizations and funders, the expectations of breast cancer support group members and other seniors, and how representations of the group and its members changed over time. These changes highlight the identity practices through which biosociality and ethnicity are coproduced within community-based organizations and among Filipina breast cancer survivors as they interface with funders and negotiate funding policies and expectations. As this group vied against other ethnically defined breast cancer support groups and services in the city for scarce resources, members struggled with boundaries around participation and what was appropriate to talk about in support group sessions. A detailed accounting of instances of frictions (Tsing, 2004) through which self- and group-making practices become visible illustrates the unanticipated defining power breast cancer foundations wield over communities (e.g., disparities populations) they seek to help. At the intersections of philanthropy and community-based organizations, ethnic identity is at times a commodity and at times a casualty.

And now back to the graduation.

Fieldnote: March 12, 2008

When Marisol got up to speak, Lenny introduced her as an important community leader. The first thing she did was to admonish people not to talk while a guest speaker is talking. "We have great speakers coming here to talk with us and it is rude to have conversations so that it is hard for us to hear them. Yesterday was a great event here, but it was difficult to hear because there was so much talking. Okay, so that is all I am going to say about that. Now about my experience with cancers. Not cancer, but cancers. I had bilateral breast cancer and a diminished spleen." She went on talking about her experiences with breast cancer treatment, which were oftentimes negative, especially with the university hospital, and said that they are continually checking her spleen to see if she has a recurrence.

When undergoing treatment for breast cancer at the university hospital, she said that she was invited to participate in a clinical trial for Femara. Initially, she agreed to participate, but then had a terrible experience with the drug. She felt that she was going to die. They had to take her into the hospital to revive her ("I almost died that day"). "But," she continued, "I kept going and I kept moving. As you all saw, before when the music was on, I was moving. I was doing my exercises. I move every day. I take two-mile walks. Moving is very important. And your diet. No meat. That's what I've been doing." She went on to advise women to keep their spirits up and take care of themselves. "That's all I have to say. Thank you" and her talk ended with applause.

Several other women got up to speak, declaring "I didn't have to have chemo or radiation, just the surgery" as if this were a point of pride, while others talked about repeated treatments. Alice stood up to say that she was on Arimidex but would probably stop taking the medicine soon. There was an alarmed intake of breath in the crowd and the question "why?" popped out in the row behind me. Alice, not noticing, continued talking in halting English and said, "I have eight years." "Oh," several voices replied, as if understanding.[2]

Soon after it was Elizabeth's turn to get up to speak. Everyone knows Elizabeth, as they all know Marisol. Elizabeth manages a low-income apartment building nearby where many of the women find housing with Lenny's help. Elizabeth said that she was a 20-year survivor of breast cancer, that her children were so little when she had it and now they are all grown. Her breast cancer has never given her any problems. She has never had a recurrence. Her problem now, she said, is her kidney. Her kidneys have stopped working and she is on the transplant list. "You look good though," a nurse sitting on the couch against the wall said. 'Yes, but today for some reason I woke up swollen, see?' She responded, kicking out her ankles for the women in front (one of whom was Marisol) to see. "I don't know why." "It could be your diabetes," one of the women in front said. "Could be," Elizabeth answered. "But that is what is giving me problems now." Marisol said, "You should have eaten better." Elizabeth looked at her and smirked, "yes, I tried to eat well," and sat down.

This conversation, very public, yet at the same time private in the sense of addressing bodily functions and personal responsibilities, reflects previous interactions I observed in the support group. About a year prior, Elizabeth commented jokingly during check in of the support group, "I have diabetes and cancer. I hope I die from the cancer, not the diabetes. If you die from cancer, people feel sorry for you. If you die from diabetes they think you liked to eat too much [i.e., it is your fault]."

The moral and individualizing aspect of self-making here, as an agent responsible for ensuring health through *eating right* and *keeping moving* form an essential part of modern biosociality. Discussed elsewhere in terms of biological citizenship, a concept that evokes not only the self-responsibility for personal health surveillance but also the rights and engagements achieved through the donning of the biological identity (Petryna, 2002; Rose & Novas, 2008), this self-crafting is responsive to the market forces that inform biomedical understandings of chronic diseases (e.g., cancer) as preventable products of lifestyle, individual choice, and decision-making. In this context the moral duty of self-regulation expands to include the need to accept, understand and act upon expert knowledge (e.g., information) on things like low fat diets and the importance of exercise. The responsibility of knowing oneself biomedically in this biosocial paradigm is a new form of labor expected of everyone (Whitmarsh, 2013).

BALANCING ETHNICITY AND THE NEED FOR CAPITAL

In mid-September I received an email from Lenny, the Filipino Community Group Director. She was nervous about the impending site visit from their major funder, the local chapter of a national breast cancer foundation. She asked what she should expect and what they would want to know. She was worried because she was well aware of the funder's concern that their monies only go to support breast cancer survivors. Her program, which ran in 10 week sessions with an educational group on Mondays, and karaoke, bingo and ballroom dancing on Fridays, was open to all Filipino seniors, as she felt all could benefit from the educational sessions and it would be inappropriate to not welcome everyone to the meetings. The following field note excerpt describes the site visit in question.

Fieldnote: December 15, 2011

The Monday meeting was held out in the hallway outside the office, which made it feel more like a party than a regular meeting. There was a long table covered with a white tablecloth and filled with chicken adobo, fried mackerel, and pinakbet (Ilocano dish of eggplant, bitter melon and okra with bits of pork) pushed against the wall and white plastic chairs were organized in tight rows. The meeting started at 1:30 with Lenny reading the "ground rules." She had asked us to keep a lookout for the Foundation representative, but we never saw him.

Before introducing the guest speaker, Lenny invited everyone present to check-in. Each participant introduced herself and talked about her experience with illness. The breast cancer survivors talked about their history of cancer diagnosis and treatment. Several mentioned whether they had had chemotherapy, radiation, or both, drugs like Tamoxifen, and their surgeries (double mastectomy, mastectomy and lumpectomy), while others spoke of their diabetes and high blood pressure. Non-cancer survivors spoke of rheumatoid arthritis, high blood pressure, diabetes and their caregiving responsibilities for spouses and loved ones with cancer.

The speaker introduced herself as a breast cancer survivor, diagnosed in 2006. She explained that she did not feel anything before being diagnosed; a mammogram revealed a problem, and so she had a biopsy of her left breast. When the cancer was confirmed she had to figure out whether she wanted a lumpectomy or mastectomy and this was a difficult decision for her as it had been for many of the women present.

A nutritionist with a national Filipino-American organization, she started her presentation with what she called a "review" of cancer (using an American Cancer Society chart that included colon, lung, prostate, breast, cervical cancer, etc.). While she had been speaking in Tagalog about her own experience, when she began this portion of her presentation she switched to English. She asked the audience what cancer meant to them. She then went on to detail different kinds of cancer and what is known about the causes. Within this review she spent more time on breast than other cancers, and ended with the conclusion that very little is known about what causes cancer, but we can see the link between cancer and food and then went on to talk about how Filipinos eat. The meeting was interactive, but full of information. By the end the participants were tired. The meeting had lasted over 3 hours.

The next day I received a call from Lenny. She was worried and upset. The site visitor, who had been in the office meeting with Lenny and her assistant during much of the presentation, had given her "feedback" and she was offended. He had sent an email to her assistant that said:

I was informed by the foundation that the subject matter for the support group meetings had to be exclusively about breast cancer and not include general health topics, as was being presented yesterday. Since the activities of the foundation are expressly for breast cancer support, their funds are not supposed to be used for other purposes. Could you work with Lenny to separate the topics so that you have different group meetings along these lines?

The conversations that followed were telling. Lenny spoke of her responsibility to approach support for her clients in a holistic sense, that separating survivors from nonsurvivors was artificial and potentially stigmatizing, and that cancer was cancer and nutrition was important for all cancers, including breast cancer. Also, she noted, her clients did not only suffer from breast cancer. They also had issues with high blood pressure and diabetes, among other ailments. Showing the importance of diet and healthy lifestyle to those illnesses was also valuable, she thought. She was defensive that the visitor felt that breast cancer was not addressed in the meeting because it was, but when it was brought up the speaker switched to Tagalog. She also felt that she was running the support group in an appropriately Filipino way, by *not* creating artificial boundaries on the basis of biological identity and that Filipinos tend to view cancer as cancer, not distinguished by site. She did not know how to respond to the criticism.

The tension evident in the site visitor's evaluation and Lenny's receipt of it reflected tensions the group had been balancing since they started receiving outside funding and collaborating with other community-based organizations and researchers. Lenny often called to ask me if they were *"doing things right"* or to strategize on how to balance supporting her other activities with the breast cancer program (in other words, how to divide up, or not, the funds, so that breast cancer survivors were included in all the programs offered and that other seniors could participate in the breast cancer educational sessions). Our participant observation over the four years of our study had shown that women in Lenny's support group attended other mixed ethnicity groups, mainly because they wanted to share their experiences. Several had been invited to participate in speaking engagements. One member had spoken at her church during Breast Cancer Awareness month, sharing her experience in order to raise awareness about breast cancer rates among Filipinos. Lenny had gathered participants together to march in local parades and to cheer, as a group, along the route of the Breast Cancer Foundation Walk for Life. At all such gatherings and events they held signs with the organization name and wore pink ribbons, scarves and sweaters, often accentuated by traditional Filipino apparel.

This identification as a breast cancer support group was not a natural occurrence. It was a social process directly related to access to funding and participation in our research study. Previously, the Filipino Community Group served the needs of poor and low-income seniors. It continues to do so. The group became identified as a *bio* (e.g., cancer) *social* (e.g., support group) collectivity partially in response to our project's need for a collaborator. As noted earlier, Lenny had been helping us identify women to interview and, through conversations with members of our research team, realized she was basically holding support group meetings already in her office so decided she should seek funding for the group. In the application process, she realized that foundations wanted to support activities exclusively *for the women with breast cancer* and she struggled with how to separate them from the other seniors. Doing so was a heuristic exercise. They all participated together in lectures, dancing, bingo and karaoke. Splitting them up along biological as opposed to ethnic lines made no sense to her. Splitting them along ethnic lines did make a great deal of sense to her and she felt strongly about that. Yet, as evidenced by the site visit, the former is what she had to do to keep her funding.

At the close of the graduation ceremony described earlier, Lenny stood at the front of the room with the microphone in her hand and said emphatically: "This is a FILIPINA group, the FILIPINA Community Support Group. There is the Chinese, and the Spanish have theirs, and now we have ours. That's why it's very important for you to support this program." Over the course of the previous four years, through the writing of a series of grant proposals, participation in breast cancer conferences, many conversations with our research team, and participation in cancer community advisory boards, she had consolidated and differentiated the group along biological and ethnic lines. While this differentiation was fluid in practice, Lenny consciously made it in her writing and speaking engagements. She utilized language to strategically position her group in relation to others in order to gain access to funding.

CONCLUSIONS

The methodological contribution of Rabinow's 1992 essay is the suggestion that we not begin our investigations with preconceived notions of what patients' groups, lay persons, or scientists are, but rather to attend to the various practices and forms through which they are assembled at different sites and at different historical moments (Novas, 2007; Rabinow, 2008). The labor the Filipino Community Group engaged in in order to acquire and maintain funding at a moment of economic scarcity and philanthropic decline comprises a series of practices, negotiations, and priorities responsive to inequality and need not previously explored in the anthropological and sociological literature on biosociality. These include organizational shifts from holding organic inclusive social gatherings to specific structured events in which breast cancer information was shared and participation was enumerated and audited. In so doing, who was able to participate and what was suitable to discuss were defined according to staff interpretations of funder guidelines (informed by direct mandates from the breast cancer foundation) rather than inherent understandings of community needs, the reason the organization was ostensibly funded in the first place. These unintended effects caused organizational transformations that changed the form of this patient group, and may impede provision of appropriate and meaningful survivorship support.

Elsewhere, researchers have discussed the consequences of biosociality as including increased sense of risk, anxiety and personal responsibility for health (Beck, 1992; Gibbon, 2007; Gibbon & Novas, 2007b; Lupton, 2013), as well as agency, engagement and impact on the group level. Steven Epstein, for example, described the ways in which AIDS activists were transformed in the process of fighting for treatment trials and the alteration of *clean* clinical trials from outsiders to insiders in scientific debates (Epstein, 1995, 2009a). They learned the language of the science, attended conferences and began to understand the PowerPoints. Many were changed in this process and began to appreciate the rules and regulations of science. Most importantly, however, they were able to alter the course of science and treatment as active participants.

Breast cancer activists constitute another powerful biosocial collectivity that has made astonishing strides in the United States in shaping both legislative and research agendas (Aronowitz, 2007; King, 2006; Klawiter, 2008; Lerner, 2003; Sulik, 2012). Harnessing philanthropic support and political clout, the largely White US breast cancer movement includes national foundations that have funded some of the major scientific breakthroughs in understanding the biology of breast cancer and its treatment (Susan G. Komen Foundation, 2014). These foundations have also succeeded in codifying a *norm* of breast cancer survivorship, which several anthropologists and activist groups have brought into question in relation to its utility and applicability to ethnic and cultural subgroups within the United States (Burke, Villero & Guerra, 2012; Mathews, 2009). As detailed herein, this norm also influences how funds from these foundations are distributed: to breast cancer survivors as a distinct subgroup. Rather than trusting the community-based organizations tasked with providing *culturally appropriate* breast cancer support to immigrant and ethnic subgroups to do so in an acceptable and sustainable manner, foundations impose their own expectations of what is *appropriate* and who should be included in designated funded activities. Thus, the labor and language of the Filipino Community Group highlights frictions between the professed logic of disparities focused funding strategies within majority-White breast cancer foundations and the indigenous logics of support and care employed by the community-based organization that prioritizes inclusion over biological distinction.

Anthropologists explored the emergence of ethnicity in the context of (im)migration in depth in the 1990s and 2000s, highlighting how, for example, (im)migrants from the culturally and linguistically diverse Philippine archipelago came to identify as a single ethnic group—Filipinos—in the United States (Cordova & Park, 1999; Cordova, 1983; Espiritu, 2002, 2003; Gonzalez, 2009; Rafael, 1997; Strobel, 2001). How these identity practices intersect with those of biosociality have been underexplored. What we have observed over the four years of our study is the insertion of elements of biosociality into a previously ethnically defined collective. Thinking through biosociality in relation to ethnicity in cases such as this provides important insights into the very active and pervasive ways ethnicity shapes and informs support and care in the current moment. Ethnicity in this sense is dynamic and meaningful. It is strongly linked to but not limited to identity. It infuses the practices, decisions and structures of the Filipino Community Group alongside financial and contractual concerns. Such an understanding provides fodder for thinking through the ways in which sociality and disparities infrastructures intersect on the ground and frame, and at times subvert and transform, breast cancer support interventions.

NOTES

1. This work was supported by the Hellman Family Early Career Fellowship, the Susan G. Komen Foundation Breast Cancer Disparities Program, and the California Breast Cancer Research Program. I thank the San Francisco General Hospital/Avon Foundation Comprehensive Breast Care Program for its support of the Filipina Breast Cancer Support Program. I thank all Filipina Foundation staff and support group members for their continuing partnership. I also thank the "Center" for their role in this study, and our Community Advisory Board members for their invaluable time and insights. I also thank Holly Mathews and Eirini Kampriani for their insightful comments on an earlier draft of this chapter.
2. Most of the women present were aware that Arimidex was taken for five years post initial treatment.

REFERENCES

American Cancer Society. (2014). *Cancer Facts and Figures 2013*. Retrieved from http://www.cancer.org/research/cancerfactsfigures/cancerfactsfigures/cancer-facts-figures-2013

Aronowitz, R. A. (2007). *Unnatural history: Breast cancer and American society.* New York, NY: Cambridge University Press.

Beck, U. (1992). *Risk society: Towards a new modernity* (1st ed.). London: Sage Publications Ltd.

Burke, N. J., Villero, O., & Guerra, C. (2012). Passing through: Meanings of survivorship and support among Filipinas with breast cancer. *Qualitative Health Research, 22,* 189–98.

Byers, T. (2010). Two decades of declining cancer mortality: progress with disparity. *Annual Review of Public Health, 31,* 121–132.

Cockburn, M., & Deapen, D. (2004). *Cancer incidence and mortality in California: Trends by race/ethnicity 1988–2001.* Los Angeles, CA: Los Angeles Cancer Surveillance Program, University of Southern California.

Cordova, D., & Park, Y. (1999). *The Filipino community in the United States.* Seattle, WA: Cross Cultural Health Program.

Cordova, F. (1983). *Filipinos: Forgotten Asian Americans* (1st ed.). Dorothy Cordova.

Epstein, S. (1995). The construction of lay expertise: AIDS activism and the forging of credibility in the reform of clinical trials. *Science, Technology & Human Values, 20,* 408–437.

Epstein, S. (2004). The politics of gender and race in biomedical research in the US. *Body and Society, 10,* 183–203.

Epstein, S. (2009a). *Impure science: AIDS, activism, and the politics of knowledge.* Berkeley, CA: University of California Press.

Epstein, S. (2009b). *Inclusion: The Politics of Difference in Medical Research.* Chicago, IL: University of Chicago Press.

Espiritu, Y. L. (2002). The intersection of race, ethnicity, and class: The multiple identities of second-generation Filipinos. In P. G. Min (Ed.), *The Second Generation: Ethnic Identity among Asian Americans* (pp. 19–52). Walnut Creek, CA: AltaMira Press.

Espiritu, Y. L. (2003). *Home bound: Filipino American lives across cultures, communities, and countries.* Berkley and Los Angeles, CA: University of California Press.

Franklin, S. (1995). Science as culture, cultures of science. *Annual Review of Anthropology, 24,* 163–184.

Gibbon, S. (2007). *Breast cancer genes and the gendering of knowledge: Science and citizenship in the cultural context of the "new" genetics.* New York, NY: Palgrave MacMillan.

Gibbon, S., & Novas, C. (2007a). *Biosocialities, genetics and the social sciences: Making biologies and identities.* New York, NY: Routledge.

Gibbon, S., & Novas, C. (2007b). Introduction: Biosocialities, genetics and the social sciences. In S. Gibbon & C. Novas (Eds.), *Biosocialities, genetics and the social sciences: making biologies and identities* (pp. 19–52). New York, NY: Routledge.

Gomez, S. L., Press, D. J., Lichtensztajn, D., Keegan, T.H.M., Shema, S. J., Le, G. M., & Kurian, A. W. (2012). Patient, hospital, and neighborhood factors associated with treatment of early-stage breast cancer among Asian American women in California. *Cancer Epidemiology, Biomarkers & Prevention, 21,* 821–834.

Gomez, S. L., Quach, T., Horn-Ross, P. L., Pham, J. T., Cockburn, M., Chang, E. T . . . Clarke, C. A. (2010). Hidden breast cancer disparities in Asian women: Disaggregating incidence rates by ethnicity and migrant status. *American Journal of Public Health, 100,* S125-S131.

Gonzalez, J. (2009). *Filipino American faith in action: Immigration, religion, and civic engagement.* New York, NY: New York University Press.

King, S. (2006). *Pink ribbons, inc.: Breast cancer and the politics of philanthropy.* Minneapolis, MN: University of Minnesota Press.

Klawiter, M. (2008). *The biopolitics of breast cancer: Changing cultures of disease and activism.* Minneapolis, MN: University of Minnesota Press.

Lerner, B. H. (2003). *The breast cancer wars: Hope, fear, and the pursuit of a cure in twentieth-century America* (1st ed.). New York, NY: Oxford University Press.

Lupton, D. (2013). *Risk.* New York, NY: Routledge.

Marks, J. (2008) Race: Past, present and future. In B. Koenig, S.S.-J. Soo-Jin Lee and S. Richardson (Eds.), *Revisiting Race in a Genomic Age* (pp. 21–38). New Brunswick, NJ: Rutgers University Press.

Mathews, H. F. (2009). Cancer support groups and health advocacy: One size doesn't fit all. In J. McMullin & D. Weiner (Eds.), *Confronting cancer: Metaphors, advocacy, and anthropology* (1st ed., pp. 43–62). Santa Fe, NM: School for Advanced Research Press.

McCracken, M., Olsen, M., Chen, M. S., Jemal, A., Thun, M., Cokkinides, V . . ., Ward, E. (2007). Cancer incidence, mortality, and associated risk factors among Asian Americans of Chinese, Filipino, Vietnamese, Korean, and Japanese ethnicities. *CA: A Cancer Journal for Clinicians, 57*, 190–205.

M'Charek, A. (2005) *The Human Genome Diversity Project: An ethnography of scientific practise*. Cambridge, UK: Cambridge University Press.

Montoya, M.J. (2007) Bioethnic conscription: Genes, race, and Mexicana/o ethnicity in diabetes research. *Cultural Anthropology, 22*, 94–128.

National Cancer Institute. (2010). *National Cancer Institute Center to Reduce Cancer Health Disparities*. Retrieved from http://crchd.cancer.gov/disparities/defined.html.

Novas, C. (2007). Patients, profits, and values: Myozyme as an exemplar of biosociality. In S. Gibbon & C. Novas (Eds.), *Biosocialities, genetics and the social sciences: Making biologies and identities* (pp. 136–157). New York, NY: Routledge.

Petryna, A. (2002). *Life exposed: Biological citizens after Chernobyl*. Princeton, NJ: Princeton University Press.

Rabinow, P. (2008). Artificiality and enlightenment: From sociobiology to biosociality. In J. X. Inda (Ed.), *Anthropologies of modernity: Foucault, governmentality, and life politics* (pp. 181–193). Malden, MA: Blackwell Publishing Ltd.

Rafael, V. L. (1997). "Your grief is our gossip": Overseas Filipinos and other spectral presences. *Public Culture, 9*, 267–291.

Rapp, R. (2003). Cell life and death, child life and death: Genomic horizons, genetic diseases, family stories. In S. Franklin & M. Lock (Eds.), *Remaking life and death* (pp. 129–164). Santa Fe, NM: School of American Research Press.

Reiter, R. R. (1999). *Testing women, testing the fetus: The social impact of amniocentesis in America*. New York, NY: Routledge.

Rose, N., & Novas, C. (2008). Biological Citizenship. In A. Ong & S. J. Collier (Eds.), *Global assemblages: Technology, politics, and ethics as anthropological problems* (pp. 439–463). Malden, MA: Blackwell Publishing Ltd.

Smith, B. D., Smith, G. L., Hurria, A., Hortobagyi, G. N., & Buchholz, T. A. (2009). Future of cancer incidence in the United States: Burdens upon an aging, changing nation. *Journal of Clinical Oncology, 27*, 2758–2765.

Strobel, L. M. (2001). *Coming full circle: The process of decolonization among post-1965 Filipino Americans*. Manila, Philippines: Giraffe Books.

Sulik, G. A. (2012). *Pink ribbon blues: How breast cancer culture undermines women's health*. New York, NY: Oxford University Press.

Susan G. Komen Foundation. (2014). *About us, our work*. Retrieved from http://ww5.komen.org/AboutUs/OurWork.html

Tsing, A. L. (2004). *Friction: An ethnography of global connection*. Princeton, NJ: Princeton University Press.

Whitmarsh, I. (2013). The ascetic subject of compliance: The turn to chronic diseases in global health. In J. Biehl & A. Petryna (Eds.), *When people come first: Critical studies in global health* (pp. 302–324). Princeton, NJ: Princeton University Press.

6 Revealing Hope in Urban India
Vision and Survivorship Among Breast Cancer Charity Volunteers

Alison Macdonald

INTRODUCTION

This chapter[1] describes particular modalities of creating hope among breast cancer volunteers in urban India. It draws on research with women who have suffered with breast cancer and now participate as *survivor volunteers*[2] in cancer charities and nongovernmental organizations (NGOs) in Mumbai. Among this group of women, I examine how vision and the strategic revelation by volunteers of their status as breast cancer *survivors* emerges as a therapeutic tool within spheres of lay activism. I consider this practice in light of anthropological studies that highlight the primacy of sight as permeating Hindu sociality and informing multiple forms of existential practice surrounding religion, spirituality and faith. In doing so, I illustrate how the *visual*, as a process of embodied interaction, precipitates a form of disease identification whereby volunteers attempt to inspire hope and courage in other cancer patients. This takes particular salience in Mumbai where the demands of accessing care within a rudimentary medical landscape together with the privileging of kinship and community relations come to frame, and often constrain, individual experiences of living with cancer in particular ways. This chapter examines how such complexities interface with the lay breast cancer activist sphere in Mumbai as it unfolds in tandem with the emergence of novel practices surrounding psychosocial support and group sharing in Western-style support groups. By charting the complexities and tensions imbued in local philanthropic efforts to increase participation in oncological psychosocial interventions, I trace ethnographically how the affective revelatory maneuver of *seeing* survivors constitutes a form of biomedical solidarity and a particular form of activist practice.

Anthropological approaches to patient activism often focus on the transformations in knowledge and identity that are brought about by the rise of new genetic knowledge, perceptions of disease risk and illness experience. Such approaches explore the way that novel biosocial constellations impact the development of scientific knowledge and research, and in turn come to shape new forms of medical governance, sociopolitical agency and biological citizenship (see for example Gibbon & Novas, 2008; Petryana,

2002; Rabinow, 1996; Rose & Novas, 2005). In particular, anthropological exploration of the role of the patient *activist* in the absence of large-scale stable state institutions has revealed the diverse modes through which individuals cope with suffering and procure necessary medication as they carve out novel forms of *therapeutic citizenship* (Nguyen, 2010) or act as *diseased citizens* (Biehl, 2007). These patient activists draw upon personal trajectories of suffering in order to enact care for themselves and for others. For instance, Nguyen (2010) eloquently describes how complexities surrounding biographic storytelling and confessional technologies in West Africa result in both the capitalization of social networks that open up for pathways for AIDS advocates to access international drugs and reveal a bias in Western assumptions that disease solidarity based upon a shared biomedical condition could result from self-disclosure. This is especially so in a setting where kinship frames the terms of solidarity and persons fear being ostracized by family and community for speaking publically about their *diseased* status.

In a similar vein, I aim to explore how survivor volunteers participating in breast cancer charities in Mumbai engage in novel forms of activist practice that are constituted by an *experiential authority* or lay expertise (Rose & Novas, 2000, 2005). Elsewhere (Macdonald, 2013) I have expanded the notion of experiential authority in relation to experiences of suffering with breast cancer and explored how this intersects with the mobilization of patient activism in Mumbai through the prism of *survivorship*. This is intended to capture analytically the way biological biographies of suffering with, and recovery from, breast cancer are subsequently imbued in and are generative of new forms of *health activist* practice as *seva* (selfless service) and changing patterns of selfhood among the survivor volunteers. In what follows, I focus on one aspect of this: the moment of *seeing* survivors. This is a practice that I observed in interactions between survivor volunteers and patients in hospitals, and it was spoken about in everyday discourse using the verb *dekhna,* meaning to watch, look or see. In what follows, I discuss how the corpothetic work of visual exchange (Pinney, 2004) and primacy of sight in Hindu sociality operate in conjunction with ideals of a *normative* cancer survivorship to create moments of biomedical solidarity. I explore this at the interface with an increasingly global breast cancer movement[3] that emphasizes the significant role of survivors in mediating cancer care and the emergence of Western-style support groups in the local, oncological clinical arena. Examining the complexities that surround practices of group *sharing* in Mumbai, both as a therapeutic *tool* and as a means to create shared *biosocial* identity, I elaborate on how this practice is subject to complex processes of accommodation and resignification in spheres of lay activism. This is not to say that group sharing and/or the narration of illness is not important in urban India, nor that group sharing and support groups are always successful in Euro-American contexts (Mathews, 2009). In my field site, stories were often uttered quietly amidst the clamor and chatter of hospital waiting rooms and bleeps of patient ticket counter machines where one hears of the long journeys from home, the pain of leaving children behind, the pain of bringing shame on one's family, and the fear that cancer will return and the money will run out. Yet given the emphasis on the therapeutic purchase of *sight* at specific and strategic times, I suggest that other modalities of creating hope and solidarity come to the fore. I conclude that it is through the work of vision that biological affiliation and social identification are (re)configured, if only momentarily, to create a form of communion between, and among, patients and volunteers.

The research that informs this paper took place in Mumbai, India, and draws upon my participant observation with two local organizations: a large professional NGO that is at the forefront of cancer activism in India, named here as the All India Cancer Trust (AICT),[4] and a small charity run by local women in conjunction with a private hospital, which I term the Cancer Clinic (CC). Here I worked specifically with Hindu volunteers belonging to a middle-income status. I spent most of my time observing these women go about their daily activities, watching them interact with patients and discussing these interactions with relevant others present. I had many conversations with patients, relatives and doctors that typically occurred more in the context of everyday events in the clinic and hospital waiting rooms rather than in formal style of interviewing. Many of these interactions took place in Hindi but English was also commonly used among NGO professionals and volunteers.

NOVEL FORMS OF CARE: SHARING AND SUPPORT FROM THE *BĀHAR*

A large proportion of voluntary activities around cancer respond to the practical aspects of managing the disease, that is, accessing and accruing funds for transportation, shelter, food and treatment. In this sense, philanthropic organizations deal with the overspill of lateral issues associated with receiving oncological treatment in Mumbai's underserved general hospitals and oversubscribed regional cancer center Tata Memorial Hospital (TMH). Volunteers also deliver what they perceive to be more *socially* minded interventions directed towards the psychosocial needs of patients. These interventions are juxtaposed against the biomedical treatment for cancer that has an inherent focus on only treating the malignancy. Health activists and medical professionals frequently discuss the benefits of incorporating a more holistic approach to healing that encompasses the social and emotional well-being of the patient and their family in addition to medical treatment of the disease. As part of this trend, in the past 10 years, some NGO professionals and oncologists (who trained in Euro-America) have attempted to implement Western-style support groups and foster the practice of therapeutic group sharing. Although these groups are slowly becoming incorporated into predominantly private, urban hospitals, their popularity at the time of this study was minimal. Medical professionals told me that the concept was "ahead of its time" in India and volunteers participating in the group often a necessity.[5] Nevertheless, the NGO professionals with whom I worked adapted their sense of Western mental health science to what were perceived to be the needs of Indian patients. The AICT, for example, train their volunteers through a specifically adapted psycho-oncology program whereas others, such as the volunteers at the CC, have loosely adopted psychosocial terminology such as the notion of *counseling*.

As part of my work as a volunteer with AICT I was asked to assist in the implementation of a breast cancer support group. Although we managed to recruit five or six women, who did participate fairly regularly in the monthly meetings, ultimately it was incredibly difficult to recruit more patients. The employees of AICT and other volunteers were sympathetic to my efforts, but even they confided in me that they would not participate in a support group. During a conversation with two senior AICT employees, one of them said, "I find better support at home," and the other commented, "Over here, social networking is better: friends and family. It's not uncaring over here." With *here* being juxtaposed to what they imagined to be over *there* in my own country, they played off India's more tightly woven and enriched familial fabric against the very need for a support group in the first place. Indeed, the role of the family in providing *madad* (support; help) is treated as axiomatic in India, which has a long tradition of collective caregiving and management of sickness in the home. I learned that *madad* from the *bajar* (outside), as it was frequently described, was rarely sought out. First, this is a straightforward matter of restricted resources. Few patients have the time, money or indeed the energy to seek out additional models of care across Mumbai's heaving and crowded metropolis. It is in this respect that cancer charities have tailored their services to mirror patient pathways by sending volunteers on outreach missions where they take their services directly to the patient's hospital bed. However, it is also readily acknowledged that counseling and seeking support from social workers or mental health specialists is also somewhat marginalized. Patients and their family members told me repeatedly that they did not need this kind of care given the availability of support from the family. In turn, counselors and social workers explained that counseling is a novel concept and that families shy away from seeking this kind of intervention. The volunteers echoed this viewpoint, explaining that it is considered a stigma to go to *those* kinds of people, and that psychiatric illness is not recognized as a real problem in India. "No one wants to admit to getting help," explained a senior member of the AICT team, "it's not like in the US where people say 'I wear Gucci, Armani, I'm so stressed, and I have therapy three times a week!' People here don't tell anyone. You are just *pāgal* (mad)."

Complexities surrounding patient participation in voluntary interventions are further compounded by the fear that surrounds cancer and the social ostracism experienced by patients. It was often said that people do not die of cancer but they die of the *dar* (fear) of cancer. This fear surrounds the synonymy of cancer with death as patients are treated by their families and the wider community as a *bechārī*, a pitied and hopeless person. Cancer is also subject to intense sociocultural interpretation and metaphorical elaboration (McMullin & Weiner, 2008; Sontag, 1991). I encountered various, predominantly malevolent interpretations of cancer. Cancer is frequently considered to be a *pāp* (sin) and/or a *sajā* (punishment) from god for unintentional / intentional moral transgressions committed in this life or the previous one. Women would often question what was in their *nasīb* (fate; luck) to have brought such misfortune into their lives, which in turn invited moral judgment from their families and wider community and aroused deep feelings of shame. Breast cancer is also considered to be contagious, described as *phaīl rahi hai* (spreading) between persons through touch, the sharing of utensils, breast milk and sexual intercourse. This also surrounds the specific risk of contagion of cancer from mothers to their daughters, whereby daughters are perceived to be more susceptible to cancer if the mother has the disease. In turn, this tarnishes the marriageability of a daughter and threatens the moral welfare and honor of the family (Macdonald, 2014).

In light of these sociocultural perceptions of cancer, patients are encouraged not to dwell upon the idea of cancer or keep it in their *dyan* (attention). The power and danger of words is a common preoccupation in contexts dealing with illness such as cancer (McMullin & Weiner, 2008; Trawick 1991). Therefore, to speak openly about cancer is considered inauspicious as it invites the disease into being. To say the word *cancer* is dangerous and it is frequently replaced in everyday conversation by the much softer sounding *gārnth* (lump), *cīz* (thing) or simply *chāti taklīf* (breast/chest problem). Thus breast cancer is a disease bound up with particular sociocultural moralities that in India are confronted from within the sphere of domesticity and community, where the stigma of suffering with breast cancer is experienced interpersonally as a biomoral problem of "connected body-selves" embedded within a network of far-reaching social and kin relations (Das & Addlakha 2001, p. 512). It is thus the moral state of the family—as both a unit of protection and preservation from the *outside* community, and the vulnerable nexus through which cancer can spread and contaminate as *connected body selves*—that is so often at stake in the context of suffering with breast cancer. As such, the benefits of self-disclosure and *stranger solidarity* fostered by the process of participating in support groups are sometimes negated by the prevalence of these wider local moralities (see also Nguyen 2010; Argenti-Pillen, 2007). Talking *about* cancer is not necessarily perceived as a cathartic and therapeutic process but rather as a risky and morally dubious venture.

BEING A *SURVIVOR VOLUNTEER*

Casting a lens to the work of the survivor volunteers one finds a radically different perspective on what suffering with breast cancer can come to mean. I was surprised to find such strong associations with a *survivor identity* in India, especially given its resonance with cancer survivorship in Euro-American biomedical, activist and public discourse (DelVecchio Good, Good, Schaffer & Lind, 1990; Kaufert, 1998; Stacey, 1997). Yet I soon came to learn that in the daily struggles to manage breast cancer in Mumbai, the survivorship of the patient turned volunteer had a certain productivity and value. These early pioneers recalled that, when they were diagnosed, there were no volunteers, no information booklets, no outreach programs, no patient rehabilitation clinics nor breast prostheses. Thus much of their charity work started while they themselves were still patients, either by just striking up conversations in patient waiting rooms, reading each other's medical files or by creating strategic alliances with like-minded oncologists that resulted in the formation of small, patient-focused charities. Furthermore, given that many of these women had treatment in TMH, they were able to mobilize their experiential knowledge as a practical pedagogical tool. By acknowledging themselves as previous sufferers in ways that had not been heard or seen before, including participation in emergent forums for the display and airing of suffering and survivorship experiences, these women were fundamental in mobilizing breast cancer as a *social* disease. With this came changes to the delivery and provisions of the oncological health care system that is now trending towards a more patient-centered approach and toward incorporating psychosocial interventions into processes of patient recovery.

Anupama's story is an apt example of this. On the first afternoon that I met her, she exclaimed in English, "I tell the world I am a breast cancer survivor!" Anupama's experience of suffering with and surviving breast cancer, as well as the trauma of losing her sister to the disease just before her own diagnosis, had transformed her entire life. She considered herself blessed, not only because of her own recovery from two cases of breast cancer, but because she was in a position whereby she could now perform *seva* (selfless service)[6] for her fellow patients. This, she claimed, in the eyes of god is what she is meant to dedicate her life to. Rather than go and "listen to some guru" or "sit at the temple for hours and hours," she considered there to be no other option after recovery than acting in the service of others. The two were inextricably linked. "By god's grace I am blessed to serve my fellow patients," she explained. "I could sit at home or I could help . . . what would I rather do?" As part of this service, Anupama readily acknowledged the lack of psychosocial support in the medical system and consistently pointed out that there was not adequate rehabilitation for women regarding, for example, how to use the breast prostheses and wigs, and how to prevent and manage lymphedema. She said, "After all the treatment is over, what happens next? No one knows! So that is when people like us come in."

In the urban milieu of treating cancer in Mumbai, women like Anupama—the survivor volunteers—are openly living their lives not only as persons once affected by breast cancer but as individuals now thriving *from* cancer. They have converted their suffering into socially sanctioned acts of *sevā* that are inextricable from their lay expertise. Thus it is their individual biographies of sickness and recovery that are contributing to the texture and tone of lay breast cancer activism in Mumbai. The work of *seeing* survivors is one aspect of this activism, derived from their own experiential authority of having recovered from cancer, which now feeds into the way the survivor volunteers and volunteers attempt to inspire hope in patients and open up a space for sharing and solidarity.

SEEING SURVIVORS

In 1971, the film *Anand* was released in India. Set in Mumbai, it charts the life story of a cynical doctor named Dr. Banerjee, played by Amitabh Bachchan, who meets a cancer patient named Anand. One day Dr. Banerjee meets a colleague in his office who sets about describing, with great severity, a patient with an incurable case of "lymphocercoma." Just as this colleague finishes speaking, a man bursts into the doctor's office shouting excitedly, *"Dost! Dost!"* (Friend). This man is Anand, the incurable patient, whose vitality, exuberance and joy undercut Dr. Banerjee's expectations of a dying, sickly, doomed fellow. This is pressed upon the audience further by the reaction of the hospital matron, who for a short while at the beginning of the film, does not realize that Anand is the incurable cancer patient. When she finally does, the soundtrack switches to an ominous melody and the camera zooms in to focus on the matron's widening eyes, horrified and shocked. Although there are endless metaphorical connections one could make between the religious, cinematic, emotional, affective and aesthetic elaborations of vision here, I cannot help but read into the cinematic gaze on the matron's widening eyes a resonance with the primacy for visual apprehension in Hindu sociality. Indeed, it is these aspects of perceiving and seeing that I found so notable in interactions between patients and survivor volunteers.

Sitting with Roopal in the patient waiting area in the basement of TMH, she explained how during her first diagnosis of breast cancer she had sought inspiration from an elderly lady who lives in her native place, back in the northern parts of Uttar Pradesh. "Twenty years she is a survivor" commented Roopal raising an eyebrow at me, "and I wanted to be like her." It is from the same sentiment that she now offers counseling to the patients she meets on a daily basis throughout the hospital. *"When I meet patients on the ward I tell them look at me; that I have survived cancer for 23 years . . . it is that sentence that makes them smile"* she said. Roopal's evaluation of her role as a survivor resonated with my daily observations of volunteers and patients. Here I frequently encountered revelations of one's status as a survivor together with an inherent emphasis on visual apprehension as a means to take *himmat* (courage) and *acchi hallat* (to improve confidence). This revolves around the ideal of *normalcy*[7] as an instantiation of the possibility of life itself whereby the very physicality of looking *thee* (normal; ok) or *acha lagta hai* (good) emphasizes to patients and their relatives that recovery from cancer is possible and everyday life can resume.

I was frequently struck more generally by the way *seeing* emerged in everyday life. Anupama often told me that one should just go and stand in TMH and watch. For one week, she insisted, one should just watch. And then, she emphasized, one would come to know real humanity and the nature of humility and God's grace. In this sense I came to learn that one could *see* the divine in anything and everything, and found many social practices are underscored by mandates to see—whether it be the new bride, the deity, the guest, the dying person or the sick. The propensity for visual apprehension as paradigmatic of social practice is considered to be particularly prevalent in Hinduism. This is aptly captured by Diana Eck (1985) who states that "whenever Hindus affirm the meaning of life, death and suffering, they affirm with their eyes wide open" (p. 11). The primacy of sight in Hinduism especially is frequently captured by the concept and practice of *darsan*; the act of "seeing and being seen." This central act of Hindu worship consists of beholding the image in which the deity is present and from which the devotee takes or receives *darsan* from the deity priest. Images or religious iconography have a sensory quality whereby it is the exchange of vision, the process of seeing and being seen, that lies at the heart of Hindu worship (Eck, 1985). Moments of religiosity and epistemological endeavors are thus arguably achieved through the sensory work of sight. Unlike visual representation or objectification of a subject that is often characteristic of the more disconnected, unidirectional perusals of images in the West, Hindu sight is described as a *corpothetic* engagement, that is, the everyday corporeal aesthetics through which embodied vision constitutes a fluid interchange of visual interaction (Pinney, 2004).

The corpothetic work of sight was reinforced every week during the postoperative classes at TMH. Here Anupama would hold classes for patients who had just been operated on that week. These classes grew out of collaboration between TMH and a small breast cancer charity, of which Anupama had been a member. As an intervention, it feeds into the emergent ethos of trying to incorporate additional social therapies into mainstream oncological treatment. This class focused predominantly on answering questions, teaching lymphedema exercises, discussing breast self-examination and handing out leaflets for patients to take back home. At the start of each class Anupama would address the women seated around her with a *namaste* and then, after introducing her name and her affiliation with the hospital, she would tell the class, "*Mai survivor hu*" (I am a survivor). "I was like you—I had a double lumpectomy, radiotherapy and I developed lymphedema." This would immediately invite questions inquiring about how many *sal* (years) she had been alive since completing treatment. At other times, Anupama was *shown* by the attending physiotherapist who would put her arm around Anupama, and ask the class, "*aap dekh sakti hai?*" (Can you see?) "This how you will become *(ho jaega)* also." Thus in the volunteers' everyday work to support and comfort breast cancer patients the primacy of revelation and vision seems to also have some kind of corpothetic resonance in terms of the way disease affiliation is reckoned with and used to inspire hope. Although the emphasis in these engagements is not conceptualized in terms of the *shared gaze* of the religious act, and indeed this is clearly something quite different from the volunteers' practices (which are not articulated as an invocation of *darsan*), it is the inherent sensory quality of the embodied vision that is of particular pertinence here, and which I explore as a therapeutic tool in more detail next.

VISION AS A THERAPEUTIC TOOL

Thus far I have explored the ways by which seeing survivors appears to have a particular kind of social resonance as a strategy deployed by survivor volunteers in order to create some kind of immediate solidarity with other breast cancer patients. In the excerpt from fieldnotes that follows, I suggest that this produces a therapeutic tool that is strategically utilized by both volunteers and survivor volunteers to create a tangible sense of hope. *One morning I was accompanying Padma, a previous breast cancer sufferer and long-standing charity volunteer, on her weekly visit to a chemotherapy wing in a local private hospital a short bus ride away from her house. We knocked on the door of a private room and asked if we could come in and speak with the patient and her family. . . . A woman was lying on a metal bed with an IV drip attached her arm. The drip hung from a rusty black metal tripod positioned next to the bed. Across from the woman sat her husband and son. We stayed chatting with the family for about an hour covering various topics including what causes cancer and why it can happen. The family was calm but as we discussed the various risk factors for cancer it was clear that the family was perplexed about the diagnosis and anxious for a speedy recovery. Speaking on behalf of his mother, the son explained that they were concerned about the effects of chemotherapy, especially the possibility of hair loss. At this point, Padma said that she had also suffered from breast cancer. Both the husband and son were astonished. Uncertain as to whether his mother had heard (she had up until this point engaged minimally in the conversation), he signaled to her saying "dekh dekh! (look!) She is also a breast cancer patient!" Padma nodded and smiled, and the woman asked her how long it took for her 'bal' (hair) to grow back. As she explained that her hair grew back quickly, Padma unclipped the black slide from the nape of her neck and let loose her long black hair over her shoulders for the woman to see.*

In a similar vein, survivor volunteers and volunteers working at the Cancer Clinic in a south Mumbai district also draw upon survivor status in moments of patient distress. The Cancer Clinic runs twice a week for breast cancer patients. Although it is housed on site in a private hospital, it welcomes patients from all over the city. The clinic is run out of two small, cramped rooms, and volunteers meet on average seven patients in each three-hour slot. One Tuesday morning, I was sitting in my usual spot on a low stool next to the examination bed. Jyoti was the attending volunteer. She was a previous patient who finished her treatment for breast cancer five years earlier. . . . The following excerpt from field notes describes what happened that day:

A patient knocks on the door. Jyoti calls to come in. The woman enters the room and she sits down in front of the small desk, opposite Jyoti. She is alone and appears very nervous, hesitant and shy. She takes out her medi-cal report from her plastic shopping bag and hands it to Jyoti, and asks her if she could explain the report. She has just had a mastectomy and has been told by the doctor she needs chemotherapy and radiotherapy but she does not know what this entails. Jyoti opens the file, looks down briefly, and starts to explain what chemotherapy is. The woman looks particularly anxious and seems distracted, and Jyoti stops mid-sentence and asks her in English: "Why are you looking very tense?" Jyoti reaches out to rub the woman's hand affectionately and the woman starts to cry. Jyoti tutts gently and says, "Nothing is going to happen to you nah?" And then continues: "I am a survivor from five years back. Look at me! Do you think I had the same surgery? No!" she exclaims. "We are the lucky ones," she continues. The woman looks astonished. Pointing to the women's medical file Jyoti continues to explain that they are both lucky because they are recipients of the latest treatment and technology. "Nothing is going to happen, be posi-tive" Jyoti urges, and she asks the woman if she is working. The woman nods and says she is a lecturer in commerce and business studies. Jyoti smiles enthusiastically, encouraging the woman to open up, which she does, a little, and the conversation ensues with more ease.

On another occasion, a woman and her husband had just been brought in to the clinic. I recorded the following in my field notes: *The woman had been crying on the ward so one of the volunteers had brought her down to meet the other volunteers in the CC. One of the volunteers, Rani (who is not a previous breast cancer patient) takes her hand. "Don't worry" she says, "there is pain but this is temporary. Don't worry. You have this trauma but it will be ok (theek hoge)." She starts to tell her about the prosthesis. "This will make you feel better," she says, as she takes out the prototype cotton prosthesis from the box and lays it in front of her. The woman is clearly distraught and tries to speak, saying something about the pain on her chest. Her husband interrupts and starts to speak but Rani cuts him off. Not looking at the husband, but focusing on the crying woman, she strokes her hand. There is silence in the room for a few moments until Jyoti opens the door and comes in. Rani looks up and says to the patient, "Look she is a survivor!" The woman looks at Jyoti in shock. Jyoti, accustomed to such bold and spontaneous introductions, smiles and says, "I am five years (paunch sal) completed. I am normal (mai theek hu)." To which Rani adds, "See, look at her. Tension mat lo (don't worry)." The woman who has still said nothing, smiles shyly and the awkward ambiance slowly dissipates and a more relaxed form of conversation starts to flow. After the clinic ended that morning, I asked Rani why she had introduced Jyoti in that way and she explained, "See, she just has to sit there. It's like a miracle working for them [the patient] mentally."*

Although Rani was not a survivor volunteer, she acknowledged, along with Jyoti and the other CC volunteers, that interactional modes of *seeing* survivors constituted a process of emotional exchange that conferred a greater impact on a patient's will to live than any amount of *talking*. Indeed, regardless of whether one was a survivor volunteer or not, it was agreed that seeing survivors was a pivotal aspect of delivering cancer care, and in this sense having the participation of survivor volunteers in your charity or NGO is considered a kind of trump card for success.

Sight and seeing are pivotal mediums through which volunteers and survivor volunteers are delivering patient care as part of their charity work in Mumbai.[8] By strategically revealing the exceptionality of surviving through appeals to visual apprehension of the vitality and normalcy of the survivor volunteers, these lay activists have found a way to make tangible, through the act of sight, the otherwise unknown and inchoate so typical of the suffering caused by cancer. I suggest that this creates a moment of biosocial identification by offering the possibility of becoming a survivor. Yet this potential of *becoming* materializes disease affiliation and *being like her* in a very concrete way. However, this process rarely results in the assimilation of patients into support groups or other forms of social identification based on a *survivor identity*. Although this is the case for those women who decided to become volunteers, the *biosociality* of their survivorship as a form of patient activism and source of changing personhood is marginalized in relation to the vast majority of women suffering with breast cancer in India. Among the patients that I met and from the interactions that I observed, living with cancer is too often marked by fear of social ostracism and familial rejection for anything profitable to be gained from mobilizing one's status as a survivor and being biosocially active (see also Bharadwaj & Glasner, 2009; Das & Addlakha, 2001). Yet in the volunteers' daily work of extending hope and care to patients, I argue that it is through corpothetic visual apprehension that disease affiliation and the therapeutic work of sharing has productive and virtuous value. In a context where group sharing is elided and talking is deemed to fail, those specific and strategic moments of seeing survivors, however fleeting they may be, offer a hope of *becoming*.

CONCLUSION

This chapter began by questioning the kinds of strategies that give rise to variants of therapeutic patient activism and has ruminated on the productivity of vision as a therapeutic modality among lay breast cancer volunteers in urban India. It has charted the complexities and tensions imbued in local philanthropic efforts to increase participation in oncological psychosocial interventions, and in turn, revealed contingencies surrounding the ways by which patient solidarity is created and maintained. In a context framed by kinship solidarity, social ostracism and demands of receiving care in a resource poor setting, less emphasis is placed on practices of talking and group sharing, and participation in patient solidarity groups is not desired. However, I have suggested that it is through the process of *seeing* survivors as a corpothetic engagement that relations of disease affiliation become salient among breast cancer patients. It is at this point that biological affiliation and social identification come to matter, and do so in ways that have some kind of therapeutic purchase for patients who meet with survivor volunteers. As figures of experiential authority, these women emerge as role models for other patients and their families. It is through the exceptionality of their vitality juxtaposed against the weight of hopelessness and fear of death that the complex moralities of suffering with breast cancer collide and are confronted via the international mode of sight. Such nuances thus highlight the divergent ways psychosocial interventions and therapeutic technologies take particular forms and are rendered meaningful in different social settings. As anthropologists working in fields of emerging diseases and their associated forms of health activism, it is prudent to be attuned to the way transnational interventions are subject to these processes of resignification. The strategies of the survivor volunteers illustrate how such forms emerge from within fields of familiarity and represent locally profound patterns of creating and attaining solace and hope. These transformations thus shape our understanding of what it means to be biosocially active in different locales where practices and sentiments take on unique biosocial resonance.

NOTES

1. Research for this chapter was carried out from March 2009 until August 2010 and was supported by an Economic and Social Research Council (ESRC) doctoral scholarship. An earlier version of this paper was presented at the Association of Social Anthropologists (ASA) conference in Delhi, India in 2012. I am indebted to the volunteers and organizations in Mumbai for their hospitality and friendship, and to Tata Memorial Hospital for kindly granting me access to conduct research. I am extremely grateful to the editors for their comments on earlier versions of this chapter.
2. Different individuals are involved in the NGO and voluntary sector around cancer in Mumbai. This ranges from persons who have not been affected by cancer, persons who have been affected indirectly as caregivers, or previous patients. In order to highlight the pivotal role of survivorship in forms of lay activism within the broader philanthropic and voluntary sphere in Mumbai, I refer specifically to previous patients turned volunteers as *survivor volunteers* and to all other persons as *volunteers*.
3. This includes a burgeoning South East Asian breast cancer forum spearheaded by the organization Reach2Recovery that emphasizes the beneficial role the

previous survivors can play in forms of patient counseling. Likewise, in Euro-America, the role for the survivor has become an iconic figure in many activist circles, biomedical discourses and medical campaigns (see also, DelVecchio Good, Good, Schaffer & Lind, 1990; Kaufert, 1998; Stacey, 1997).

4. For the sake of anonymity, all names of organizations and persons have been changed.

5. The few groups that I did encounter were structured like question/answer forums, peppered with patient testimonies that focused less on the act of narrative sharing or confessions and more on the acquisition of knowledge to dispel misconceptions about cancer and to clarify medical uncertainties.

6. The fact that charity work is conceptualized as *seva* (selfless service) is significant in understanding the kind of activism of these women. As self-proclaimed *volunteers,* many of these women do not refer to themselves as *activists.* They do not conceive of their charitable work as *activism* in the sense that activism is perceived to have state level public policy impact. Rather, performing charity as *seva* is intimately bound to Hindu spiritual and cosmological frameworks through which these women conceive of, and have come to understand, their suffering and subsequent recovery. As such, serving humanity as a cancer volunteer is ultimately to serve god in spiritually inflected acts that are inextricable from the pious subjectivities that these women seek to harness in life after recovery from cancer (Macdonald, 2013).

7. Certainly in other spheres of breast cancer charity that I encountered, the *normalcy* around survivorship correlates to typically middle and upper class/caste and thus privileged viewpoints of a minority group of women experiencing breast cancer in India. However, although normalcy can at times reinforce the viewpoint of a hegemonic few, in this specific context, it does not detract from the fact that the desire for normalcy is so often articulated by patients and their families.

8. It is significant to note that both volunteers and survivor volunteers emphasize and mobilize around the ameliorative work of *seeing* cancer survivors. Although volunteers cannot draw on any kind of experiential knowledge, they frequently point to the figure of the survivor volunteer in their interactions with patients as a means of creating hope.

REFERENCES

Argenti-Pillen, A. M. (2007). Mothers and wives of the disappeared in southern Sri Lanka: Fragmented geographies of moral discomfort. In Skidmore, M., & Lawrence, P. (Eds.), *Women and the contested state: Religion, violence and agency in South and Southeast Asia* (pp. 117–138). Notre Dame, IN: University of Notre Dame Press.

Bharadwaj, A., & Glasner, P. (2009). *Local cells, global science: The rise of embryonic stem cell research in India*. London: Routledge.

Biehl, J. (2007). *Will to live: AIDS therapies and the politics of survival*. Princeton, NJ: Princeton University Press.

Das, V., & Addlakha, R. (2001). Disability and domestic citizenship: Voice, gender and the making of the subject. *Public Culture,* 511–531.

DelVecchio Good, M. J., Good, B., Schaffer, C., & Lind, S. E. (1990). American oncology and the discourse on hope. *Culture, Medicine and Psychiatry,* 59–79.

Eck, D. (1985). *Darsan: Seeing the divine image in India*. Chambersburg, PA: Anima Books.

Gibbon, S., & Novas, C. (2008). *Biosocialities, genetics, and the social sciences: Making biologies and identities*. London: Routledge.

Kaufert, P. (1998). Women, resistance and the breast cancer movement. In M. Lock & P. Kaufert (Eds.), *Pragmatic women and body politics* (pp. 287–309). Cambridge, MA: Cambridge University Press.

Macdonald, A. (2013). *Breast cancer survivorship in urban India: Self and care in voluntary groups.* Thesis (Unpublished doctoral dissertation), University College, University of London, London.

Macdonald, A. (2014). Situating breast cancer risk: Gender, temporality and social change. In S. Gibbon, G. Joseph, E. Kampriani, J. Mozersky, A. zur Nieden, & S. Palfner (Eds.), *Breast cancer gene research and medical practices: Transnational perspectives in the time of BRCA* (pp. 83–94). London: Routledge.

Mathews, H. (2009). Cancer support groups and health advocacy: One size doesn't fit all. In J. McMullin & D. Weiner (Eds.), *Confronting cancer: Metaphors, advocacy, and anthropology* (pp. 43–61). Santa Fe, NM: School for Advanced Research Press.

McMullin, J., & Weiner, D. (2008). *Confronting cancer: Metaphors, advocacy, and anthropology.* Santa Fe, NM: School for Advanced Research Press.

Nguyen, V. K. (2010). *The republic of therapy: Triage and sovereignty in West Africa's time of AIDS.* Durham, NC: Duke University Press.

Petryna, A. (2002). *Biological citizenship: Science and the politics of health after Chernobyl.* Princeton, NJ: Princeton University Press.

Pinney, C. (2004). *Photos of the Gods: The printed image and political struggle in India.* London: Reaktion Books.

Rabinow, P. (1996). Artificiality and enlightenment: From socio-biology to biosociality. *Essays on the anthropology of reason* (pp. 91–111). Princeton, NJ: Princeton University Press.

Rose, N., & Novas, C. (2000). Genetic risk and the birth of the somatic individual. *Economy and Society, 29,* 485–513.

Rose, N., & Novas, C. (2005). Biological citizenship. In A. Ong & S. J. Collier (Eds.), *Global assemblages: Technology, politics and ethics as anthropological problems* (pp. 439–463). Malden, MA: Blackwell Publishing.

Sontag, S. (1991). *AIDS and its metaphors.* London: Penguin.

Stacey, J. (1997). *Teratologies: A cultural study of cancer.* London: Routledge.

Trawick, M. (1991). An Ayurvedic theory of cancer. *Medical Anthropology,* 121–136.

Part II

Cancer and the Sociality of Care

Intimacy, Support and Collective Burden-Sharing

7 Love in the Time of Cancer

Kinship, Memory, Migration and Other Logics of Care in Kerala, India

Kristin Bright

INTRODUCTION

In his novel, *Love in the Time of Cholera*, Gabriel García Márquez (1988) compares the affliction of his protagonists' lovesickness with that of cholera, and then makes a further allusion to the anguish (*cólera*) of economic and political divisions in late 19th century Colombia. It was during the summer of 2005 as I was reading this book that I started speaking with women undergoing treatment for breast cancer in Kochi, a city of roughly two million people on the Malabar Coast of India's southernmost state of Kerala. Their words about the current of emotions that followed diagnosis (shock, fear, anger, worry) echoed the sentiments of García Márquez's protagonists, and I realized that their suffering grew out of a similar intersection of material and relational concerns.

For the women I met in Kochi, affliction and regard were intertwined: a circuit of hope, despair, caring and being cared for. All of the women had cared for seriously ill relatives, many of whom had died. As they described their own cancer diagnoses, they made allusions to sisters, brothers, daughters, sons, parents and neighbors: a steady compilation of the self through the telling of others' concerns. More than affect or empathy, their narratives grew out of and comprised a number of social and cultural structures: the composition of a family, its makings and undoings; the shape of a person who holds a secret about her diagnosis, and the shape she becomes after telling others; the making of a self in place, time, sociality and solitude. Their voices shined with gratitude for family in Dubai who helped to pay for treatment, and churned with the anguish of having to sell one's marriage necklace or a parcel of farmland to cover the costs of care.

This chapter investigates how structures of kinship, migration and capital influence the way women approach and engage with cancer treatments. My analysis draws from fieldwork that I conducted at a large specialty hospital in Kochi that I refer to here as Neelam Medical Center (or "Neelam")[1] and ethnographic data that I collected through participant observation, medical chart and database review, and in-depth interviews with women undergoing clinical treatment for breast cancer, their family members and oncology providers.[2] What I want to examine here is how women approach and experience cancer care, less in terms of what oncologists have called stages in a *continuum of care* (NCI, 2014) and rather in terms of what I will call *relational logics*—spatially diverse and nonlinear structures of shielding, sharing, persuasion, reproach and support—that have specific and powerful effects on clinical events (presentation, diagnosis, therapy) and when and how those happen.

In the sections that follow, I make a multi-part argument. First, I consider some of the ways that care and care seeking are relational, drawing a distinction between the *cultural* aspects of relationships, that is, the ways in which they reflect socially inherited norms and meanings, and the *individual* aspects, that is, particular concerns unique to a person. In looking at relationships, especially in terms of specific actors, it is important to keep in mind that the cultural models and norms of kinship, while important, are not the only things that impact the practice and experience of treatment. Individual histories of things, like place and movement, matter. Migration to and from the Persian Gulf, for example, crucially impacts relational care, not only in terms of the use of "Gulf money" to pay for treatment or the use of return travel by migrants to seek care, but in the ways people's sense of self is transformed by participation in such activities.

A second part of my argument examines some of the implications of relationships and individual histories for how cancer treatment is practiced in India. The complexity of the factors that shape decisions about treatment, for example, mean that improving outcomes cannot be achieved by anything as straightforward as increasing access. The final part of my argument looks more closely at relationships and what holds them together. Specifically, I examine how culturally particular meanings of love shape practices of care, making cancer treatment in Kerala something more complex than an emotional impulse or tactical effort, but both of these things and something more (Lutz & Abu-Lughod, 1990).

THE CONTEXT OF CANCER TREATMENT IN KERALA

Founded in 1998 by a popular spiritual leader in South India, Neelam Medical Center, according to its website, follows a philosophy of "love, discipline, and humanity." One of the largest medical centers in India, Neelam sits on a campus of 125 acres, thick with palm trees, and consists of a 1450-bed hospital; 25 operating theaters; schools of medicine, nursing, dentistry, and pharmacy; and an average of 3000 patient visitors a day. Neelam is open to any patient regardless of ability to pay, although one must go through a lengthy process to apply for a treatment waiver. Typically, one must be very poor to qualify for a waiver, with no cash on hand and no assets to sell (e.g., property, jewelry). Even then, waivers may cover the cost of surgery, radiation and chemotherapy, but do not cover tests (mammography, biopsy, blood work) or drugs (hormonal therapy), which must be purchased from outside vendors.

When Neelam established its cancer center in 2004, there was already a phalanx of guesthouses along the border of campus, available for weekly and monthly rates. Alongside these, chemists' shops, internet booths, tea stalls and tailors line the narrow, undulating roads. Next to a pillared archway that marks the entrance to Neelam, local trains and buses make regular stops throughout the day. The campus reflects a design of "maximum greenery in mind," the cancer center director Dr. Gopinath explained to me one day. This was something I grew to appreciate while staying in Kochi—Neelam had less traffic and air pollution than other parts of the city. It was a feature that Neelam's publicity department clearly understood as well. On a webpage for international patients, they describe Neelam as being in "one of the world's most beautiful travel destinations." (Although providers are also careful to attenuate this status, as I discuss later, not wanting Neelam to seem *too* far from home.)

In 1954, Jawaharlal Nehru proposed that hydroelectric dams would be the "temple, mosque, and gurdwara" of modern India (Khilani, 1999, p. 61). Today, specialty medicine has to some extent taken over the mantle as one of the key signs of modernity, from assisted conception and childbirth (Bhardwaj, 2006; Ram, 2001; Van Hollen, 2003) to gerontology and psychiatry (Cohen, 1998; Ecks, 2005; Jain & Jadhav, 2009). Kerala, in particular, is touted as a state with some of the highest rates of literacy, gender equity and life expectancy in India.[3] Although in general its medical system is deeply stratified, consisting of boutique hospitals for the rich and government hospitals for the poor, Neelam does not exactly fit this typology. Because it is administered as a philanthropic trust, it is neither private nor public. Although nationally regarded for its specialty care, it does not have the same aesthetic of India's new mega-hospitals or *medical cities,* vast hospital complexes that cater to local elites and medical tourists in larger cities such as Mumbai and Delhi (Solomon, 2011).

Neelam is a pay-for-care facility, yet 90% of women who come for breast cancer care do not have health insurance. There is no government insurance for the elderly or the poor in India, and employer coverage is rare; only a few patients are covered by a healthcare plan supplied by the government to military families. The women I interviewed are in some ways similar to most oncology patients in India (i.e., uninsured). Money or its lack is a consistent facet in their approach to treatment, but the impact of money is also filtered through various relationships and local particularities of disease. For example, in a pattern resembling other urban cancer centers in India (Ali, Mathew & Rajan, 2008; Yeole & Kurkure, 2003), women present more often at Neelam with locally advanced breast cancer (LABC) than any other stage. LABC includes stage 2B-3C, where the tumor is more than five centimeters in diameter but localized to the breast, and axilla, the most advanced stage still potentially curable with surgery, radiation and chemotherapy

(Simos, Clemons, Ginsburg & Jacobs, 2014). Among the women I interviewed, 20 were diagnosed with LABC and 12 with earlier stage disease (stage 1–2A). Thirty women had self-discovered a lump in their breast, and 2 had lumps detected through mammography. The size of a lump at presentation varied from 2 centimeters in diameter (the size of a walnut) to 14 centimeters (the size of a grapefruit), with an average diameter of 5 centimeters.

To understand how these data compare with the broader picture at Neelam, student research interns and I put together a retrospective database of breast carcinomas seen at Neelam in 2008–2010. Of the 416 cases we reviewed, 33% were locally advanced and 10% were metastatic tumors. This stage burden corresponds with national level data where LABC is estimated to be the most common stage of breast cancer in India (Leong, et al., 2010) and in other low-resource countries (El Saghir et al., 2011). Oncology centers in rural areas in India may see a higher burden of advanced disease than urban hospitals. Ahktar, Akulwar, Gandhi and Chandak (2011, p. 404) found that LABC accounts for 50.7% of new breast diagnoses at a specialty center in rural Maharashtra. By comparison, LABC comprises only 4% of new breast cancer diagnoses in the United States and 8% in Europe (Allemani et al., 2013).

On the one hand, Neelam's proportion of advanced breast cancer cases appears to reflect a global problem, that is, that treatment delays may be correlated with treatment cost, even among the "financially comfortable" middle class. On the other hand, cost barriers do not sufficiently explain why advanced stage breast cancer would represent 43% of cases, or why a person with advanced stage cancer would experience an average nine-month delay from when she first detects a symptom to when she arrives at Neelam.[4]

Although studies are available on the correlation between treatment delay and stage of disease (Ali, Mathew & Rajan, 2008; Bright et al., 2011), few studies in cancer health have considered what delay *means* (for example, the cultural categories people use to define or structure time) or the social norms people use to assess when it is "too soon" or "too late" to make a visit to a physician. Mathews and colleagues offer one of the first analyses of delay from the perspective of women's own narratives and lived experiences of etiology, time and the body (Mathews, Lannin & Mitchell, 1994). How are symptom discovery and care seeking in Kerala similarly shaped by cultural particularities of migration, kinship and the self?

To assess what delay means to women (and whether that is even a sufficient category to understand how people apprehend or live with a disease), I spent several months at Neelam between 2005 and 2010, gathering ethnographic data in the form of field notes; chart and database review; and interviews with 32 women, 12 of their family members, and 10 clinicians and administrators. Oncology staff at Neelam as well as student research interns from New York University School of Medicine assisted me in collecting and translating interviews from Malayalam to English. Interviews with women and family members were conducted in a separate wing from where treatments take place at Neelam, and interviews with providers were conducted in their offices.[5] I clustered questions into three interview guides (patient, kin member, provider) and then used follow-up probes to explore individuals' perceptions about care settings (i.e., home, hospital) and associated care practices; the role of family and other social networks in symptom discovery and treatment; opportunities and barriers to care; and meanings associated with kinship, migration and care. I used a similar set of themes to code the interview transcripts and field notes.

Because the situation at Neelam is one in which patients think about oncologic treatment as therapeutically and ontologically contiguous with relational care (including, for example, the treatment decisions that family members make together, or the financial support that relatives provide for chemotherapy), my goal in the next section is twofold. First, I want to offer an analysis of the ways women use relational logics to struggle through the highly personal situation of being sick. Second, I want to look at the interaction of individual situations and cultural narratives in shaping the ways people engage with the clinic. Let me start with an explanation of the kinds of relationships that go into care in the first place.

RELATIONAL LOGICS OF CARE

What do women define as good care? According to the women, family and clinicians whom I interviewed, good care consists of relational care, clinically effective care and (in another blending) a clinical space that seems like home. Towards these ends, administrators at Neelam have gone to some length to organize the cancer center in a way that simulates features of domestic life. In addition to guesthouses along the campus perimeter, facilities include a canteen with low-cost meals for patients and families, and an ashram, with free-of-charge accommodations for families who qualify based on need. In the recovery ward where patients stay after surgery, there is one cot for each patient and an additional cot for a companion.

In medical anthropology, clinical "spaces" are generally understood less as physical destinations than as settings in which physicians and patients struggle to communicate and negotiate different ideas of health, illness and care (Kleinman, 1988). For example, whereas clinicians at Neelam described to me in interviews how they see the campus as a quiet, green refuge that resembles home (e.g., ashram, companion cots, prayer rooms) patients and their kin tended to describe it as physically and socially distant from home, even if this was to some extent mitigated by the presence of family members accompanying them to treatment.

How are expectations about where, how and with whom treatment takes place (and *whether* it takes place) filtered through particular understandings of propriety, mobility, privacy or support? If we want to understand why people delay presentation, we need to understand the influence of a variety of sociocultural relationships on care. Some individual cases can give a sense of the kind of things I am talking about here. "I sat on the news," said Devaki, after getting the results back from her fine-needle biopsy. "I couldn't tell anyone. Not even my husband. I couldn't afford to be sick." It was only after considering the news for a week that she decided to tell her spouse but not her 10-year-old son. Across the interviews, women expressed fears about debt, job insecurity and income loss during the months of treatment. Sandya (age 34) explained that her husband's family had "sold some properties" (parcels of farmland) to pay for her care. Kalyani (age 45) described how she had a bakery that went out of business, so she had "borrowed money from agencies" to cover costs. "Until now," Kalyani said, "we never had to worry as no one in the family has fallen sick or needed treatment."

Pratima explained how she, like Devaki, kept the news of her diagnosis to herself, not telling anyone other than her two daughters and husband. "I don't like telling everyone," she said. "I don't like publicizing to all the people. If that [cancer] is what the fate has for me, let it be like that. Whatever it is, whether good or bad happens to me, I don't want to publicize it."

Unlike Devaki, Pratima did not hesitate more than a day before she went to the hospital. She explained that social support (her daughter Sachi works in Dubai and is able to cover her treatment costs as well as accompany her to treatment), as well as her son's death from metastatic cancer at an early age, prompted her to want to go to the hospital "without delay." Aditi (age 73) spoke to still another side of diagnosis. "My dear girl," she said, "when you have a disease, only you will understand it." She had tried for six months to ignore the walnut-sized lump in her breast. But then, several weeks before our interview, she had decided to show her sister. Her sister notified the rest of the family and, within days, Aditi's closely guarded secret had become a matter of shared concern. "I went to the hospital only on my family's insistence."

Devaki, Pratima and Aditi's experiences of coming to treatment disrupt the expectation that relational care is only about "solidarity." Care emerges out of a variety of transactions among people. Each person's actions expressed a different meaning of *relational* and how that fuses with care. Devaki compared her "sitting" on her news to the way she could only "move" on that news later. Aditi juxtaposed the solitude of her illness with the affinity that comes for people with the same disease ("when you have a disease, only you will understand it"). Although family members could be generous in their support (caring for Aditi at home or at Neelam), they did not have access to her experience, not in the way she does. This, I argue, has a key implication for how we understand care seeking and treatment in Kerala. Mutual support and mutual understanding do not need to coincide for care to happen. People can be involved, indispensible even, in the care of others while unaware of the private experience of illness—or in this case, what it means to shield others from the reality of one's diagnosis.

WHAT'S RELATIONAL ABOUT RELATIONAL CARE—AND WHAT'S NOT

In her work on diabetes treatment in the Netherlands, Annemarie Mol (2008) draws a distinction between a logic of choice, where the focus is on an individual patient's ability to differentiate treatment options, and a logic of care, based on a model of mutual regard among diverse agents. At Neelam, care and choice are not opposed in the way they are in the "neoliberal" context that Mol describes. Because choices are made by a family group, decisions about treatment, for example, are made within a logic of mutual care.

Trends in the design and administration of biomedicine in India manifest in highly various ways, as a number of anthropologists have shown (Ecks, 2005; Pinto, 2011; Solomon, 2011). I found that women's narratives in Kochi revealed similarly complex things about the therapeutic encounter that exceeded neoliberal logics of choice, autonomous decision-making or rational consumption. It is difficult to boil down disparities in cancer treatment to a political economy of access, even though researchers tend to emphasize economic gaps as the first axis of difference: that is, "low," "middle," and "high" resource settings (Anderson et al., 2011; WHO, 2002).

Political economic factors, that is, resources, certainly have an impact on treatment seeking in Kerala. The effects of transnational migration on people's experiences with care are a good example of this. That migration leads to more resources is undeniable. Remittances (i.e., bank transfers) to spouses and other relatives contributed nearly 40% of Kerala's GDP in 2013 (Viswanath, 2013). But Gulf capital flows unevenly, and only 17.1% of households in Kerala received any remittances in 2011 (Zachariah & Rajan, 2012, p. 61). Furthermore, in the context of kin making in South Asia, transnational flows of people and capital affect kinship and gender relations of labor in asymmetrical ways (Gamburd, 2000; Osella & Osella, 2000).

But migration involves more than harnessing new resources; it changes what people do and therefore who people are. Kerala has seen a steady rise in labor migration since the 1970s. The Gulf is by far the most popular destination, and 90% of emigrants live in countries such the United Arab Emirates and Saudi Arabia.[6] Most transnational migrants are men (86%) whereas women tend to migrate more often within India, for example, to seek higher education (Zachariah & Rajan, 2012, p. 47). While most emigrants to the Gulf work in construction, they also work as electricians, mechanics, drivers, cooks and health care workers. A small yet increasing number of migrants work as engineers, computer technicians, physicians and nurses (Zachariah & Rajan, 2012, pp. 56–60).[7]

When families including migrants seek care, the impact of the migrants is not exclusively the greater financial resources they might make available. Both the kinds of jobs they do abroad and the cosmopolitanism engendered by international travel cause these people to develop new forms of social identity and class consciousness. These in turn affect the way they seek health because the kinds of care people choose to seek is not only an attempt to cure an illness but is a reflection of their self-understanding with regard to class identity, work, modernity and family. As I explore in the ethnographic examples that follow, women's stories reveal that *how* a person interacts in a health system is not simply a functional question of what's available or how things work (health care funding, infrastructure, access to care). A woman's desire to seek care, or to remain in care, is also contingent on how she draws on particular cultural resources—as well as the extent to which the medical system, in which she is member, is able to recognize her membership in other systems (i.e., kinship, migration) not visible in the continuum of care model (NCI, 2014). My claim is that if we want to look at the political economy of health, we need to look at things other than health and things other than economics. Political economy is precisely about relating health to the broader social and political organization of society, not simply the facilities in which health is treated.

TRANSNATIONAL RELATIONSHIPS AND CARE

Among the aspects of the broader organization of society relevant to cancer care in South India are connections people have to other places. Some of the women and family members I interviewed have relationships with trading partners and work opportunities in the Persian Gulf that span several decades. Transnational networks provide information and monetary support that women draw from in making decisions about treatment. Fathima (age 50) has 10 children, 6 of whom live with her and her husband. In addition to helping to care for a large household (several of her daughters also have children and husbands), Fathima works as a day laborer on a farm. Two months before coming to Neelam, she discovered a lump in her breast. Although her doctor recommended that she consult a surgeon for a fine-needle biopsy, the idea of the procedure terrified her and she opted instead to consult a *hakim*, a practitioner of Unani (Greco-Islamic) medicine (Bright, 1998).

"I went on my own interest," Fathima said. Her family did not support her decision, but she was able to convince them to take her anyway. But, then, she had to convince the hakim to treat her as he was concerned that the lump might be cancer. He advised her to consult a specialist for a biopsy, but Fathima demurred. "I was so scared that it might be serious. I said to him, 'please cure me soon'." Although the hakim was reluctant, he advised her to take a course of herbal therapy.

Meanwhile the lump in her breast continued to grow. The hakim advised her a second time that she get a biopsy. "So, we went and they took an FNA [fine needle aspiration] and they said you have the problem. So my children came to know . . . and they all started to call. And I started feeling bad [worried]." She decided to call her nephew Farooq who lived in Dubai. "He is working in a hospital, so we decided to call him with the results." When Fathima and her husband reached Farooq via Skype, he offered to speak with the physicians in his department about treatment centers in Kerala. A couple days later, he called back and said that one of the doctors (a fellow migrant from Kerala) recommended that Fathima go to Neelam immediately.

Although we have only indirect knowledge of Farooq, it seems reasonable to conclude that his job in a hospital has acclimated him to a different set of understandings about treatment than Fathima and to see him as having mediated her relationship (and that of her husband and other household members) to those norms. When Fathima expresses reluctance to travel and seek care at Neelam, Farooq uses another transnational loop to call his parents who in turn notify the extended family in Kerala. Although Fathima tries to put them off by proclaiming the absence of any pain and refusing to cut back on her farm work, her relatives convince her to start treatment at Neelam. One week later, accompanied by her husband and daughter, she takes the five-hour train trip from their home in Calicut to Kochi.

Relationships and care are even more complexly intertwined in the case of transnational migrants who come home for treatment in Kerala. Relationships at once determine the location of care and are strengthened by travel. In the early 1990s, Sabah moved to Abu Dhabi to work as an engineer for a state-run power company. Each summer, she returns to Kerala with her husband and children to stay with her parents for a month. It was during one of these trips that she learned she had cancer. In this excerpt, I focus on Sabah's relationship with her mother. Unlike Pratima and Fathima who have relatives in the Gulf, Sabah is herself settled there, and this raises questions about treatment among nonresident Keralites. Although generalizability is limited by the fact that Sabah is just one person among 2.3 million migrants, her experience reveals how, even for transnational subjects, the meanings that a person attributes to illness and the decisions they make about treatment are mediated by relationships at "home" (in this case, Abu Dhabi and Kochi).

Eight months before I met her for our interview, Sabah had a minor accident in Abu Dhabi, bumping the left side of her body into a doorframe. That evening, she felt a lump on her breast. During her nightly telephone call with her mother, Sabah's mother, Asma, expressed concern. "She said that I should get the lump checked out. So, I went." But after a physical exam and ultrasound, Sabah's gynecologist in Abu Dhabi could find nothing wrong, and suggested that the lump was "just a thickening, and nothing to worry about." Sabah returned to her life as usual. A month later, the lump was still there, a rock hard grape just beneath her left armpit. "The lump kept developing and I was under the impression that it was because of that hitting-of-the-door. I never imagined it to be cancer."

Sabah flew back to Kerala for her summer visit with her parents, and within a week, she and her mother were sitting in a consultation room at

Neelam, waiting for the biopsy results. After learning of her diagnosis of locally advanced breast cancer, Sabah was devastated. "I was thinking, why? Why did it have to happen to me? Was I such a horrible, evil person that it had to happen to me?" She paused, and looked across the social workers' office where we sat on a pair of upholstered chairs. On the far wall of the office hung a brightly illustrated calendar, a picture of some children playing with a cat. Sabah stared at the calendar for a few moments.

"How does this affect your life right now?" I asked her.

"It's affected my life in all the ways," she said. "Because our return is fixed for the 25th. I have two children studying there. So, then, maybe I'll have to stay back and extend my leave [from work]. My husband may have to take care of the children. Everything is being upset. But then, I think everything will be taken care of."

"How so?" I asked. Sabah again mentioned her mother, this time describing her parents' home in Kochi in more detail. This is where she planned to stay after surgery, she explained, and during chemotherapy. She described how she and her mother kept a garden together, read some of the same books, how they deliberated over the meaning of her disease, spending hours discussing why she might have gotten sick, whether the lump was there because she had only breastfed her second child for six months. "I had to go back to work. So I stopped [breastfeeding]. But now I wonder whether that was the reason this happened to me."

At another point in the interview, I asked her, "Do you have a term or a name for the problem you're having with your breast?" Sabah paused. "Name . . . ? Well, I think maybe God wanted me to think in a different way. Maybe after this problem, I'd be a different person."

It could have been a miscommunication, or perhaps Sabah was still thinking about her response to the previous question "why do people develop this kind of lump?" but I find it interesting that rather than describing her cancer as a "lump" or "thickening" (the terms she used during our interview), she chose a more philosophical response, and questioned the origins and effects of her disease rather than pigeon-holing her experience into any one term.

Sabah shared another snippet of a conversation with her mother. They were deliberating about the cause of her cancer. Had she done something wrong, carried out some transgression? Had she eaten the wrong foods, consumed alcohol? They discussed every angle. "I don't know why this happened to me. I find that people who deliberately hurt others, walk about nicely, without any problems." It was on this note, Sabah explained, that she and her mother had arrived at a mutually agreed-upon reason for her illness. "Bad things happen to good people."

Sabah and Asma's interactions reveal a few things about the influence of individual histories and relational logics (i.e., migration, kinship) on care seeking. First, there are ways that Sabah and her mother produce a relationship across time and space (flights to and from Kerala; nightly phone conversations). Second, there are the ways they use speech, both in the sense of shared language (Malayalam and English) and speech acts (idioms, moral explanations). Then there are the social roles they play: daughter and mother, sufferer and confidante, speaker and sounding board. Lastly, there are the ways Asma physically cares for Sabah: she picks her up at the airport, takes her to Neelam and attends to her while she is recovering from treatment.

INDIVIDUAL HISTORIES AND THE RELATIONAL SELF

Beyond what Sabah and her mother's relationship reveals about perceptions of cancer, I am interested in what their interactions (e.g., phone calls, shared hobbies, mutual attempts to reconcile the meaning of a disease) produce as a social project of kin making (Bright, 1998; Cohen, 1998; Pinto, 2011; Ramberg, 2013). Despite the distance between Abu Dhabi and Kochi, Sabah and her mother's relationship is impressively close. Their interactions recall a question I used to frame this chapter: what are the cultural and individual aspects of relationships and how do those impact on treatment? On the one hand, Sabah and Asma's link is structurally similar to that of Pratima and Sachi, and to Fathima and Farooq—all three consist of one person who lives in the Gulf and one in Kerala who, despite that gap, manage to share a number of things—most particularly, a *cultural* shared-ness of meanings, norms and language.

On the other hand, each relation is distinct in tone and effect. Sabah and Asma's discussion about motherhood, fallibility and self-improvement is structured by their upper-middle class position and gendered dynamic as mother and daughter, whereas Fathima and Farooq's interaction consists of more tactical concerns, like where to go for treatment and whether they can afford it. The individual histories of things, like place and migration, matter. Sabah's comment "it's affected my life in all the ways" applies not only to the way culture impacts care seeking but equally to the ways individual history does so; culture affects everything about cancer—from the ways it is narrated and lived by people (Gordon & Paci, 1997; McMullin & Weiner, 2009) to the social relations of its treatment (Livingston, 2012) to the metaphysics of its time, space and chronicity, and the impact of those on people's ideas about life and death (Manderson & Smith-Morris, 2010)—but especially in the case of relationships, cultural norms are always instantiated in individually distinct ways.

As Lawrence Cohen (1998) demonstrates in his ethnography about old age debility in India, types of familial practice "structure a universe of discourse in which larger collectivities are continually materialized" (p. 171). Farooq's insistence that Fathima go "immediately" to Neelam is a good example of this materialization of group norms about treatment. But Fathima's response, her insistence that she is doing fine and her refusal to give up her farming jobs, is not outside the transactional expectations of being a person. There is a way in which even the meaning of Fathima's refusal is structured by the relational system because the private side of her illness is, in her words, about shielding her family from suffering. "What I earn is already not enough to feed my family," explained Fathima, "so [taking time away from work] is going to be difficult."

In considering the ways people's economic realities intersect with relational systems, I build on Cohen's critical rereading of anthropological and psychological depictions of the "Indian self" as hierarchically arranged (Dumont, 1980) or essentially relational (Roland, 1991). Whereas the self in these accounts is primarily structured through its relations with other selves (i.e., kin members) positioned *before* the autonomous or interiorized action of individuals, cases like Fathima's concession to seek care and Sabha's self-evaluation suggest a more complicated use of the self in relational systems. Fathima's concession is relational, not because of its opposition to a "Western" or "non-relational" self—or because of an internally consistent quality of selfhood that is "Indian"—but because of how it indexes norms and relations of treatment in Kerala (and the Gulf) about disease and treatment. Furthermore, the process of becoming relational in the first place involves a certain amount of social effort and conciliation (e.g., the willingness to travel from Abu Dhabi or Calicut to Neelam).

> Becoming one's family entails two linked processes: political marginalization and performative centralization. One must be unable or unwilling to assert a subjectivity that maintains a distinction between oneself and the family.
>
> (Cohen, 1998, p. 179)

Veena Das (1996) makes a similar argument that suffering can sometimes only become relational through the body—that it is the body, with all of its capacities for expressing the extraordinary and ordinary, where personalized concerns get to matter as culture. For Devaki and Pratima, "sitting" (*irikku*) and "moving" (*poku*) on the news of their biopsies were individual performances of the self that helped to translate suffering, through common idioms of the body, into culturally legible terms. Alison Macdonald's chapter in this volume makes a similar argument about the use of bodily signs in cancer advocacy in Mumbai: among survivor volunteers, the body is a site where the experience of individual suffering (e.g., surgery-induced lymphedema) can be translated into culturally recognizable forms of advocacy (showing new patients how to prevent lymphedema).

So far, I have focused a good deal in this chapter on the pragmatic aspects of relationships, particularly the role that kinship and migration play in opportunities for treatment. But relationships are affective too. Just as treatment is produced within culturally particular forms of care, these forms of care are also shaped by culturally particular forms of love. Following on those who have tried to find a place for an anthropology of love within social scientific discourse (Ahearn, 2001; Cole & Thomas, 2009; Hirsch & Wardlow, 2006; Orsini, 2006; Trawick, 1992), I want to identify some of the ways women use cultural relations of love to make sense of illness and to struggle through treatment.

WHAT'S LOVE GOT TO DO WITH IT?

Sachi takes a two-month leave from her job in Dubai to accompany her mother Pratima to her treatment appointments at Neelam. Aditi and Fathima decide that a biopsy is not worth pursuing if it will only result in news that depletes their families' savings accounts. Aditi and Fathima's children, shaken by the realization of their mothers' illnesses, insist on taking them to Neelam. What are the culturally structuring effects of love on care? These narratives reveal love to be something more than an emotional impulse or show of solidarity. I propose that what this love looks like is a complex scenario of mutual persuasion and regard, embedded in norms of kinship, migration and capital that enable it to have social uses and effects in things like cancer treatment. It this sense, love is *like care*, but with a key distinction. Love is the place where individual and cultural aspects of relationships *meet* (or divide) and make care un/tenable.

Marshall Sahlins (2013) asserts that kinship is not structured as a shared substance (e.g., blood, ancestors, food, land) but rather a *mutuality of being*. "Kinfolk are persons who participate intrinsically in each other's existence; they are members of one another" (2013, p. ix). In a vivid demonstration of this, Aditi described how her husband persuaded her to see a doctor.

> I was sitting outside on a chair [when] my husband came and sat next to me. He doesn't usually do this. He asked me to not get angry . . . but to listen to what he was saying. Even while I was listening to him, I felt angry. . . . I didn't want to trouble my husband or children anymore. My husband is also old, he is about 80. He loves me a lot and has undergone a lot of hardship because of me. We don't fight. We don't have any problems at home. I felt bad that someone who loves me so much has to go through a lot of hardship just because of me.

Relations of love, like care, are not segmented from treatment but are intimately linked to its very possibility (including, for example, whether a person decides to go to Neelam, how she gets there and whether she returns for treatment).[8] People who care for one another, as in Aditi's narrative and others I discussed earlier, do so less because they share a "substance" (like land or blood) and rather because they are part of the same cultural entity. As Dr. Vaniathan explained in an interview: "the family goes through treatment, too."

The mutuality of being evident in Aditi and her husband's interaction was echoed in clinicians' descriptions of their encounters with patients. Dr. Sundar explained the process by which he explains a diagnosis. First, he avoids using the English word "cancer." Instead he uses Malayalam words for lump, mass or disease. In conversations about prognosis, he assesses what information he will give to a patient and her family based on what he thinks they are prepared to handle. This presents an interesting contrast with the logic of choice that Mol (2008) describes, where a patient is expected to assimilate as much information as possible and then select her preferred option.

In another interview, I asked Dr. Vaniathan for whom consent forms regarding participation in clinical research are designed. He responded: "I don't think it's for the patient. It's more for the family. Decisions are made by the family as a group. Or at least one or two members of the family. Then the patient signs. But this is only after the family gives the green signal." For Vaniathan, a consent form was an artifact and not a starting point in a conversation about treatment. In this sense, the socially recognized goal was not individual choice but a mutually considered decision.

SECRECY, SHARING AND THE MUTUALITY OF BEING

Aditi's memory of the day when she noticed her lump is hazy, but she remembers that she was taking a bath. Six months passed. Then, one day her youngest sister came to visit, and Aditi asked her to promise to not tell anyone and showed her the lump. "She was shocked and extremely upset. . . . She said that she would be doing a great crime if she didn't tell [my daughters]." Both daughters came to the house the next day, but Aditi was angry and told them to "look after their own affairs." Aditi gazed down at her hands. "But they were insistent and said they wouldn't leave until I told them what was wrong." She paused and drew a slow breath. "We had already spent so much money on my treatment [hospitalizations for two surgeries and a heart attack]. This money was supposed to be for my children."

The desire to put aside money for one's children (for educations and marriages) came up frequently in interviews, as women described their feelings of anxiety and conflict about the cost of treatment. It was a major point of contention for the clinicians. As Vaniathan explained: "People will take out a loan or sell their gold jewelry or property to come up with the payments for treatment. Only families who can establish that they are very poor [with no cash on hand and no assets to sell] are eligible for a waiver." He expressed frustration that some of his patients would forego treatment to save money for their children's weddings:

> Some people want to wait until their daughters are married before beginning treatment. My feeling is that if they [patients] could just create a

modest health savings account, the same way that they save and save for their wedding savings account, they would not have to worry so much about money for treatment. But people are much more interested in putting aside money for happy things.

But, weddings are not just happy things. They are socially recognized goals. They involve expectations of ritual transformation and material success. Aditi's narrative opens up several things, importantly, about the cultural uses of concealment (Gordon & Paci, 1997) as a form of love. On the one hand, her efforts to "not trouble" her family and to save money for her children's weddings and educations are group-sanctioned ambitions, not individual attempts to deny norms. On the second hand, her use of shielding as a relational logic of care (what parents do for their children) exceeds the reach of psychosocial measures such as *denial* or *avoidance* (see for example Aggarwal & Rowe, 2013). These are imprecise descriptions of women's behavior and norms, in the much the same way that Mathews, Lannin and Mitchell (1994, p. 799) demonstrate *fatalism* to be an incomplete and unfortunate explanation of African American women's relationships with breast cancer treatment seeking in North Carolina.

CONCLUSION

Anthropologies that come to chronic disease from the perspective of individual, social and cultural aspects do more than help us to think about how people make meaning or struggle through complex life events like cancer. They are also an important way to question public health discourse and its approaches and outcomes (Manderson & Smith-Morris, 2010). Part of my analysis in this chapter has been to look at the powerful and culturally structuring effects of kinship, migration, capital and love in women's approaches to cancer treatment. In doing so I have addressed the question 'how are kin networks and households significant to people's perceptions or uses of clinical care?'

Kin relations flow within and between households in Kerala and the Gulf. Regardless of geographic distance, they are integral to treatment because they provide a possible basis of mutuality of being (Sahlins, 2013) through which the interests of a person/s can be tenable for another as Aditi's husband demonstrated, in his gentle, yet persuasive, conversation with Aditi outside their house. Love is affective and it makes care effective. But as Trawick shows (1992), love is also more than just emotion. As with space and time and kinship, love flows through the structuring practices and norms of culture.

This is particularly evident in the conversations that Sabah recounts having with her mother. These nightly phone calls may seem, at first glance, to be the kinds of exchanges and solidarities a daughter and mother might have. But the *kinds* of questions they ask (e.g., what did Sabah do wrong, what can she do to make things better?) and the mutual consensus they reach at the end ("bad things happen to good people") suggest that these conversations do certain things for Sabah beyond the social and personal aspects of relationships; they link her to a shared history, and to norms and meanings about life, illness, morality and parenting. In other words, Sabah and her mother do more than express affect. They search together for a way to understand something that (because they have mutuality of being) has afflicted them both.

Whatever the status of this as a generalization, it captures something important about how disease and treatment are understood in South India. Devaki, Aditi and Fathima's attempts at concealment stem from a complex set of desires to save money for their children, to shield their families from suffering and to pursue socially recognized goals for success. These are intricate negotiations and not the automatic result of structural inequality. Therefore when we talk about "health system factors" (e.g., structures of funding, access, treatment) we should really be taking another step back before the moment that a women walks across the threshold of a clinic to consider the social, cultural and political "system factors" through which she lives in the world.

Although person-focused ethnography may not (or fully) answer broader system questions, issues of how access happens in one way for one person and in a different set of arrangements or struggles for another person are important, as those particulars help to show how people are distinctively and culturally situated in the political and economic life of healthcare. Significant to this is the argument that although relational care is often familial, the way familial relationships work out in practice is governed not only by the logics of the kinship "system" but by the intersection of these with other logics of space, migration and individual history (e.g., Farooq's treatment advice, Sachi's work leave to accompany her mother to treatment).

How does a "system barrier" appear in the context of logics of migration or mutuality? How do expectations about propriety, shielding or success alter the shape of a barrier? Aditi was determined to never leave her house, vowing that her prior hospitalizations had caused her family "too much stress." Months later, after her family had convinced her to go to Neelam, Aditi's mind changed. She was "determined," she said, to "keep going with treatment." In this, her older decision that she was a "burden" receded, and another intention came into play. Her decision to pursue treatment, scraping together enough cash to cover treatment, did not mask or remove her from the structural reality of high treatment costs or a low farming salary; but things shifted with her family's position on the matter.

Narratives like Aditi's provide an important window into how kin relations, as disparate as they may seem, powerfully impact on systems of treatment. As women use cultural structures of bodily meaning, delay, persuasion, migration and home in everyday practices of symptom assessment and care seeking, they also detail how these structures come together to inform, buffer, undo or eventuate treatment. Hearing these narratives (letting these women speak) is something ethnography can contribute to local and international analyses of cancer.

Research and programs aimed at building new capacity and addressing the rising incidence of breast cancer in India will go some way towards improving mechanisms for earlier detection and more comprehensive treatment, particularly if existing clinical resources and skill can be better distributed into free or low-cost care (Goss et al., 2014; Pal & Mittal, 2004). Anthropologies of cancer are crucial in this regard for the attention they give to ordinary things, like family, labor and home, and the uses of these in cancer care. Perhaps more than anything, we need anthropologies of cancer that draw closer to Edith Turner's recommendation:

> The purpose of anthropology is to supply humankind with information about itself. However, *humanistic* anthropology draws nearer to the living human being. It seeks to give humankind an understanding of the heart of the human being in relation to his or her fellows.
>
> (Turner, 2007, p. 108)

What women's narratives reveal about the heart of health behavior is that logics of kinship, love and migration are neither natural to, predictive of, nor divisible from treatment, but are cultural ways of being that powerfully inform how health and illness are defined and lived out.

NOTES

1. All personal names in this chapter have been changed to ensure participant confidentiality. Neelam Medical Center is also a pseudonym.
2. This work would not have been possible without the insight and candor of patients, family members, and clinicians at Neelam Medical Center. I also wish to thank the oncology department at Neelam, especially Dr. Vaniathan and the social work team for their assistance with interview coordination and translation. Research interns Juliana Eng, Shimoli Vyas, Sonia Dutta, Marra Katz, Kylie Birnbaum, Ilina Datkhaeva and Arthur Winer contributed vitally to medical chart review, database compilation and interview gathering. This work was supported by a grant from the Breast Cancer Research Foundation. I am deeply grateful to Holly Mathews, Nancy Burke and Daniel Rosenblatt for their keen insight and comments on earlier drafts of this chapter.
3. According to the Government of India Human Development Report (2011), Kerala ranks highest among India's 29 states on the Human Development Index (score 0.790), with the highest literacy rate (95.5%), the highest sex ratio (1,084 women per 1,000 men) and the highest life expectancy (almost 77 years).
4. In a separate retrospective study we did at Neelam on breast cases seen between 2004–2007, breast cancer patients (N = 300) overall experienced an average 6-month delay between symptom discovery and presentation at Neelam. However, LABC patients experienced an average 9-month delay as

compared with non-LABC patients whose delay was 4 months. Univariate regression analysis showed that this duration time difference was significantly (p = .026) associated with late stage presentation. A multivariate regression analysis controlling for demographic variables showed that duration time was still significantly (p = .028) the independent variable driving advanced stage at presentation.

5. The consent process consisted of an oral consent that we read aloud in Malayalam including a thumbnail description of the study aims and research protections including confidentiality. All study materials were translated into Malayalam and pre-approved by ethics committees at Neelam and NYU.

6. Zachariah and Rajan define emigrants as "persons who are usual members of a household in Kerala, but living outside [India], not the same as persons of Kerala origin or the Diaspora" (2012, p. 18). According to the latest census, Kerala has a population of 33.4 million (Census of India, 2011) and 2.28 million Keralites live abroad, compared with 1.36 million in 1998 (Zachariah & Rajan, 2012, p. 4). The majority of migrants (85%) are age 25–40 years, with an average age of 33.6 years. Muslim Keralites migrate to the Gulf more often than Hindus or Christians, comprising 44.3% of Gulf migrants but only 26% of Kerala's population, while Hindus make up 36.4% of migrants and 56% percent of Kerala's population (Zachariah & Rajan, 2012, p. 27).

7. Over the 2000s, the wage gap between laborers in Kerala and the Gulf narrowed (wages for construction workers were significantly higher in the Gulf 10 years ago but are more or less the same in Kerala and the Gulf today). Other factors including the cost of air travel are thought to be leading to a migration slowdown among working class laborers, although the high value of oil continues to draw people to the Gulf. The number of migrants who returned to live in Kerala in 2011 was significantly less (511,000) than in 1998, when nearly twice as many migrants (959,000) returned to Kerala (Zachariah & Rajan, 2012, p. 46); this may be the result of larger numbers of professional workers settling abroad.

8. As we found in a separate study in 2010 on breast cancer treatment seeking and completion, accompaniment has an important impact on whether women opt to pursue treatment after diagnosis and whether they discontinue treatment once they have started. When we reviewed 416 cases recommended for treatment at Neelam, we found that 43.8% of patients did not complete treatment and 41% were lost to follow up within six months. When we spoke with some of these women (N = 60) via phone interview to explore why they had not returned, financial difficulties and lack of family support (i.e., accompaniment to Neelam for appointments) ranked as the two most common reasons, along with the desire to complete treatment at another medical facility in Kerala.

REFERENCES

Ahearn, L.M. (2001). *Invitations to love: Literacy, love letters, and social change in Nepal.* University of Michigan Press.

Aggarwal, N., & Rowe, M. (Eds.). (2013). Denial in patient-physician communication among patients with cancer. *New Challenges in Communication with Cancer Patients* (pp. 15–25). New York, NY: Springer.

Akhtar, M., Akulwar, V., Gandhi, D., & Chandak, K. (2011). Is locally advanced breast cancer a neglected disease? *Indian Journal of Cancer, 48,* 403.

Ali, R., Mathew, A., & Rajan, B. (2008). Effects of socio-economic and demographic factors in delayed reporting and late-stage presentation among patients with breast cancer in a major cancer hospital in South India. *Asian Pacific Journal Cancer Prevention, 9,* 703–707.

Allemani, C., Sant, M., Weir, H.K., Richardson, L.C., Baili, P., Storm, H., . . . & Coleman, M.P. (2013). Breast cancer survival in the US and Europe: A CONCORD high-resolution study. *International Journal of Cancer, 132,* 1170–1181.

Anderson, B.O., Cazap, E., El Saghir, N.S., Yip, C.H., Khaled, H.M., Otero, I.V., . . . Harford, J.B. (2011). Optimization of breast cancer management in low-resource and middle-resource countries: Executive summary of the Breast Health Global Initiative consensus, 2010. *The Lancet Oncology, 12,* 387–398.

Bharadwaj, A. (2006). Sacred conceptions: Clinical theodicies, uncertain science, and technologies of procreation in India. *Culture, Medicine and Psychiatry, 30,* 451–465.

Bright, K. (1998). The traveling tonic: Tradition, commodity, and the body in Unani medicine in India. Doctoral dissertation, University of California, Santa Cruz.

Bright, K., Barghash, M., Donach, M., Gutiérrez de la Barrera, M., Schneider, R., & Formenti, S. (2011). The role of health system factors in delaying final diagnosis and treatment of breast cancer in Mexico City, Mexico. *The Breast Journal, 20,* S54-S59.

Census of India. (2011). Government of India. Retrieved from http://www.census india.gov.in/

Cole, J., & Thomas, L.T., (Eds.). (2009). *Love in Africa.* Chicago, IL: The Chicago University Press.

Cohen, L. (1998). *No aging in India: Alzheimer's, the bad family, and other modern things.* Berkley, CA: University of California Press.

Das, V. (1996). Language and body: Transactions in the construction of pain. *Daedalus, 125,* 67–91.

Dumont, L. (1980). *Homo hierarchicus: The caste system and its implications.* University of Chicago Press.

Ecks, S. (2005). Pharmaceutical citizenship: Antidepressant marketing and the promise of demarginalization in India. *Anthropology & Medicine, 12,* 239–254.

El Saghir, N.S., Adebamowo, C.A., Anderson, B.O., Carlson, R.W., Bird, P.A., Corbex, M., . . . & Cazap, E. (2011). Breast cancer management in low resource countries (LRCs): Consensus statement from the Breast Health Global Initiative. *The Breast, 20,* S3-S11.

Gamburd, M.R. (2000). *The kitchen spoon's handle: Transnationalism and Sri Lanka's migrant housemaids.* Ithaca, NY: Cornell University Press.

Gordon, D.R., & Paci, E. (1997). Disclosure practices and cultural narratives: Understanding concealment and silence around cancer in Tuscany, Italy. *Social Science & Medicine, 44,* 1433–1452.

Goss, P.E., Strasser-Weippl, K., Lee-Bychkovsky, B.L., Fan, L., Li, J., Chavarri-Guerra, Y., . . . & Chan, A. (2014). Challenges to effective cancer control in China, India, and Russia. *The Lancet Oncology, 15,* 489–538.

Hirsch, J. S., & Wardlow, H., (Eds.). (2006). *Modern loves: The anthropology of romantic courtship and companionate marriage.* The University of Michigan Press.

Jain, S., & Jadhav, S. (2009). Pills that swallow policy: Clinical ethnography of a community mental health program in Northern India. *Transcultural Psychiatry, 46,* 60–85.

Khilnani, S. (1999). *The idea of India.* New York, NY: Farrar, Straus and Giroux.

Kleinman, A. (1988). *The illness narratives: Suffering, healing, and the human condition.* New York, NY: Basic Books.

Leong, S.P., Shen, Z.Z., Liu, T.J., Agarwal, G., Tajima, T., Paik, N.S., . . . & Foulkes, W.D. (2010). Is breast cancer the same disease in Asian and Western countries? *World Journal of Surgery, 34,* 2308–2324.

Livingston, J. (2012). *Improvising medicine: An African oncology ward in an emerging cancer epidemic*. Durham, NC: Duke University Press.

Lutz, C. A., & Abu-Lughod, L. E., (Eds.). (1990). *Language and the politics of emotion (studies in emotion and social interaction)*. Cambridge: Cambridge University Press.

Manderson, L., & Smith-Morris, C. (Eds.). (2010). *Chronic conditions, fluid states: Chronicity and the anthropology of illness*. Piscataway, NJ: Rutgers University Press.

Marquez, G. G. (1988). *Love in the time of cholera*. New York, NY: Alfred A. Knopf.

Mathews, H. F., Lannin, D. R., & Mitchell, J. P. (1994). Coming to terms with advanced breast cancer: Black women's narratives from Eastern North Carolina. *Social Science & Medicine, 38*, 789–800.

McMullin, J. M., & Weiner, D. E. (Eds.). (2009). *Confronting cancer: Metaphors, advocacy, and anthropology*. Santa Fe, NM: School for Advanced Research Press.

Mol, A. (2008). *The logic of care: Health and the problem of patient choice*. New York, NY: Routledge.

National Cancer Institute. (2014). "Continuum of care." Dictionary of cancer terms. Retrieved from http://www.cancer.gov/dictionary?cdrid=561395

Orsini, F., (Ed.). (2006). *Love in South Asia: A cultural history*. New York, NY: Cambridge University Press.

Osella, F., & Osella, C. (2000). Migration, money and masculinity in Kerala. *Journal of the Royal Anthropological Institute, 6*, 117–133.

Pal, S., & Mittal, B. (2004). Improving cancer care in India: Prospects and challenges. *Asian Pacific Journal of Cancer Prevention, 5*, 226–228.

Pinto, S. (2011). Rational love, relational medicine: Psychiatry and the accumulation of precarious kinship. *Culture, Medicine, and Psychiatry, 35*, 376–395.

Ram, K. (2001). Modernity and the midwife: Contestations over a subaltern figure, South India. In L. H. Connor & G. Samuel (Eds.), *Healing powers and modernity: Traditional medicine, shamanism, and science in Asian societies* (pp. 64–85). Westport, CT: Bergin & Garvey.

Ramberg, L. (2013). Troubling kinship: Sacred marriage and gender configuration in South India. *American Ethnologist, 40*, 661–675.

Roland, A. (1991). *In search of self in India and Japan: Toward a cross-cultural psychology*. Princeton, NJ: Princeton University Press.

Sahlins, M. (2013). *What kinship is—and is not*. Chicago, IL: University of Chicago Press.

Simos, D., Clemons, M., Ginsburg, O. M., & Jacobs, C. (2014). Definition and consequences of locally advanced breast cancer. *Current Opinion in Supportive and Palliative Care, 8*, 33–38.

Solomon, H. (2011). Affective journeys: The emotional structuring of medical tourism in India. *Anthropology and Medicine, 18*, 105–118.

Trawick, M. (1992) *Notes on love in a Tamil family*. Berkley, CA: University of California Press.

Turner, E. (2007). Introduction to the art of ethnography. *Anthropology and Humanism, 32*, 108–116.

Van Hollen, C. C. (2003). *Birth on the threshold: Childbirth and modernity in south India*. Berkley, CA: University of California Press.

Viswanath, C. (2013, October 13). Kerala migration survey to begin soon. *The New Indian Express*. Retrieved from http://www.newindianexpress.com

World Health Organization. (2002). National cancer control programs, policies and managerial guidelines. Retrieved from http://www.who.int/cancer/media/en/409.pdf

Yeole, B. B., & Kurkure, A. P. (2003). An epidemiological assessment of increasing incidence and trends in breast cancer in Mumbai and other sites in India, during the last two decades. *Asian Pacific Journal of Cancer Prevention, 4,* 51–56.

Zachariah, K. C., & Rajan, S. I. (2012). Inflexion in Kerala's Gulf connection: Report on Kerala migration survey 2011. Centre for Development Working Papers, no. 450. Trivandrum, Kerala: Centre for Development. Retrieved from http://www.cds.edu

8 Cancer Crisis and Treatment Ambiguity in Kenya

Benson A. Mulemi

In her recent ethnography of a cancer ward in Botswana, Julie Livingston (2012) writes that cancer in Africa is an epidemic that will profoundly shape the future of global health. Low- and middle-income nations now bear the majority of the worldwide cancer burden; yet, even though two-thirds of the world's cancer patients live in developing countries, less than 10% of cancer care resources are available to them (Murray, Grant, Grant & Kendall, 2003, p. 4). This chapter presents a case study of the cancer ward of the Kenyatta National Hospital (KNH), the largest public referral hospital in Nairobi, Kenya, to illustrate the negotiations and challenges that emerge as people attempt to deal with cancer in a low-resource setting where profound inequities exist in access to care. For many of those diagnosed with the disease, cancer becomes a collective burden shared within families.

Patients and their caregivers struggle to navigate a complex referral system to attain a diagnosis, secure treatment, find relief for pain and assign meaning to their experiences. In the cancer ward, ambiguities of cancer treatment shape the experience of suffering at three levels: 1) the disease itself generates uncertainty because of its unknowable aspects and ambiguity is directly related to medical uncertainty about how best to treat cancer; 2) this lack of knowledge combined with the painful side effects of treatment when it is available confound patients' attempts to understand the meaning of the cancer experience and their own suffering; and 3) the prevalence of late-stage diagnoses combined with a lack of cancer specialists and hospital treatment resources means that most patients are not guaranteed the restoration of health or even a better quality of life. As a result, patients and families must cope with catastrophic disruptions to their social and economic lives while struggling with the emotional consequences of the disease. Ironically, cancer care in the Kenyan public hospital both alleviates and increases suffering.

CANCER CARE AND NATIONAL HEALTH SYSTEMS IN AFRICA

While much of Africa must confront a growing cancer burden with limited resources, there are significant variations in treatment options and patient experiences depending upon the ways that national values and political influences structure overarching health care systems. Livingston (2012) reports that Botswana, in southern Africa, has enjoyed a stable democracy and an established system of functioning social welfare programs for many years. Health care, including oncology, is provided as a public good for citizens under a program of universal care (p.17). However, patients are not able to access the oncology clinic directly, but must be referred by a physician at a primary or provincial hospital where staff lack training in cancer detection and diagnosis. As a result, patients arrive at the oncology ward after a long process of seeking care and usually with advanced stage disease (p. 75). Yet, because Botswana has a collective ethos and a commitment to the equitable distribution of services, bed space is only open to patients who can be treated (p.102). Those who are too far along at diagnosis and those for whom treatment is no longer working are sent home to suffer and die, usually without palliative relief from pain (p.158). Paradoxically, care in Botswana is a universal right, but delays in diagnosis along with broken equipment, uneven staffing and uncertain supplies mean that many patients receive little of the assistance to which they are entitled.

Alternatively, access to health care is becoming privatized in other parts of Africa, and many nations have hybrid systems with differing mixes of public, private and internationally supported treatment options. This chapter examines cancer care in Kenya, a large nation in east Africa, with a health system that differs dramatically from the one found in Botswana. While cancer patients in both places experience some common issues stemming from scarce resources and poverty, many of their forms of suffering are contextually shaped by national health care structures and local cultures. A country of approximately 37 million people, Kenya has struggled to build a health system that could effectively deliver services to its population (Turin, 2010). Health facilities are distributed regionally in a hierarchical structure. At the top of the system are the national, referral and teaching hospitals, including the one presented in this case study. The next level of care is in provincial hospitals, followed by subdistrict hospitals. Finally, at the local level are health centers and dispensaries staffed by public service nurses and additional personnel from some community health organizations.

Turin (2010) notes that there are stark disparities in care both vertically, between the different levels of care, and horizontally, from facility to facility by region. At the health center level and below, a minimal level of care is available and serious conditions are referred to the nearest hospitals. Hospitals also offer a mix of public and private services. For example, the Kenyatta National Hospital (KNH) has both public and private wards (referred to as the *private wing*, or *amenity wards*), attended by the same physicians. A patient in the public ward can be expected to experience long waiting times and even to share a bed with another patient. These patients are grouped into large, open rooms with little privacy, but the cost is minimal compared to private wards, where physicians are paid more for attending to the patients.

Employed workers with a certain income level contribute to a national health insurance fund to cover care; others pay as they go for health services.

The Kenyan health care system is also strongly impacted by the work of nongovernmental organizations (NGOs), including faith-based organizations, which may offer free care for small segments of the population. In addition, there is a private, for-profit sector operating 34% of the country's facilities (Turin, 2010). As a result, the two major barriers to finding care in the Kenyan system are cost and the availability of suitable facilities within a reasonable distance for patients.

In this context, the growing cancer burden in Kenya presents a system already overwhelmed with profound challenges with the prevalence of communicable diseases such as HIV/AIDS, tuberculosis and malaria. Cancer is presently the third leading cause of death in the nation after infectious and cardiovascular diseases; however, the statistics are likely underestimated due to a lack of functional population-based cancer registries in the country. Hospital based registries indicate that the incidence of new cancer cases per year is about 28,000 and that annual mortality due to the disease is over 22,000 per year (Republic of Kenya, 2011). Most of those affected (over 60%) are below the age of 70, in the prime of life, and they face a high risk of dying from cancer before age 75.

The five most common types of cancer among men in Kenya, in order of incidence, are esophagus, prostate, non-Hodgkin's lymphoma, liver and stomach cancers (Mutuma & Ruggut-Korir, 2006). High rates of HIV/AIDS have increased the prevalence of Kaposi's sarcoma, which is more common in men than in women. Breast and cervical cancers with incidence rates of 19% and 10% top the list for women followed by esophagus, stomach, ovarian and non-Hodgkin cancers. A review of patient records at KNH indicated that new cancer cases in Kenya had doubled over a short period of time. This rapid rise in cancer cases likely results from changing lifestyles and increasing life expectancy (Parkin et al., 2008). Exposure to risk factors such as the use of tobacco, alcohol and environmental pollutants along with high rates of poverty accelerate the prevalence of specific cancers. In addition, a threatening synergy is emerging between HIV and viral cancers such as non-Hodgkin's lymphoma and cervical cancer. Patients on antiretroviral drugs in Kenya, as in other parts of Africa, add to the complexity of vulnerability to cancer due to immune system suppression (see Livingston, 2012).

Until passage of the Cancer Prevention Control Bill by Parliament in 2012, the government of Kenya had never formulated a program to address the increasing crisis. Yet despite national attention to cancer, funding for the disease lags in the health budget, which still emphasizes the politically visible conditions of tuberculosis, malaria and HIV/AIDS. As a result, a large proportion of the cancer cases seen in lower-level and referral hospitals are diagnosed at advanced stages when treatment cannot significantly alter the prognosis. The lack of screening services and diagnostic facilities and poorly structured referral networks contribute to this problem (Republic of Kenya, 2011). Kenya has few cancer specialists and they are concentrated in the capital city of Nairobi. Public hospitals lack adequate treatment technologies, medical supplies and essential drugs for pain management. Whereas wealthy Kenyans can travel abroad to access cancer therapies, the majority of the population, especially those in rural areas, lack access to basic health services.

ETHNOGRAPHY OF CANCER TREATMENT IN KENYA

I collected ethnographic data for 12 months between August 2005 and July 2006 in the cancer ward and treatment center clinic at Kenyatta National Hospital (KNH) in Nairobi (Mulemi, 2010a), which is the only public national hospital that offers better-quality cancer treatment technology and expertise in Kenya. The adult cancer ward had five rooms with a bed capacity of 32. It admitted patients with head and neck, breast, cervical, colon, colorectal, prostate, esophageal, and gastric cancers. Chemotherapy, radiotherapy and supportive management are administered to those in the unit as well as to out-patients at the cancer treatment center. Supportive management includes intravenous feeding, wound treatment and palliative care. The Hematology, Obstetrics and Gynecology units elsewhere in the hospital manage the other types of cancer. The average hospital stay is between 7 and 15 days, but some patients stay for over a month.

I observed interactions in the cancer ward and treatment center and engaged patients in informal conversations. I also recruited a purposive sample of 42 patients (27 male, and 15 female), 11 relatives, 3 doctors and 11 nurses for focused, in-depth interviews as well as informal conversations on multiple occasions. I took the position of a nonparticipant, listening to narratives about cancer treatment and help-seeking efforts among patients and their relatives. This approach was based on the awareness that attempts by ethnographers to conduct participant observation in medical settings often lead to role ambiguities and ethical dilemmas (Goodwin, Pope, & Smith, 2003; Mulemi, 2010b). Therefore, my participation was limited to activities and conversations in which ethnographers without biomedical training could engage. I also made follow-up home visits with 10 purposively selected patients to explore how they and their families coped with the disease and recovery process. Seven of these lived in rural areas up to four hours from the study hospital. Three of them had temporarily moved to live with relatives in Nairobi city. I conducted thematic analyses of interview and observations transcripts to describe the trajectory of help seeking in which experiences of cancer treatment were situated. All the respondents mentioned receiving multiple referrals for their symptoms and delayed diagnoses and medical treatments.

MULTIPLE REFERRALS AND TREATMENT DELAYS

Mr. Jabari,[1] 49 years old and a father of four, was admitted to the cancer ward in February 2006 to treat cancer of the colon; he told me:

> The problem began in 2002 . . . they did not discover the disease. I had problems with the stomach and eating . . . Doctors kept giving me more

drugs for malaria, typhoid, and amoebas . . . In 2003, I was admitted in five different hospitals, but they could not diagnose the disease. They just gave drugs . . . painkillers . . . I returned to Mater Hospital in Nairobi and they discovered that I had a problem with the colon. They did an operation . . . but they "did not see the cancer" . . . A piece of flesh from the colon at the point it had blocked was removed for examination . . . I was allowed to return home and I remained there for two years. . . . At the end of 2005 I started feeling the problem again . . . a CT scan showed a mass . . . I had to be operated again in Nakuru to remove the mass; it was taken to Aga Khan Hospital in Nairobi for diagnosis . . . They found that there were some cancer cells and they advised us to come and follow up the matter here.

(February 10, 2006)

All the patients who participated in the ethnography reported variations on this theme of long referral paths and the severe impacts from the socioeconomic burdens of earlier unsuccessful treatments. Rural health facilities or even district hospitals in Kenya do not have cancer diagnostic technologies and adequate cancer expertise. Moreover, only a very small fraction of poor cancer patients are able to obtain a referral to the National Hospital for specialized treatment, and not all those who are referred make it there.

Studies of cancer management in Kenya emphasize the negative effect of late presentation for medical treatment and poverty on treatment and recovery (Onyango & Macharia, 2006). A few studies (e.g., Murray, Grant, Grant & Kendall, 2003; Onyango, Omondi, Njiru & Awange, 2004) highlight the intensity of suffering as families struggle to care for cancer patients, particularly the terminal cases, in homes, and the inadequacy of regional hospitals in helping them do so. Shortages of pathologists and oncologists and an inadequate supply of cancer medicines, effective analgesics and technology in regional health facilities and referral hospitals worsen adverse experiences of patients and their families. The long help-seeking paths contribute to the prevalence of incorrect diagnoses, undertreatment and delays in accessing appropriate treatment.

FUTILITY OF DIAGNOSTIC REFERRALS

On January 18, 2006, Mr. Khasi, a 64-year-old patient from western Kenya, told me:

After tests here [at KNH], I was just told it is tumor; they had written "cancer," in brackets . . . It was in the left leg and now it has come on the right leg . . . Before it was discovered that I have this disease, I tried many places . . . It was in 1999 that [I] started suffering . . . feeling heaviness at the back . . . When I walked and slept the leg seemed heavy . . . So I went to see my doctor, in a local hospital near home. They would tell me "oh, [it is] malaria" . . . then they referred me to the District Hospital, where they told me "oh, [it is] typhoid" . . . this and that . . . Then it was swollen here on the collar bone; the swelling became distinct in 2004. Now they told me . . ."go and check with the bone specialist" . . . [The specialist] . . . Dr. Mulimo used to work here at KNH. I went to him and he sent me for X-ray examination in the government laboratory. . . . I asked him to check the X-ray results that I already had and he said there was an ailment there on the bone . . . He referred me to the Moi University [teaching and] referral [hospital] in Eldoret. . . . The doctor who was attending to me at this hospital exclaimed "no! This Dr. Mulimo is a qualified doctor! I cannot dispute what he has written in his diagnosis . . . there is nothing to add." So . . . he did not help me. He said, "So let him (Dr. Mulimo) do the way he has decided, because he taught me in Nairobi University!"

As Mr. Khasi's experience narrated here illustrates, subsequent referrals for cancer patients in Kenya do not necessarily add value to previous diagnoses. Such referrals may instead add to patients' suffering as they delay treatment and entail further social, financial and psychological burdens. With regard to this, Mr. Khasi added:

I wanted him [the doctor] even to see what the referral required, or even to go and examine me on another machine that would be a little more refined than the one used in the district hospital . . . he instead referred me to another doctor, back in Bungoma District Hospital . . . the doctor in the district hospital said . . . "I can see from this X-ray film that there is a defect on the bone." He said "I agree with the recommendation of the other doctor that you just need to go for surgical operation and we will see the disease" . . . When he cut open the place he did not see the disease! Even a little . . . He took a small piece of flesh from the spot back to Moi referral [hospital] for further medical investigation. . . . He took it to doctor Akrohauf . . . a Russian, because he was the one who "was good at looking" [analyzing samples]. . . . The results came after two weeks and he told the other doctor . . . "The flesh [biopsy sample] you removed has [revealed] *nothing at all* [emphasis] like disease in it. Then he said; "ah, now this is becoming hard. Now what you will do?" [I responded] "I can't get tired" . . . He said "I will write for you (another referral note) because we don't have CT scan machine here. You go for some CT scan examination . . . back at Moi referral hospital . . ."

Other participants similarly recounted multiple referrals that were fraught with misdiagnoses, inappropriate treatments and drastic interventions, such as surgical operations, mastectomies and amputations. Some patients interviewed felt that cancer treatment initiatives were erroneous and inflicted undue anguish. Indeed, some therapeutic and hospital release decisions turned out to be the result of medical errors and hospital staff subtly expressed such recognition. Mr. Khasi noted this when he said:

> That machine in Bungoma [District Hospital] is very bad! Even the doctor had told me: "I wronged you so much; I operated on you, yet you did not have a disease there." He said there is flesh which has grown from the back and it seems to have come to obstruct the heart here. In fact when I touched here, the heart was not beating, the growth had gone over it. So the doctor told me "return to Eldoret [referral hospital] very quickly; this is not something that can be operated here. I will send you to the doctor who deals with the heart . . . Professor Ashuluda . . . When he operates you he will tell you whether this flesh (growth) affected the heart or not . . ."

TREATMENT FUTILITY AT THE NATIONAL HOSPITAL

Although arrival at the national referral hospital in Nairobi may instill hope, most patients come with advanced stage disease, requiring intensive, arduous and expensive therapies. Similarly, immediate treatment is not guaranteed on arrival as it is the only facility accessible to the public, hence its capacity is overstretched. The cancer clinic is often full, with long queues of desperate and uncertain patients seeking admission, treatment or routine outpatient reviews. People travel from across the country, some as far as 600 kilometers for treatment, but only a few are able to gain admission or even outpatient treatment. Once denied the chance to start treatment, most are unable to return for future appointments. Doctors may cope by sending some patients back home "to rest" or to visit health facilities in their local areas for indefinite *supportive care*. Hospital personnel explained in the following conversation taken from my fieldnotes how they often assisted patients to leave the hospital when they could not be treated successfully or afford care:

CONSULTANT:	". . . we used to help patients in ward 39 and 40 abscond hospitalization . . . If we found that they could not pay, we would help them abscond treatment . . . If the patient could not pay and we were 'not doing anything for him', we would discharge him or her. We would even give them (bus transport) fare and escort them to the bus stop! We would tell them to go home and rest. . . . You can help such patients to abscond . . ."
WARD PORTER:	"Then people would remain writing statements [to explain why the patient left before completing treatment]."
PHYSIOTHERAPIST:	"If you do that today, you will be indicted . . ."
RADIOGRAPHER:	"That is very bad . . . It is very dangerous . . ."

CONSULTANT: "That would save the hospital a lot of money . . . There is no need to keep the patient . . . We are doing nothing for him, yet he is eating . . . you end up discharging him anyway, but who pays the bills? You can help the hospital to save a lot if you help such patients abscond" *(Field notes, June 2006).*

Multilayered cancer treatment delays affect the process of recovery and the patient's quality of life. Barnes-Josiah, Myntti and Augustin (1998) proposed a three-tiered framework for understanding maternal mortality in Haiti, which is also useful in characterizing cancer treatment delays in Kenya. These include delays in deciding to seek appropriate medical help, reaching appropriate medical facilities and receiving adequate care at the correct facility. With regard to such delays and their implications for cancer treatment at KNH, some hospital practitioners attribute responsibility for poor prognosis to the patients. Physicians may suggest that patients (and their relatives) are to blame for the advanced stages of cancer illness (Hunt, 1998, p. 306). Such placement of blame may also extend to explaining vulnerability to cancer as the result of interruptions of treatment by patients when they could not afford services. Mr. Khasi, for example, reported ". . . Dr. Ashuluda saw that thing and said, 'ah! This is too much, when this flesh was growing, where were you? . . . It has grown so big . . .' Then he said 'what do you want, do I got to operate on you?'" Ms. Souda similarly complained:

I didn't know what I was suffering from. I bled for three years . . . since 2001; continuously . . . I was in (sanitary) pads all these years . . . day in, day out, until this year (2005), in February, when I collapsed in town! A friend took me to a clinic . . . I was not happy with the doctor . . . he mistreated me. He thought I was aborting, because I was bleeding . . . I think he is just one of these quacks who are making money . . . He didn't know what to do. I was bleeding and almost getting a blackout [fainting] in his clinic. And then he got scared . . . He referred me to St. Mary's [Hospital] . . . When I came to KNH, a doctor dropped a bombshell when he said bluntly, "Souda, your cervix is rotten . . ."
(Ms. Souda, age 39, October 3, 2005)

Hospital staff and patients' relatives and friends at times unwittingly impute suffering to the cancer patient's personal responsibility. Ms. Souda, for instance, added:

My relatives thought I was (HIV) positive and I was trying to conceal it . . . You know, when they hear that you are a single parent, they think you are just "out there" . . . So they were not ready to help me pay my bills . . . I stayed in Nairobi Women's (Hospital) for three days . . . The medication had to be terminated; as per their policy you have to pay a deposit within 24 hours for your treatment to be completed. . . . It was my brother who paid for my first admission here (at KNH) . . . I was so surprised . . . because when I told him . . . he told me "what?" "You are suffering from cancer of the cervix? What brings it? Is it an infection or what?" . . . It was "loaded" . . .

(Ms. Souda, October 3, 2005)

Hospital workers on occasion asked "where patients had been" up to that point, because the disease was so advanced. Such interrogation reflects the popular assumption among health care professionals, researchers and family care givers that patients' ignorance and inappropriate or negative health beliefs underlie the presentation with late stage disease and inconsistent adherence to hospital appointments or schedules and abandonment of treatment exacerbate the vulnerability to cancer (Mostert et al., 2014, p. 705).

INVISIBILITY OF CANCER

Livingston (2012) argues that cancer as defined in the West has been largely invisible in Africa because precancerous and early stage disease does not exist in areas where palpable lesions are the defining symptoms of cancer (p. 52). Therefore, in many ways, cancer is more visible in Africa than in the West because, as study participants claimed, cancer could only be seen later or at KNH when it had "already eaten someone." Cancer is invisible in the Kenyan public consciousness, yet visible in the form of advanced disease, due to inadequacies of the public health care system and its emphasis on the treatment of communicable diseases. Although the Kenyan government seemed to have realized the need to address the increasing cancer burden by 1994, the long-awaited Cancer Prevention and Control Bill it envisaged was only formally introduced for discussion in parliament in October 2011 and passed in June 2012.

Patient experiences of cancer treatment and recovery in Kenya, therefore, must be understood against the backdrop of historical invisibility of the disease. A doctor at KNH's cancer ward, for instance, observed: ". . . we are not given the resources and facilities we are supposed to receive. . . . We are just seen a ka-peripheral (diminutively peripheral) unit compared to other departments like surgical, obstetrics, gynecology and medical department for HIV/AIDS."

ACCESS TO TREATMENT EXPERTISE
AND TECHNOLOGY

The Kenyan cancer treatment context entails complex dynamics of local, national and global circumstances of health care inequalities, including the glaring disparities in the way cancers affect rich and poor people (Knaul et al., 2012, p. 3). Public hospital management in Kenya, for example, is linked to the state, which in turn seeks services of other national and international corporate actors. Most of these actors, such as international pharmaceutical companies, have an interest in the health care sector for financial profit. Although Kenya has the largest number of pharmaceutical firms in sub-Saharan Africa, imports still provide the majority of drugs within the country. Shortages often result, and when they do, patients bear the burden for trying to procure drugs on the open market, but ineffective regulation has resulted in a flood of substandard and counterfeit drugs on the market (United Nations Industrial Development Organization, 2010). Mr. Jabari talks about the issues he faced with medications:

> You have to pay the hospitalization fee, and buy medicines. There are no medicines in the hospital now, so I bought both medicines at about 9,000 Shillings . . . I should forecast ahead to see how many times I will come . . . I was speaking to a patient from the other room out there; he said he came for two courses, or three of [chemotherapy], but did not have the money. . . . Since he didn't have money, he had already stayed for three months without coming to the clinic. . . . As he looked for money, he said the [cancer] sickness spread from the esophagus and to the liver . . . If it is a loan you want to borrow from an agency for treatment, you arrange to get the entire loan together so that you can foot the bill without interrupting treatment. For those of us who come from far we also have to organize bus fares and other expenses . . .
>
> (Mr. Jabari, March 21, 2006)

The Kenyan public health system includes revenue collection policies, which contributes to reduced accessibility to affordable cancer treatment for the poor. Turin (2010) writes that the cost of care remains a paramount issue in Kenya where 44% of ill people surveyed reported the high cost of care as a reason for not seeking treatment. He reports that funding by the national government for the health sector has been inadequate, ranging from 6–8% of total government spending in recent years. As a result, funding for the health sector is financed primarily by the private sector, with 36% of funds originating from household through out-of-pocket spending. These intersecting structural barriers affect patients, contrary to what some health professionals and researchers (e.g., Mostert et al., 2014) report. Mr. Joji, a 34-year-old nasopharyngeal carcinoma patient, for example, noted:

> When you come here . . . and someone tells you that the drugs are not available, you go and buy them in the streets. . . . where do I get the money? There are people who are so poor, they have borrowed some transport fare to come here. How do you help such a person? So [we would be happy] if the ministry [of health] could help us, to increase the money allocated to cancer care, it can help us.
>
> (Mr. Joji, March 22, 2006)

Unequal distribution of medical resources and stringent procurement rules may limit access to essential cancer drugs and treatment technology. The national referral hospital in Kenya, for instance, relied on only two radiotherapy machines and one of them was permanently put out of service after my research in 2005. Whereas some patients succumb to cancer complications before receiving treatment, the procedures often become too arduous for many others to endure, which increases suffering and patient awareness that a cure is unlikely. This often contributes to treatment abandonment and non-adherence. The following excerpt from Ms. Souda's narrative recorded on March 3, 2005, partly illustrates this. Ms. Souda had been admitted intermittently for treatment of very advanced cervical cancer.

MS. SOUDA: ". . . unfortunately radiotherapy could not help . . . So he [the doctor] had to put me on chemo [therapy]. . . . but the doctor mentioned yesterday that I am supposed to finish with the chemotherapy, then go back to radiotherapy and go for further treatment in Uganda . . . I understand the [brachytherapy] machine here is broken down. So my final destination is Uganda after all this! I was diagnosed in St. Mary's (hospital). They referred me here for radiotherapy because I couldn't go through an operation . . . yet, they don't have a radiation machine . . . many people are coming here. We even had a case from Sudan . . . but I am on transit to Uganda. . . . So when I was asking my doctor why I have to go to Uganda, she showed me, a machine in the radiotherapy room . . . the machine is broken down. And I was so surprised there is nobody to repair it here in Kenya! Somebody has to come all the way from Canada!"

ETHNOGRAPHER: "Why not go to Nairobi hospital, for example?"

MS. SOUDA: ". . . Maybe they are also considering financial status, because I can imagine it can be damn expensive in Nairobi hospital . . . So it could be cheaper in Uganda . . ."

Drug shortages, faulty medical technology, side effects and poor responses to treatment interrupted therapy for many of the patients who participated in the Kenyan ethnography. This contributes to fatigue, hopelessness and disappointment during hospital treatment of cancer.

FATIGUE, DISSATISFACTION AND DISAPPOINTMENT

The lives of cancer patients and their families eventually rotate around clinics, battery of medical tests, and quests for medicines and special diets. There were many cases in which patients stopped treatment because they could no longer bear debilitating side effects. Several resisted "medicines that hurt," and were unable to adhere to prescribed diets that turned out to be expensive. Others would stop taking prescribed medicines and decided not to return to the hospital for scheduled appointments because of the perceived futility of medical attempts to restore their deteriorating health. Ms. Stella, a breast cancer patient, had been hospitalized for over five months for recurrence and metastasis. She decided not to buy the prescribed medicine for the next course of chemotherapy and did not intend to go back to the hospital when I visited her at her daughter's house in a Nairobi slum area. She observed:

> Perhaps the next hospital visit is for "enhancement chemotherapy" . . . But I fear the medicines will kill me. I am tired. Why is chemotherapy endless? I am forced to have two sets of meals, one for myself and the other for other family members, yet it is not affordable. I will stop the chemotherapy and continue with Chinese [medicines].
>
> (Ms. Stella, age 47, October 8, 2005)

Some patients' families and other caregivers acted on the illness through continued treatment, even beyond the stage when it was useful. However, many people in Kenya are not fully aware that upon completion of prescribed cancer therapy courses, such as chemotherapy and radiotherapy, regular follow-up clinic visits are required to monitor the disease. For the few patients who reach this stage of treatment each subsequent hospital appointment revives the thought about suffering due to cancer, past treatment adversities and related emotional burdens, which further contradict treatment expectations (Shaha, Cox, Talman & Kelly, 2008, p. 62). Unfortunately, most of the study participants always hoped for a full recovery, which to their disillusionment never materialized. A male nasopharyngeal carcinoma patient observed:

> My expectation is that I will be well after the sixth session. But it seems that now the tumor is not disappearing completely . . . It has gone a long way and I am happy . . . I can enjoy life. I can laugh . . . I am able to lead a normal life again . . . But it is just sad that it has not disappeared as I expected. I thought that . . . I will have recovered by the time I finish the chemo's . . . In the near future, I expect that I will heal. But it seems that the fight is not over . . .
>
> (Mr. Samagi, age 34, September 19, 2005)

Anticipation of Recovery and Cure

Popular narratives in the Kenyan hospital ethnography associated cancer treatment processes with stepping up debility and suffering. Some patients blamed their suffering on medical personnel for "touching the cancer and spreading it," or medical "interference with the cancer" and the inability of clinical personnel to fix it effectively. Ms. Stella was bitter about her biopsy and subsequent mastectomy as she believed that these interventions were unnecessary. She also reported about fellow patients "going down and gradually dying in the ward due to chemotherapy." She said: "they all come here when they are much better and energetic, eating on their own, but they gradually wear out and just die."

Some nurses expressed reservations about cancer chemotherapy. One of them referred to chemotherapy as "toxic substances," which they would rather replace with the harmless food supplements promoted by some of her colleagues in the hospital. The nurses had difficulties coming to terms with the reality that commencement of treatment apparently coincided with either gradual or rapid physical deterioration of patients. Negative side effects of chemotherapy, such as vomiting, diarrhea, loss of appetite and weight increased doubts among patients, nurses and family members about treatment utility and success. Low survival rates of cancer inpatients and those discharged from the hospital further contributed to this sense of uncertainty about clinical regimens. Some patients and nurses perceived a relationship between frequent deaths and *toxic* chemotherapy or *lethal* radiotherapy popularly referred to as *kuchoma* (burning). A male patient expressed fear of antagonizing hospital staff who he said could punish "bad patients" by treating them with "risky unverified trial medicines." The patients perceived the risks of hospital treatment of cancer, which contributed to their construction of treatment ambiguity. Admission to the hospital exposes patients to new risks, unpleasantness, general iatrogenic morbidity and patient care errors, which nurses and doctors should be aware of (Raik, 2003; Roth, 1972). The perceived uncertainty about hospital treatments for cancer in Kenya highlights the need for medical personnel to allay fears about medical errors, improve pain management and develop initiatives for offering optimal care.

Treatment circumstances in the Kenyan public hospitals and homes undermine prospects for recovery and improvement of patients' quality of life. Poor nutrition, comorbidity and opportunistic infections, for instance, increased unpleasant experiences of cancer treatment. Previous futile multiple referrals pave the way for the most intensive and expensive—yet uncertain—treatment for those who arrive at the national referral hospital. Treatment at different levels of the public health care system entails cumulative and catastrophic disruption of livelihood, social and emotional stability of many patients and their families. Mr. Katsembe observed:

> In life, people plan what they have to achieve . . . But we don't plan that at a certain time . . . maybe I can be sick. You just plan . . . that by such a time I should have achieved this, without saying I will be sick . . . This sickness was very abrupt. It came when I had a number of projects to attend to . . . I was just settling down . . . I discovered

cancer is a very expensive disease to manage. Whatever resources I had put aside . . . were diverted to treatment . . . I finished all the finances; I had to go back to people to do some harambee (fund raising) so that I come to complete the treatment. It created a psychological imbalance; it shot down my ambitions and plans . . . I narrowed my focus on treatment. I am unable to pursue the things I wanted to pursue in life, I have postponed them to deal with the treatment first . . .

(Katsembe, age 34, March 22, 2006)

Patients' silenced concerns coincide with the medical personnel's unspoken uncertainty about cancer treatment. The stigma of having cancer and participating in treatment of the disease is often implicit. To some hospital staff deployment to the cancer ward and treatment center was stigmatizing and demoralizing as they were being asked to treat and care for patients "whose prognosis was already determined." However, clinical practitioners' and patients' views and expectations regarding successful cancer treatment varied. Medical professionals' attempts at objective diagnoses may not capture all the aspects of suffering as experienced by particular patients. Reports about health improvement or positive response of the disease to medication by doctors, for instance, often contradicted patients' lived experiences (Mishel, 1988). A patient on treatment for bone marrow cancer, for instance, said:

I did not feel pain after radiotherapy, but I become weak. . . . I feel very bad after chemotherapy . . . It starts again paining the back very much. . . . This medicine is very bad . . . I do not have appetite, it makes me very tired, I am just sleeping and can't even walk and fulfill my "conjugal responsibility"(*kufanya kizazi*).

(Adelo, age 28, November 2, 2005)

Pessimism arising from unpleasant treatment experiences blurred anticipation for recovery and cure. Reactions by caregivers indicating that cancer "is the ultimate and dangerous disease" contradicted further the treatment efforts. Paradoxically, some patients tended to appreciate knowing from the beginning of the treatment process that cancer is "incurable and dangerous." They were therefore ambivalent about the value of hospitalization and medical treatment:

They said it is a dangerous disease which cannot be cured quickly; even it cannot get finished quickly. It is a very dangerous disease . . . That disturbed me a bit . . . [But] it is the doctor who will decide whether I have completed the required treatment, or he gives me further medication and my expectation is that I get cured.

(Adelo, age 28, December 3, 2005)

Cancer treatment tends to be indefinite for many patients in Kenya and other developing countries. Each session appears to undermine a patient's welfare and quality of life. Thus some patients begin to miss appointments, fail to comply with medical directives or drop out of the treatment system altogether, due to inadequate disclosure regarding their condition and outcomes.

Uncertainty and Disclosure Issues

Where the medical staff succeed in "naming the disease," ineffective disclosure of treatment options and outcomes contradict the hope hospital workers instill in patients. However, hospital staff members feel morally obliged to help patients sustain hope for treatment success (Mulemi, 2014). They try to protect patients' determination and motivate them to endure by retaining nondisclosure as a cultural norm in patient care. Doctors and nurses are morally compelled to sustain patients' high expectations about restoration of health through reassurance that "something can (still) be done," in spite of apparent poor treatment outcomes. Physicians and oncology consultants end up ordering many burdensome tests in both private and public health facilities hoping to discover a more quantifiable basis for treatment plans (Padgett & Johnson, 1990, p. 206).

Inadequate disclosure obscured and silenced patients' concerns about the clinical processes and prognoses. However medical practitioners in the Kenyan Cancer Treatment Center held different views on treatment. This could account for contradictory therapeutic strategies and drug regimens to deal with uncertain prognoses. One respondent complained that colleagues were practicing oncology depending on what they learned, without sharing their knowledge with others. Clinical personnel positioned further up the chain of command overruled their colleagues' decisions on several occasions and this caused further treatment contradictions and ambiguity.

Patients and their families struggled to obtain test results, some of which could not be traced at the time they were needed, necessitating repeat exams. Similarly they weighed the usefulness of required tests against their overstretched financial abilities, especially when there was a lack of clear explanation and justification for the tests being ordered. In this regard, the struggles to cure cancer tend to obscure individual patient care needs. One patient, for instance, noted:

> They told me "this disease of yours is defeating the doctor . . .," but they kept me in the ward . . . I spent my little money on tests . . . I told that doctor, "you are a big [high ranking] doctor. Tell me the things you must tell me . . . If you see it is the [deadly] disease . . . and that I will die . . . I will go home to die! I am waiting for nothing here! . . . If you know I will recover tell me . . . I will stay well . . . I will pray . . ."
> (Mrs. Ndunduri, age 54, March 21, 2006)

Pursuits of Cure Versus Care for Suffering Patients

Subjective individual patient experiences are important in the search for comprehensive cancer management initiatives. The struggles to cure cancer need to consider experiences that may increase emotional suffering and perceived vagueness of treatment. Uncontrollable side effects, such as pain, nausea and vomiting, diarrhea, loss of appetite and hair, mouth sores and reduced body function particularly undermine the perceived value of treatment. Ms. Stella, for example, narrated of the gradual deterioration health of fellow patients on the cancer ward:

> They come when they are a bit strong . . . But all of a sudden, there is change; they diarrhea, vomit, refuse to eat. . . . and pass away . . . The lady who was here was eating well . . . I thought she will be alright . . . and I can't understand whether there is no medicine . . . or they delayed in buying the correct medicine . . . It is a bit difficult to know. You come when you are a bit strong, but you gradually exhaust . . . and you just pass away "peacefully . . ." The nurses say chemo's [chemotherapy drugs] are just chemicals, which are killing patients. They produce sores and loss of hair, we suffer, and the treatment is killing us . . .
>
> (Ms. Stella, age 47, October 8, 2005)

Health care providers often overlook patients' personal experiences of pain and other forms of suffering and tend to medicalize such experiences (Scheper-Hughes, 1990; Padgett & Johnson, 1990). Cancer ward physicians in the Kenyan hospital often seemed disgusted when they realized that they could not follow patients' expressions of suffering. The ward physician's communication with patients, for instance, typically took the following pattern:

DR. WARIO: Are you feeling any pain?
MR. SONY: Yes . . . but there is a lot of air in my stomach. . . .
DR. WARIO: (interrupting callously) Are you feeling pain or not? That is what we want to know . . . Are you feeling any pain today?
MR. SONY: (after a little while of silence) Yes, but not much today.
DR. WARIO: Okay, we will give you painkillers and other medicine . . .

The experience of pain and eating difficulties were the main aspects of cancer in-patients' embodiment of suffering (Mulemi, 2010a). This suffering tends to increase with duration and frequency of hospitalization. In addition, life in the cancer ward entailed a daily struggle to cope with pain, reduced ability to eat well and social isolation. However, medical staff routinely asked patients about pain as the main physical symptom to which they directed their insufficient treatment efforts. There was dual difficulty in alleviating patients' physical suffering. First, available medicine did not relieve pain symptoms, eating difficulties and treatment side effects. Second, some patients felt that some staff did not empathize sufficiently to respond to their concerns appropriately. Conscious or unconscious attempts by medical professionals to separate disease from personal experiences often contribute to the failure to address patients' perceived treatment uncertainty. Medical care may be an important resource to patients in times of distress and pain, but it may also constrain their search for the deeper meaning of illness experience (Bury, 1982).

Murray, Grant, Grant and Kendall (2003) contrast the experiences of cancer in the Meru South district of Kenya with the experiences of patients in Scotland, a developed nation that provides free primary and secondary health care and a comprehensive social security system. They report that cancer patients in Kenya have considerable unmet physical needs and that pain dominates their experiences of the disease. The *Kenya Cancer Strategy 2011–2016* aptly acknowledges the scarcity of some essential drugs for pain management in most public hospitals. Absence of clear cancer treatment guidelines and policies concerning terminal pain management, supportive and palliative care compound the ambiguity of treatment. One key informant noted:

> We do not have enough time with the patients. I have only seven minutes per patient. They are always looking for a place to empty their problems. They are looking for somebody to tell about their misery. They want someone who is ready listen to them. Patients have many problems that they bring along to the hospital. Some of the problems may be about their homes . . . Perhaps things were not working well there. Due to this the patient may think that the world is too heavy to carry, and just need somebody who can pay attention . . .
>
> (Intern Hospital Chaplain, July 12, 2006)

Legal restrictions on the use and availability of opioid analgesics add to other factors such as lack of awareness, and shortage of financial and human resources, which make cancer treatment experiences extremely unpleasant. In the face of perennial livelihood struggles, lack of health insurance and inadequate government subsidies for hospital treatment, chronic disease causes further impoverishment and catastrophic livelihood insecurity. In the Botswana cancer ward studied by Livingston (2012), pain was also the key issue of 64% of respondents. She found reluctance on the part of administrators to allow nurses to prescribe opiates even though nurses were the ones to staff rural health centers (p. 125). But she also points to the lack of expectation of chemical palliation that shaped patient demand. When patients did not expect help, they were less likely to demand it even though morphine, codeine and peethidine are easily available for low cost from the generics industry (p. 125). Livingston faults the emphasis from international quarters on evaluating African health systems in terms of public health metrics related to communicable disease. Pain relief is not prioritized and pain management comes to be seen as a luxury (p.126). Because the system in Botswana is committed to the equal distribution of health resources, shortages affect all cancer patients. In Kenya, however, those who can afford pain management have a greater chance of obtaining it either through private care on the black market.

CONCLUSION

The incidence of cancer in Kenya as in many sub-Saharan countries today is an increasing public health problem. The status and practice of cancer treatment remains largely ambiguous in a national system that prioritizes communicable, infectious diseases and where cancer care is situated in a confusing hybrid structure of public and private facilities with great inequities in access to care. Cancer remains a politically invisible disease in Kenya, and cancer specialists and pathologists are scarce in peripheral public hospitals, which serve the majority of low-income people. Narratives and experiences from patients depict local images of silenced uncertainties about cancer treatment and the hope for recovery.

Ambiguity of treatment at three levels complicates the cancer crisis in Kenya. First the disease itself generates uncertainty due to its unknowable aspects, and medical uncertainty in dealing with the disease. Second, low awareness about the disease and the experience of treatment side effects confound patients' quest for meaning. Finally, cancer treatment in Kenya often coincides with accelerated deterioration of health, which further entails catastrophic disruptions to livelihood, social networks and emotional health. The completion of each treatment course hardly guarantees restoration of health as patients and their families expect. This is the core of cancer treatment ambiguity in Kenya—it both alleviates and increases suffering among patients and their families. Moreover, the contexts of suffering for both patients and care providers are multilayered, constructed through interactions within the health care system. Whereas the process of cancer diagnosis and treatment is designed to alleviate the patients' distress and improve physical health, the lack of care facilities, trained medical personnel, diagnostic technologies and medications often paradoxically intensifies the emotional anxiety, financial distress and physical pain experienced by patients. As patients become more debilitated and less certain of cure, their perceived unwillingness to comply with treatment increases the sense of ambivalence among clinic personnel and frustrates their attempts to instill hope and provide cure. As Murray et al. (2003) point out, these contexts of suffering and the needs of patients that develop from them are very different in the developing and developed world. Patients in medically underserved areas characterized by a shortage of services and extreme levels of poverty share certain similar experiences. In both Botswana and Kenya, for example, cancer is a low priority disease. Those who suffer with it in these countries have great needs for basic treatments to alleviate pain and provide basic assistance meeting daily needs. In the developed world, where systems are in place to diagnose and treat cancer, the context of suffering shifts to high-light the psychological and spiritual needs of those facing death in a medical system designed to preserve life at all costs.

In 2009, Paul Farmer and colleagues formed the Global Task Force on Expanded Access to Cancer Care and Control in Developing Countries. This task force, composed of leaders from the global health and cancer care communities, is dedicated to challenging the assumption that is widespread among public health organizations that cancer will remain untreated in poor countries. As they note, the humanitarian rationale is clear—more than 4 million people will die from cancer each year in lesser-developed nations, many without any access to basic palliative care. They call for including cancer treatment in national health insurance coverage, strengthening primary health care systems, improving cancer detection at the local level, training more oncological specialists, and working with developed nations and pharmaceutical companies to correct the inequity in the distribution of resources to treat cancer (Farmer et al., 2010, p. 1188). Although the focus of this chapter has been to illustrate the unique context of suffering created by treatment ambiguity in Kenya, Farmer and colleagues note that researchers and policy makers must no longer differentiate between diseases of the poor and the rich and adopt a bold agenda to fill the gaping voids in cancer care and control worldwide (p. 1192). In the interim, Murray et al. (2003) argue from data similar to mine from Kenya, that it is an essential first that pain control be improved for humane end-of-life care. They argue that flexible methods of essential drug dispensing, distribution and payment should be developed, which recognize poverty in patients (p. 4). Similarly, Brennan, Carr and Cousins (2007) have called upon the World Health Organization to make pain management a worldwide priority. My data also indicate that while there is clearly a need in Kenya for additional resources and personnel to treat cancer, it is also important that the management of the ambiguity of cancer treatment be a component in the discussions among and training of health care providers at all levels of the system. Provision of adequate information, support and patient-centered treatment is necessary for minimization of negative effects of treatment ambiguity on quality of life and therapeutic relationships, while systemic structural reforms are needed to make cancer care more affordable and accessible to the majority of citizens.

NOTE

1. I use pseudonyms for the anonymity of study participants.

REFERENCES

Barnes-Josiah, D., Myntti, C., & Augustin, A. (1998). The "three delays" as a framework for examining maternal mortality in Haiti. *Social Science and Medicine, 46,* 981–993.

Brennan, F. D. B., & Carr, M. C. (2007). Pain management: A fundamental human right. *International Anaesthesia Research Society, 105,* 205.

Bury, M. (1982). Chronic Illness as biographical disruption. *Sociology of Health and Illness, 4,* 167–182.

Farmer, P., Frenk, J., Knaul, F., Shulman, L., Alleyne G., Armstrong, L., . . . Seffrin, J. (2010). Expansion of cancer care and control in countries of low and middle income: A call to action. *The Lancet, 376,* 1186–1193.

Goodwin, D., Pope, C., Mort, M., & Smith, A. (2003). Ethics and ethnography: An experiential account. *Qualitative Health Research, 13,* 567–77.

Hunt, L. M. (1998). Moral reasoning and the meaning of cancer: Causal explanations of oncologists and patients in Southern Mexico. *Medical Anthropology Quarterly, 12,* 298–318.

Knaul, F. M., Gralow J. R., Atun, R., Bhadelia, A., Frenk, J., Quick J., Shulman, L., & Farmer, P. (2012). Closing the cancer divide, overview and summary. In F. M. Knaul, J. R. Gralow, R. Atun, & A. Bhadelia, (Eds.), *Closing the cancer divide: An equity imperative* (pp. 3–36). Cambridge, MA: Harvard University Press.

Livingston, J. (2012). *Improvising medicine: An African oncology ward in an emerging cancer epidemic.* Durham, NC & London: Duke University Press.

Mishel, M. H. (1988). Uncertainty in illness image. *Journal of Nursing Scholarship, 20,* 225–232.

Mostert, S., Njuguna, F., Langat, S. C., Slot, A. J. M., Skiles, J. M. Sitaresmi, N., . . . & Kaspers, G. J. L. (2014). Two overlooked contributors to abandonment of childhood cancer treatment in Kenya: Parents' social network and experiences with hospital retention policies. *Psycho-Oncology, 23,* 700–707.

Mulemi, B. A. (2010a). *Coping with cancer and adversity: Hospital ethnography in Kenya.* Leiden: African Studies Centre.

Mulemi, B. A. (2010b). On being 'native' and 'outsider' in hospital ethnography. *Viennese Ethnomedicine Newsletter, 12,* 6–14.

Mulemi, B. A. (2014), Technologies of hope: Managing cancer in a Kenyan hospital. In R. Prince & R. Marsland (Eds.), *Making and unmaking public health in Africa: Ethnographic and historical perspectives* (pp. 233–261). Athens, OH: Ohio University Press.

Murray, Scott A., Grant, E., Grant, A., & Kendall, M. (2003). Dying from cancer in developed and developing countries: Lessons from two qualitative interview studies of patients and their carers. *British Medical Journal, 326,* 1–5.

Mutuma G. Z. & Ruggut-Korir, A. (2006). *Cancer incidence report; Nairobi 2000–2002.* Nairobi: Nairobi Cancer Registry, Kenya Medical Research Institute.

Onyango, J. F., & Macharia, I. M. (2006). Delays in diagnosis, referral and management of head and neck cancer presenting at Kenyatta National Hospital, Nairobi. *East African Medical Journal, 83,* 85–91.

Onyango, J. F., Omondi, B. I., Njiru, A., & Awange, O. O. (2004). Oral cancer at Kenyatta National Hospital, Nairobi. *East African Medical Journal, 81,* 318–321.

Padgett, D., & Johnson, T. (1990). Somatizing distress: Hospital treatment of psychiatric comorbidity and the limitations of biomedicine. *Social Science and Medicine, 30,* 205–209.

Parkin, D. M., Sitas, F., Chirenje, M., Stein, L., Abratt, R., & Wabinga, H. (2008). Part I: Cancer in indigenous Africans—burden, distribution, and trends. *The Lancet Oncology, 9,* 683–692.

Raik, B. G. (2003). Hospitalization can be dangerous. In E. L. Siegler, S. Mirafzali, & J. B. Foust (Eds.), *An Introduction to Hospitals and Inpatient Care* (pp. 79–88). New York, NY: Springer Publishing Company.

Republic of Kenya. (2011). *National Cancer Strategy 2011–2016.* Nairobi: Ministry of Health and Sanitation and Ministry of Medical Services, Government Press.

Roth, J. A. (1972). The necessity and control of hospitalisation. *Social Science and Medicine, 66,* 425–446.

Scheper-Hughes, N. (1990). Three propositions for a critically applied medical anthropology. *Social Science and Medicine, 30,* 189–197.

Shaha, M., Cox, C. L., Talman, K., & Kelly, D. (2008). Uncertainty in breast, prostate, and colorectal cancer: Implications for supportive care. *Journal of Nursing Scholarship, 40,* 60–67.

Turin, D.R. (2010). *Health care utilization in the Kenyan health system: challenges and opportunities. Student Pulse, 2,* 1–3. Retrieved from http://www.studentpulse. com/articles/284/health-care-utilization-in-the-kenyan-health-system-challenges-and-opportunities.

United Nations Industrial Development Organization. (2010). *Pharmaceutical Sector Profile: Kenya.* 2010 Global UNIDO Project. Vienna: United Nations Industrial Development Organization. Retrieved from http://www.unido.org/fileadmin/user_media/Services/PSD/BEP/Kenya_Pharma%20Sector%20profile_TEGLO05015_Ebook.pdf.

9 From Part to Whole

Gender Roles and Health Practices in the Experience of Breast Cancer in Northeast Brazil

Waleska de Araújo Aureliano

INTRODUCTION

Suffering is the central experience that underlies the responses of coping and caring. A diagnosis of cancer is potentially life altering as individuals must readjust their concepts of self and respond to the shifting labels attached to them by family, friends, co-workers and medical personnel. Bury (1982) was the first to suggest that biographical disruption, such as that caused by chronic illness, lies at the heart of suffering because it causes a threat to the individual's established self-image, sense of agency and vision of the future. Suffering emerges from the meaning that individuals in particular contexts assign to the importance of such disruptions and the extent to which these are viewed as causing pain or loss. Bell (2012) finds that psycho-oncology in the United States and Canada is moving toward a view of cancer as beneficial trauma because it paves the way for those who experience suffering to undergo a positive transformation and become better selves.

Such discourse is absent from the mutual aid groups I studied in Brazil, where a cancer diagnosis is something women seek to disguise or hide from view. This article explores the role of cultural context in shaping definitions of and responses to suffering. Crucial to understanding identity practices is a consideration of how the symbolic and social representations of the body and appropriate roles behaviors in specific cultural environments impact the illness experience.

Data from research with two groups of working class breast cancer survivors in the city of Campina Grade in northeast Brazil demonstrate how women stressed the management and uses of the body through work, including housework, as a way to normalize the experience of cancer in everyday life. In the process, they inverted and challenged dominant discourses about female sexuality as the core of women's identities and resisted fragmentary representations of the body by emphasizing, instead, the importance of the whole person. In other contexts, however, in an effort to provide for their families, women adopted the label of "disabled" in order to qualify for government assistance. These findings illustrate how conceptions of individual, social and political bodies are interrelated (Scheper-Hughes & Lock, 1987).

BACKGROUND

In Brazil, nearly 50,000 cases of breast cancer are diagnosed each year. Information from the Cancer Registries Population Base (RCBP), available in 16 Brazilian cities, shows that in the 1990s breast cancer was the most common type of cancer in the country. According to statistics from the National Cancer Institute (INCA),[1] Brazil's large urban centers present the greatest rates of the disease, with the southeast region having the highest incidence: up to 65 new cases annually for every 100,000 inhabitants. Mammographic screening is currently the main tool for controlling the disease in Brazilian public health (Brasil, 2004, 2009).

Despite these numbers, breast cancer as a disease has been seldom addressed by the social sciences in Brazil. When I started my master's research in 2003, there was only one published anthropological work on breast cancer (Carvalho, 2002). One year after the completion of my M.A. thesis, the first Ph.D. dissertation on the topic was defended by a social scientist (Britto, 2007), although in a public health program.

Although breast cancer is considered a pathology related to the processes of urbanization, with high incidence in developed countries and in women with higher socioeconomic status (Brasil, 2009), most of the socio-anthropological studies about breast cancer in Brazil have focused on working-class women,[2] as access to patients with this type of cancer is often granted by public hospitals, the major centers for treatment of the disease in the country[3]. Initiated in hospitals, support groups and patient associations become privileged places for contact with women with breast cancer. One of INCA's recommendations for the treatment of breast cancer involves the formation of such groups in hospitals (Brasil, 2004). In addition, there are independent groups formed by patients and/or physicians.[4]

One recurring issue in these studies, including mine, is how perceptions of the female body, particularly as regards the management of daily life and the relationship of women to the world of work, are triggered by working-class women as they negotiate biomedical directives. The bodily changes caused by the surgical removal of the breast (mastectomy) strongly affect female sexuality, and also become highly relevant in labor dynamics. This is particularly true for the working-class women who identify themselves as *homemakers* or who, apart from working outside home, are also identified as family members responsible for the care of home and family.

Most of the women who took part in my research study came from working-class families, were identified as *homemakers* and did not work outside home. Others were retired, civil servants or autonomous workers. The management of body use in work, including housework, was reported by many of these women as a way to normalize daily life after the cancer experience and to avoid being seen as victims by family members. In this process women inverted and challenged biomedical understandings about appropriate health care after breast cancer and the fragmentary representation of the female body underlying these biomedical recommendations. Women adhered to these gender roles not as a form of subjugation to culturally established gender models, but rather as a way to maintain a positive identity in the world of work and autonomy in the use of their bodies. In these ways they avoided being labeled as ill or an "invalid."

On the other hand, women sometimes needed to emphasize their limitations as cancer patients in order to claim a government pension. Even without a formal profession, any person can contribute to social security in Brazil and claim a retirement for the time of contribution and/or age, as well as for total or partial disability due to accidents or diseases. Although Brazilian legislation guarantees this benefit, it is often difficult for people to claim it. They must receive medical certification and pass through a series of tests while submitting appropriate documentation to the appropriate government agencies. For women who need these pensions to survive, the status and identity of cancer patient must be embraced, at least temporarily, in order to demonstrate that the disease interferes with normal activities to such an extent that government support is warranted.

The research informing this chapter was conducted with women from two support groups in the city of Campina Grande (PB), in the northeast of Brazil. I systematically followed the activities of these groups between the years 2003 and 2005. One of the groups studied (group A) was a physical therapy group based in a public hospital, a complementary part of the post-surgical treatment of breast cancer in that institution.[5] The therapist running the group encouraged mutual support and some women continued to attend the group even after the end of their treatment. Women who attended group A were almost entirely working-class, were served mainly by the public health system and had no formal professional or gainful employment.

The second support group (group B) was explicitly a support group for women who had undergone mastectomy. Although founded by a breast specialist and a physiotherapist, it was not linked to any medical institution. Both experienced breast cancer after the group was founded. The composition of group B was more heterogeneous than that of group A in terms of income, employment and education. The group included women of higher socioeconomic status, with cars and jobs outside the house, as well as a significant number of working-class women brought to the group by one of its founders who worked in both private clinics and the city's public hospitals.

... AND GOD CREATED WOMAN: A BRIEF HISTORY OF THE FEMALE BODY IN THE WEST

To understand the social and symbolic representations of the female body, a brief analysis of the historical construction of discourses of the female body and the creation and establishment of certain female roles still present in Western societies is necessary. I highlight the historical role of biomedicine in this process, particularly the strategies for the medicalization of the female body in the 18th and 19th centuries. This historical perspective illustrates the powerful role of biomedicine in the creation of norms, standards and practices on bodies, although not without generating new readings, resistance and conflict.[6]

When analyzing the formative period of what we call social medicine, Foucault (2000) depicts the trajectory of the establishment of biomedicine in the 18th and 19th centuries as a form of scientific knowledge, showing its political role in the formation of European states (mainly Germany), and its pragmatic role as a system of medicine to treat the problems created by increased urbanization (analyzing the case of France) and the medicalization of the poor where it was used as an instrument to control the working classes (in the case of England). Biomedicine developed as a medical system for the care of individuals—via welfare programs to the poor—and of the greater population through vaccination, sanitation in cities and the control of epidemics. In this way, biomedicine's foremost representative—the doctor—became invested with the power to supervise and determine not only individuals' health, but also the organization of populations and how they should live socially.

According to Foucault, the disciplining power of biomedicine would necessarily be present in the social construction of human bodies, specifically in determining *bodily conduct* and the *morality of bodies*, for both men and women. It is important, however, to keep in mind that the production of medical and scientific knowledge during the consolidation of biomedicine as a science was essentially masculine; discourses about the female body and its medicalization carry a morality that defines women as primordially "natural" and "organic," as opposed to men, who are "cultural" and "historic" (Matos, 2003).

Vieira (2002), analyzing the discourses of Brazilian medical schools in the 19th century, demonstrates how the figure of the doctor and the knowledge he represented were consolidated through the need for sanitation in the large urban centers undergoing transformation in this period of population growth. Biomedical discourse argued for the eradication of sanitary dangers (making cities more hygienic), the sanitation of public spaces and the ordering of family life. On this last point, women were called upon to fulfill a role that, according to 19th century medicine, would be consistent with her "nature."

The woman came to be valued as a wife and a mother and acquired greater power within the home, within private spaces, from the moment she was designated caretaker of the children and administrator of the domestic sphere. Matos (2003), analyzing medical discourse on the representations of the male and female body in fin-de-siècle São Paulo, notes that doctors viewed women as products of their reproductive system, which formed the basis of their social function and behavioral characteristics. The uterus and ovaries determined female behavior, which resulted in individuals incapable of engaging in complex reasoning, abstractions and intellectual activity. "The combination of these attributes, combined with an emotional sensitivity, prepared women for the procreation and raising of children" (Matos, 2003, p. 115).

This "biological determination" of women subscribed them to the private home space and maternal and domestic functions. Her "emotive nature" was considered ideal for generating and caring for children. Maternity appears in these discourses as a "biological obligation." It was not a choice, but an organic determination. Men, on the other hand, were inherently social and intellectual creatures. Not being determined by procreative functions, although being an essential part of them, men were elemental to the "rationalized" universe of culture and able to completely develop their intellectual capacities (Martin, 1989).

Thus, the western medical discourses of the 18th, 19th and the early 20th centuries enclosed women within their *biology*, minimizing possibilities of being completely autonomous cultural subjects. Social roles were defined and uses of the body determined according to this logic, provoking an alienation of women in relation to their own body.

Martin (1989) places the fragmentation and alienation of the female body in a more recent era. Analyzing the impressions of North-American women of reproductive health procedures, Martin depicts the manner in which the gynecological exam fragments the female body, as the preparation for the exam separates the woman from her genitalia and from the person who examines her. Martin also highlights the use of metaphors of industrialization (e.g., images of machines and factories) in American medical discourse around menstruation and reproduction. These same metaphors, however, are absent in the classification of the male reproductive system.

Londa Schiebinger (1994) evokes a longer timeline in her depiction of the historical and social origins of the definition of the term "mammals." In 1758, she argues, Carolus von Linnaeus introduced the term *Mammalia* to define a class of animals comprising humans, apes, elephants, whales, bats and all other organisms with hair, three ear bones and a four-chambered heart. Linnaeus made the female breast the icon of this class of animals, known as "mammals" still today. The new nomenclature provoked arguments, even criticism of Linnaeus. Opponents argued that another term ought to be chosen to define such bodies, because the breasts were a feature in only some members of this class, namely the females, and during only a certain period of time (lactation); furthermore, in the absence of pregnancies and births the breasts lack organic functionality in the life of the female.

Schiebinger examines, then, the cultural-historical moment during which Linnaeus developed the term *Mammalia*, an era of the political, medical and moral movement in Europe to valorize the figure of the woman as responsible for the care of the children and organically determined to fulfill the maternal role (see Ariés, 1978; Donzelot, 1986). Combining this discourse with a scientific definition for the classification of the species Linnaeus reinforced women's connection to the "natural" and "organic" world, because the breasts' function is the same for all females of the many species of mammals. Simultaneously, Linnaeus's definition of the term *Homo sapiens* distanced the male from this "natural" world, distinguishing men from other animals by his power of reason:

> This term—'man of wisdom'—was used to distinguish humans from other primates (apes, lemurs and bats, for example) . . . From a historical point of view, however, the choice of the term *sapiens* is highly significant. Man had traditionally been distinguished from animals by his reason; the medieval apposition animal rationale, proclaimed his uniqueness. Thus, within Linnaeus terminology, a female character (the lactating mammal) ties humans to brutes, while a traditional male character (reason) marks our separateness from brutes.
>
> (Schiebinger, 1994, p. 191)

The history of the origin of the term *Mammalia* shows us how scientific concepts emerge from complex social and cultural matrixes that become naturalized with time, overshadowing the political construction behind the most apparent categories that are established and shared in the society.

Despite the continual influences of these historical threads on women's roles and symbolic constructions of the female body, my experience in the field demonstrated a range of conflicting discourses with this historically constructed model. While I noticed on the one hand a discourse and demeanor of shame, due to the loss of a symbol of the female body (the breast) and the social representations contained within it, I also observed a rejection of such a fragmented vision of the body. At the same time, social roles assigned to the "female condition" (mother, homemaker, wife), even if challenged by the experience of cancer and mastectomy, proved to still be present for my interlocutors. Furthermore, the body revealed itself as an arena of struggle and negotiation with biomedical knowledge; women questioned the representation of their bodies and medical prescriptions and challenged ideas about care and health proposed by biomedicine.

THE PART AND THE WHOLE IN THE EXPERIENCE OF BREAST CANCER

The impact that mastectomy has on perceptions of the female body and how this mutilation is signified in the development of women's social identities cannot be denied. Cancer represents a disruption to the self and causes both physical and psychic suffering for those attempting to adjust to the diagnosis. After the experience of the disease new discourses will be developed to normalize the perception and performance of this body. In the beginning of my research, I noted the disruptive impact of breast cancer and mutilation in participants' narratives, as the women experienced the stigma associated with representations of a body sick and mangled. This was especially evident during chemotherapy and afterwards as women resignified their bodies through such statements as *"I'm more than my breasts"* or *"I'm the same person as before."* It was also present in their performance of daily tasks in the constant quest to normalize the body's uses, evident principally in the search for a positive identity in the world of work, be it paid, voluntary or in the home.

The majority of my interlocutors, as I have stated, were working-class homemakers. Because they did not engage in remunerated work outside the home, it might be expected that these women would suffer less from the impact of the disease in relation to work. However, I found that they suffered greatly from perceptions of uselessness stemming from physical limitations imposed by the disease. The domestic work performed by a homemaker requires more of the body than the work of a doctor, for example. After surgery women experienced, in their daily, repetitive activities of washing, ironing, sweeping, etc., new restrictions: one cannot ring out a pair of jeans, remove food from an oven without protection or care for plants without gloves. Even washing a glass required great care, because a slip up and a deep cut can lead to lymphedema.[7] Their domestic work did not become impossible to carry out, but they did undergo significant changes that caused women to experience a loss of autonomy in the domestic sphere. Many began to need help, to limit daily tasks and to make some activities less fatiguing, even as they struggled against being seen as "worthless" and "not good for anything anymore."

> At home I still don't wash heavy clothes, just light clothing. When there's some heavy clothing or a bedspread, I ask my sister and she does it. I've called a girl to come wash, to do the dusting—these things, I don't do. I wash the floors and walls, and my son dries them.
>
> (M., 52, group A)

As the home is her domain, women who identified as *homemaker* experienced deeply the changes brought about by breast surgery, for home and work were for them one and the same. These changes also affected the family. Because women administer the domestic arena, their limitations required family members to mobilize and take on "responsibilities" that were previously theirs. This did not sound to women in my study as a democratization of domestic work; for many, it foregrounded their feelings of uselessness due to disease and gave them an identity they did not want: that of an invalid. The inability to carry out activities done before diagnosis (washing, ironing, cooking, cleaning) was not seen as a relief or respite from fatiguing chores, but rather as a loss, leading to self-devaluation and a sense of uselessness.

They struggled against this view of themselves and attempts by others to view them as victims by not adhering to medical recommendations:

> I do everything: cook, wash clothes, iron—my fingers ache sometimes here in the joints, but Dr. G. says that it's not cancer, it must be arthritis. Then I do physical therapy to get better.
>
> (B., 50, group A)

> Look, I want you to tell me how a homemaker can live without washing, without ironing, without cooking. In theory it's easy, but in practice it's altogether different! (Question asked during a group meeting when one of the coordinators, a physiotherapist, directed the women to avoid the heavier domestic chores.)
>
> (S., 51, group B)

Some women complained that they did everything in the house, even after the surgery, which limited their movements, but others were proud that even with limitations, they managed to continue "taking care of the house and not becoming useless." Britto (2007) observed the same attitude among women who took part in her research, who were proud to be able to continue taking care of their families and, thus, felt productive and healthy. She argues that conventional medicine's logic of self-care goes against working-class women's logic of caring for others, which, far from being perceived as a form of subordination, is rather a means of normalization of everyday life and a demonstration of autonomy and health.

This issue of taking care of one's home and children, and the role (or "responsibility") of women in caring for the family came up in a direct way in the narrative of a patient who underwent a bilateral mastectomy. This patient started dating sometime after the mastectomy. She said that her boyfriend claimed he did not care that she did not have breasts. But she took the initiative to end their relationship:

> I didn't take very seriously that relationship, you know. [Why, didn't you like him?] Because I didn't want to date, if there was no chance of getting married and being able to take care of my husband. I said, "you know what? I'll just act like I'm dating," and so I let him know I didn't want anything serious, and he gave up, you know? And these days we're friends. [So, you didn't want to keep going, not because of him, but because if it became something more serious, if you wanted to get married] . . . Yeah, getting married, taking responsibility for making food for my husband, doing the laundry—those kinds of things, and I'm in no condition for that, so that's why.
>
> (S., 44, group A and B)

At first, I regarded this comment as submission to culturally established female roles (homemaker, mother). However, upon further analysis of the points she made and taking into account other field data, I realized that for working-class women with mastectomies and no other outside paid employment, working in the home was a way both of remaining independent and of protecting a positive identity within the world of work. Challenges to such positive identifications from disease caused psychic distress and a strong desire to return to the normal and valued status by carrying out domestic work as if no physical limitations existed.

For those who had a career outside the home, its interruption was not the only problem. When women expressed their reasons for taking time off in the workplace, they directly felt stigmatized as sick and disabled. Upon returning to work, they had to deal with the gaze of others on their bodies.

> It was interesting: I was teaching high school and I used to always wear polo-style shirts, but one day I had on a more low-cut blouse, and when I was like this [leaning over the table], writing something, I think, a student saw. Because I was like this [leaning] and the bra with the prosthesis gets straight when we go like this [leans over]. Girl, when she saw it—I realized that she saw, she went "Aaannhh"—you know that shock?
>
> (D., teacher, 52, group B)

> At work I always used to tell people I had a nodule, I used to say "I have a nodule, I need to go to the doctor." And they used to ask "you went to the doctor?" I said "Yes, I am going to do a surgery," because the doctor had said already that I was going to do the surgery. Then if I said I was going to do a surgery on the breast the people already commented that it was cancer. I found it interesting, even though I didn't say "I have cancer" because I didn't say it was cancer, I said that it was a nodule and the people looked at me with a pity, this made me feel very bad . . . Then I used to say to everyone at work that I was fine, everything was ok because I did not want anyone to look at me with a pity face, saying that I had a cancer and thinking that I was going to die.
>
> (L., 47, group A)

Those who had to totally abandon their activities, because they started to be considered "too heavy," did it with a great regret:

> I liked to work a lot, it is not more the life I used to have before, is it? [Did you work before?] I did, I was washerwoman, I washed outside clothes, now I cannot do it anymore because of the arm. [And inside the house in your everyday life what has changed due to the care for the arm?] I take a lot of care of my arm, always . . . I sweep the house slowly, I wash my clothes slowly, but the heavy services, warming the fire, I don't do. [Do you miss these activities?] I miss them because I have worked all my life, initially I cried a lot because I wanted to do the things and I could not . . . Now no, now I manage to do more, now I got used [to it].
>
> (E., 57, group A)

[And are you working today?] No, not now, because I can't anymore. My job was making snack food. I made fried pies, baked pies, and savory snacks, because I owned a snack shop, and I was the one that made the food, and you know, kneading and mixing dough is hard, right? [moves her arm as if stirring a pot] and now after surgery I can't . . . [And how was it for you, used to working, having to stop?] I kind of got a bit depressed, because you're used to going out every day, you work, then you suddenly become dependent on other people for everything, you don't do anything for yourself anymore, you don't do a single thing! At some point my mother and my sister said, "Don't be like this, there's a right time for everything," and I realized they were right. I'll relax, but I was really worked up in the first months after surgery, not doing anything and used to working hard.

(L., 47, group A)

L. retired in November 2005, but looked for an activity to compensate for the work at her shop. In group A, she learned how to make macramé (a technique for making textiles using knots) from another group member. In one group meeting she thanked her macramé teacher for the lessons. She said the craft had changed her life because now she was a "useful person again," someone who "could do something useful." In this case, it was not just the financial issue that mattered to this woman who had to retire, but, above all, it was the functional and productive character of the work that protected her from the stereotype of the "ill person."

It could be argued that other types of physical impairment or chronic diseases would equally affect the performance of a woman's professional or household activities, such as the loss of an arm or a leg, perhaps even more so because of the resulting limitations on the performance of certain physical activities. However, the mutilation caused by breast cancer is distinct from other forms of amputation: a mastectomy produces a "disability" whose visibility is controlled; therefore, in principle, it is not evident and cannot be easily identified and, thus, socially legitimated. The negotiation of this visibility of the modified body permits many women safe transit within the different social spaces they frequent without making obvious their mastectomized condition. Thus, they avoided social situations in which the revelation of their physical difference could lead to stigmatization, either because of the mutilation, or because of cancer's association with death.

However, the legitimacy of this disability became an issue when they needed to use it in other contexts. In certain moments and situations, the much-desired normality was renegotiated in order to reclaim the rights of women with mastectomies as cancer patients:

Because once we remove anything from our chests we're disabled, I changed all of my documents to disabled; buying a car costs half the price, we don't pay to change license plates, don't pay taxes, don't pay a thing.

(R., 72, group B)

Although Brazilian legislation guarantees access to a pension for retirement or disability, it is not that simple for women with breast cancer to claim this benefit, because women who ask for this type of retirement needs to pass through successive medical examinations to assess their physical condition and the type of activity they could return to practice after breast surgery:

> The doctor says that I can work, doing everything, that his mother had this disease and she does everything, then I said "look, doctor, I do not know your mother, all I know is the doctor who operated on me said I can't work, I'm disabled—you're looking at his note right there—is he somehow mistaken?" It makes you want to take off the breast [the prosthesis] and throw it in his face, You see this, can I work without it?
>
> (M., self-employed businesswoman, 52, group A,)

Thus, although most of my interlocutors desired to be seen as productive, taking care of the more difficult household chores (like washing clothes) and trying not to relax their efforts as caretakers of home and family, they represented themselves as invalids, sick or disabled when they had recourse to a pension or assistance from the National Institute of Social Security (INSS). In this process, ambiguous and conflicting discourses arose in relation to body alterations from mastectomy: sometimes the women said they were "like any normal person," whereas other times they labeled themselves "disabled" and pursued their rights as people with physical disabilities.

The ambiguity of the discourses of being (the same) as before and being disabled was clearly present in the testimonies of homemakers and self-employed women, usually from more economically challenged families. This ambiguity becomes comprehensible when we see that the disease as a strategy makes possible for these women what may be the only consistent income in a family where the main providers (usually the men in the house) work odd jobs in the informal sector. Apart from this, counting on this form of support could give these women a financial independence never experienced before and, consequently, reposition them in the family structure in the moment when they change their condition from that of an ill person and/or homemaker to one who has her own income and is the provider at home. Among the strategies for the presentation and representation of this new body, breast reconstruction is a surgical intervention capable of giving back to the woman a female body closer to its *original form*. However, what I observed with many of my interlocutors was that reconstruction, far from being considered a key procedure for the rebuilding of a mutilated body, was instead perceived as another mutilation (when performed with muscle and belly tissue). According to some it represented needless suffering, because it would be not for reasons of health but aesthetics and vanity.[8]

Because exposure to the breast can be controlled, many women said that "they did not care since no one could see it anyway." This position makes us think of how the body is represented in this gaze built by others, which was also their own gaze upon themselves. However, there were negotiations regarding this gaze in the moment of sexual relations or in situations of great exposure, such as going to the beach. When showing indifference to breast reconstruction, some women argued that their partners "did not care about this," "did not mind" before even thinking if they themselves minded or not. They even expressed it humorously:

> My man does not even mind, the part that interests him is there untouched (laughs).
>
> (M., 52, group A)

> In this question he always supported me, he never minded this, it was me who kept away, I don't like it.
>
> (A., 37, group A)

The visibility of the breast and its *utilitarian functions* (breastfeeding and seduction) acted as parameters to limit or deny the importance given to the breasts and, as such, formed the basis of an argument often used by women unable or unwilling to undergo breast reconstruction surgery. If the functional aspect of that organ no longer existed, why rebuild it?

> When the doctor said I would have to undergo four surgeries to do the reconstruction, I said, 'Forget it. At this age I'm not going to go parading around anymore, I'm not going to be a beauty queen . . .
>
> (R., 72, group B)

> Early on, I asked him [the doctor] if it was possible to remove just a part. I didn't like seeing myself without a breast, but then when I left his office, I left thinking, my God, the Bible has a verse that says, "If your right eye causes you to sin, gouge it out and throw it away. It is better for you to lose one part of your body than for your whole body to be thrown into hell." I remembered this verse and began to think I'm going to lose a breast at my age; I'm not going to have any more children, I'm not going to breastfeed anymore, and here I'm crying because of this breast, when I can remove it and the Lord can heal me.
>
> (J., 58, group A)

> *[patient who did not complete the whole reconstruction]* I did not even make the nipple after, I was hesitating, took a long time and in the end did not go to make the nipple, because in order to make the nipple I needed to use a little bit from another breast, for it to be of the same size and to remove skin from one nipple to make the other one, to make it properly. But the time was passing and I did not go anymore, I said "I will not breast-feed, I will not pose for Playboy, I will not even use topless, just leave it as it is" because I am a person who has already

done ten surgeries, you know? And we get stressed with this, right? So another one without a real need, since a surgery for the necessity is ok, but not for aesthetics. Then I said I will take some time and this time was passing and I did not finalize the reconstruction.

(C., 62, group B)

In both support groups there were cases of women who had complications after the breast reconstruction surgery, which made others in the group refuse this surgical intervention. The functionality attributed to the breasts in terms of their sexual and maternal representation was present in the narratives of group members who were 50 years and older. In my research study only one participant was less than 40 years old and, although affected with a deep depression due to the loss of breast, this patient did not desire to have breast reconstruction. She was afraid of having complications caused by the surgery that could lead to removal of the second breast and new traumas.

Thus, I observed that, while denying their reduction to a "breast" and thereby refuting the valuation of their *parts* in detriment to the *whole person*, women who participated in this research sought to retain certain roles recognized as appropriate for women in the performance of housework and family care. They represented this practice as a form of resistance to breast cancer and the limitations it brings about rather than subjection to a culturally established model.

Finally, it is interesting to note how women, mainly those from the working class, challenge biomedicine's individualizing values that emphasize the importance of caring for one's body and health. For most of the women in this study, it was more important to remain active in the home, to care for children and the household, and to present a healthy, active and productive body, than it was to follow biomedical prescriptions to rest from work, by "doing nothing" or as little as possible.

Whereas the doctors I interviewed saw the women's noncompliance as a sign of not understanding the severity of cancer and its sequelae, the women themselves considered their attitudes of perseverance with household chores as a demonstration of strength, overcoming difficulties and health. In order to continue positioning themselves actively in the domestic sphere, these women created strategies and adaptations for their tasks in a constant process of negotiation through which they built new relations and modes of living with the body and the limitations left by cancer.

On the one hand, such a position can be taken as a submission to certain historically and socially established gender roles; on the other hand, it can be analyzed as a form of agency in the construction of social identities, in order to avoid being submitted pathological labels such as "invalid," "disabled" or "with cancer," categories that women strategically mobilized in the fight for their rights/access to financial resources for themselves and their families.

CONCLUDING REMARKS

Nancy Scheper-Hughes and Margaret Lock (1987) proposed the unification of the individual, social and political bodies and suggested research address emotions, going beyond the dichotomies of body/mind, individual/society and nature/culture. The experience of mutilation through mastectomy, the social stigma of cancer and the physical limitations (permanent or temporary) brought about by the disease lead women to try and return to the normal body's utility through work, whether paid or not, to negotiate the body's presentation in society and to sometimes demand rights because of the body's transformation due to cancer. All of these complex processes reveal the concatenation of individual, social and political elements in ways that women experience bodily transformations through suffering breast cancer.

For the working-class women in this study, the experience of breast cancer presented a profound disruption to their normal routines and self-definitions as productive individuals. In an effort to avoid stigma and alleviate psychic distress, these women expressed a strong desire to return to a normal and valued status by carrying out domestic work as if no physical limitations existed. They also embraced their roles as caregivers for others, even while they themselves were suffering, because such roles made them feel useful.

Western biomedical models of self-care, which emphasize rest and withdrawal from everyday activities for those with cancer, do not translate well in this working-class context and were not meaningful to the women who encountered such ideas in the clinical setting. Although the women studied strove to remain useful and avoid the stigma of illness, when the context shifted to negotiating access to disability payments from the state, their views changed. Patient identities, thus, are not static but rather dynamic, with different attributes foregrounded as individuals respond to shifting pressures at home, in the clinic and in the civic arena.

Also crucial to understanding identity practices is a consideration of how symbolic and social representations of the body and appropriate role behaviors in specific cultural contexts impact the illness experience. Although the women in this study expressed more concern about limitations on their working lives, the effects of the loss of a breast and its symbolic aspects related to sexuality and maternity were still felt by many. One way that these working-class women minimized such feelings of loss was to discuss the breast as an organ of limited functional importance.

On the other hand, as a mutilation of highly negotiable visibility, the mastectomy placed women in ambiguous situations with regards to the perception and performance of their bodies within their relational universe. While controlling the visibility of the loss of a breast allows the woman to exercise information management regarding her body, it makes difficult the social legitimization of her limitations brought by the mastectomy.

In this context, work, either domestic or not, becomes an important part in the processes of management and normalization of daily life after mastectomy. This agency of and around the body should make us question biomedicine's universalizing standards in defining health, because often such a definition becomes irrelevant and ineffective when it fails to recognize the particularities of the relational universe of people with chronic diseases and the different ways they conceptualize health and healthiness with the intention of going on with their lives with, and beyond, the disease.

NOTES

1. INCA is the main Brazilian agency for research on cancer and is part of the Ministry of Health. The Institute has four major hospitals, all in Rio de Janeiro, specializing in cancer treatment (one is a center for palliative care) and a marrow transplant center. All care provided by INCA hospitals is free and the institution is maintained by the *Sistema Único de Saúde* (SUS), a federal, universal and free health care system for all Brazil. In most Brazilian cities there are hospitals specializing in cancer treatment within SUS, and cancer control is part of public health strategies in Brazil. However, for patients who live in small Brazilian cities, especially in the northern, northeast and central-west regions, access to cancer treatment generally requires travel to the state capital or to other states.
2. The term working-class here refers to social groups characterized by low family income preventing or restricting access to certain goods of cultural, social and/or material value, such as formal education and private health care.
3. However, I should mention that not only working-class women receive treatment in public hospitals. In many cities, treatment in public hospitals is the only option for cancer patients, regardless of their financial situation. Because the costs of treatment can be very high and, in some cases, private health plans require co-payment in cancer treatment, people from higher socioeconomic levels also seek treatment in the public health care system. According to statistics from the Ministry of Health, 300,000 people with cancer receive treatment in SUS hospitals per year.
4. I will be using the term "support groups," the preferred term for speaking of the groups serving chronic patients, as it more adequately explains the relational and collective character of these groups' practices, whereas the term "self-help group" has a more individualistic connotation (Williams, 1989).
5. Almost all the women who took part in my research removed axillary lymph nodes to prevent metastasis. The removal of lymph nodes limits the arms movements after the surgery and affects the immune defense of the operated side. Physiotherapy is then prescribed to help in normalization of the arm movements and to orientate the women who had breast cancer as constant care needs to be taken to avoid lymphedema (arm swelling).
6. I would like to emphasize here the role of medicine in this process of construction of the female body on the West. However, other forms of cultural production took and take part in the construction of sexual and gender differences such as religions, arts, pornography and media in general.
7. A swelling, due to the build-up of lymph (the fluid carrying white blood cells) in the soft tissue, in this case in the arm.
8. It would be interesting here to recall the observations of Luc Boltanski (1979) on the perception of medical need in different social classes and the criticism, in the working classes, of those who turn to medicine "out of vanity," or "without necessity," noting that necessity is constructed within social groups and not determined by financial access to biomedical technology.

REFERENCES

Ariès, P. (1978). *História social da criança e da família*. Rio de Janeiro: Zahar Editores.

Aureliano, W. A. (2006). *Compartilhando a experiência do câncer de mama: Grupos de ajuda mútua e o universo social da mulher mastectomizada em Campina Grande (PB)*. Dissertação (Mestrado em Sociologia) – Programa de Pós-Graduação em Sociologia, Universidade Federal da Paraíba, Campina Grande, PB.

Bell, K. (2012). Remaking the self: Trauma, teachable moments, and the biopolitics of cancer survivorship. *Culture, Medicine and Psychiatry, 36*, 584–600.

Boltanski, L. (1979). *As classes sociais e o corpo*. Rio de Janeiro: Edições Graal.

Brasil, Ministério da Saúde. Instituto Nacional do Câncer. (2004). *Controle do câncer de mama: Documento do consenso*. Brasília: Ministério da Saúde. Retrieved from www.inca.org.br.

Brasil, Ministério da Saúde. Instituto Nacional do Câncer. (2009). *Estimate/2010: Incidence of cancer in Brazil*. Rio de Janeiro: INCA. Retrieved from www.inca.org.br.

Britto, R. H. de S. (2007). *De peito aberto: Câncer e gestão do cotidiano entre mulheres*. Tese (Doutorado em Saúde Coletiva) – Instituto de Medicina Social da Universidade do Estado do Rio de Janeiro.

Bury, M. (1982). Chronic illness as biographical disruption. *Sociology of Health and Illness, 4*, 167–182.

Carvalho, J. C. (2002). *Corpo feminino e mutilação: Um estudo antropológico*. Goiânia: Editora UFG.

Donzelot, J. (1986). *A polícia das famílias*. 2ª ed. Tradução de M. T. da Costa Albuquerque. Rio de Janeiro: Edições Graal.

Foucault, M. *Microfísica do poder*. (2000). Rio de Janeiro: Edições Graal.

Martin, E. (1989). *The woman in the body: A cultural analysis of reproduction*. Milton Keynes: Open University Press.

Matos, M. I. S. (2003). Delineando corpos: As representações do feminino e do masculino no discurso médico. In M. I. S. Matos & R. Soihet (Eds.), *O corpo feminino em debate* (pp. 107–127). São Paulo: Editora UNESP.

Scheper-Hughes, N. & Lock, M. (1987). The mindful body: A prolegomenon to future work in medical anthropology. *Medical Anthropology Quarterly, 1*, 6–41.

Schiebinger, L. (1994). Mammals, primatology, and sexology. In R. Porter & M. Teich (Eds.), *Sexual knowledge, sexual science: The history of attitudes to sexuality* (pp. 184–209). New York, NY: Cambridge University Press.

Vieira, E. M. (2002). *A medicalização do corpo feminino*. Rio de Janeiro: Editora FIOCRUZ.

Williams, G. (1989). Hope for the humblest? The role of self-help in chronic illness: The case of ankylosing spondylitis. *Sociology of Health and Illness, 11*, 135–159.

10 "As God Is My Witness . . ."

What Is Said, What Is Silenced in Informal Cancer Caregivers' Narratives

Natalia Luxardo

Cancer patients, especially those who are in the final stages of life, have multifaceted needs including disease and treatment monitoring, symptom and pain management, medication administration and assistance with personal care, daily activities of living, and emotional distress (van Ryn et al., 2011). In private, for-profit health care systems, such as the ones found in the United States and in parts of Europe, much of this care has been moved from the in-patient arena to outpatient and ambulatory settings, with a shift in responsibility for the day-to-day care of patients from institutions to their families (Given, Gien & Kozachik, 2001; van Ryn et al., 2011). Informal caregivers in the global north are most likely to be spouses or female relatives who provide these services without pay and often without training or assistance from medical personnel. Hayman et al. (2001) estimate the financial value of the labor provided by US caregivers, 62% of whom are female, for elderly cancer patients at 1 billion dollars annually (p. 3223). Although this unpaid labor helps support the profitability of health systems, it comes at great costs to those providing the care, who are at higher risk of depression, cardiovascular disease and mortality (Schultz & Sherwood, 2008). Much of the strain of caregiving as well as the suffering of patients is intensified by the relative social isolation of the nuclear family. The caregiver often not only feels responsible for caring for the physical needs of the patient, but also for trying to help the patient emotionally and spiritually.

In other high resource nations with systems of universal health care, governments may provide institutional options like hospice with trained medical personnel to care for those dying of cancer. Yet, as Harris notes in her chapter for this volume, dying patients in Scotland often feel lonely and isolated, cut off from family and friends, and unable to talk about their fears of dying with anyone. Although physical needs are met, patients often have unresolved emotional and spiritual concerns as they face death (Murray, Grant, Grant & Kendall, 2003).

Few studies examine the issues facing informal caregivers and patients dying of cancer in middle resource nations with hybrid national systems of care. This chapter attempts to do so by exploring the circumstances and issues faced by family members providing care to cancer patients dying at home or in a hospice setting in Argentina. Specific topics include the pathways into caregiving, the roles and burdens of caregivers, the psychodynamics of what is said and unsaid in the caregiving relationship, and recommendations for future policy and support of caregivers in Argentina. This chapter will outline the political and social contexts in which caregiving is embedded and deliberately focus on the dark side of caregiving to give visibility to caregivers' narratives of suffering and frustration as a first step toward achieving social transformation.

THE ARGENTINIAN HEALTH CARE SYSTEM

Argentina has developed a mixed health care system, which is composed of three sectors: an extensive and centralized public sector (mostly financed by taxes); the social security sector, that is, the delivery of medical care to people formally employed (with funds contributed by employers and employees through obligatory social security schemes); and the private sector (financed by voluntary insurance schemes) used mainly by middle-upper and upper classes. These are overseen by the Ministry of Health, which sets regulations, evaluates the system and collects statistics. According to Belmartino (2000), the country spends approximately 8–10% of GDP on health annually.

Penchaszadeh, Leone & Rovere (2010, p. 351) pointed out that: "during the economic crises of the 1980s and 1990s, the International Monetary Fund and the World Bank imposed privatizations that weakened the public system by successive fragmentations, decentralizations, and dilution of responsibilities, while the social security and private systems hybridized and increased their complexity, to the benefit of the profit-seeking sector." As a result, health services were further privatized and transferred to the provinces, increasing their fragmentation, segmentation and inequity.

Since 2001, the number of Argentines relying on public services has seen an increase, in part also because of the financial crises the nation has experienced in that time. Although medical care is free in the public sector, there are often long waiting lists for services. As a result, this hybridized system provides different types and levels of care to people, depending upon their occupations, personal financial resources and geographic location (Belmartino, 2000, p. 57).

According to the International Agency Research on Cancer Report (WHO/IARC, 2008), Argentina is one of the countries in Latin American and the Caribbean experiencing the greatest cancer burden. Like most countries in the region, it is undergoing an epidemiological transition, facing what is known as the double burden of chronic and infectious diseases. Specifically, the public health system faces the following issues in providing cancer care: the need to improve access, availability and quality of cancer treatment centers; limited access to affordable cancer drugs; and the need to increase the public health priority and resources for cancer in the public health agenda. With regards to palliative care, there are wide disparities in the capacity, resources and infrastructure dedicated to the care of people with life-limiting illnesses within the nation.

RESEARCH GOALS AND METHODS

After several years of studying the impact of cancer as a social phenomenon, I began to explore what would happen if the secondary aspects were treated as the main issues. Instead of focusing on the patients' voices and experiences, this study emphasizes the voices and perspectives of the people who stand by and support them day after day all through the cancer trajectory: feeling shocked with the first diagnoses of cancer, suffering the difficulties of dealing with symptoms and treatments, and fearing the uncertainty of the future when facing a terminal prognoses. These significant others, the caregivers, became the main interlocutors of the healthcare system.

This research was carried out with two sets of people: families attended to in a Palliative Care Service of a general hospital and families cared for by a hospice located in Buenos Aires province. Colleagues and I conducted previous research in both institutions on the complex interrelationships among patients, caregivers/families and healthcare teams at critical care times, recording what the experience of caring was like for caregivers of patients with advanced, life-threatening, noncurable disease (cancer in most of the cases). This chapter draws on data from these two previous studies, on which I served as the principal investigator (Luxardo, 2011), and turns a critical interpretive eye to use these data to answer new questions.

Participants included caregivers of a dying cancer patient receiving palliative care services at home and caregivers of dying persons receiving hospice care services also at home. Families included in this study were either caring for a terminal patient, or within six months of the death of the patient. Data were collected using semi-structured interviews conducted in patients' homes, and in some cases with open-ended, tape-recorded interviews. The biographical forms filled by the staff during the last year, recording the interventions for patient and family assessment, are another important source of data along with letters of recognition, complaints and other correspondence written by relatives to the hospice or palliative unit.

In the first institution, the Palliative Care Service at the hospital Instituto A. Lanari, the research was conducted during 2007 and 2008. This study included 50 families. In these families, 84% of the caregivers were women, most of them over 60, and more than 74% were spouses or daughters. In the second institution, Hospice San Camilo, the research was conducted during 2010 and 2011. For this study, we included 40 families, in which 70% of the main caregivers were women. Out of this 70%, three-quarters of the time the female caregiver was either the spouse or the daughter of the patient. Both groups of respondents were relatively homogenous in socioeconomic status (middle and middle-low class). More difficult economic conditions were more common among families attended to at the hospice.

Data were analyzed through repeated readings and listening to tapes, comparing among them, and identifying emergent themes. A form of constant comparative analysis was used to generate three main themes: the process of becoming a caregiver; the consequences in caregivers' lives, including perceptions and feelings aroused by the burdensome implications of caring; and the role played by structural forces in configuring the caring situation. Patient narratives were considered as open-ended and uncertain, always shifting, configurations of unfolding stories over which they had only partial control (Mattingly, 2010). People living with cancer and relatives in a caring situation will be referred to throughout the text as patients and caregivers, respectively.

TURNING INTO A CAREGIVER

"Who's the caregiver?" He doesn't have any, we couldn't afford it. He's only with me, I'm in charge of everything, from 7 am to 7 am . . . Well, what to do? I'm his wife.

First, it is important to clarify why I use the term caregiver when it is often ignored by subjects themselves. Heaton (1999) locates the emergence of discourses on informal caregivers in the 1970s. Before then, only the patient had been the focus of interest for scholars (Ellis-Hill & Payne, 2001) and policymakers (Twigg & Atkin, 1994). The incipient literature on this social group was characterized by two main preconceptions: care understood as a difficult and debilitating activity, and policy initiatives that emphasized alleviating the *burden of care* through interventions based upon therapeutic models. During the 1980s another vision arose that highlighted the potential of care to be a satisfactory activity and a source of identity, thus, positive caregivers' responses were also reported (Davies, 1980; Nolan, 2001). Yet, most research that emphasized the value of informal caregivers viewed them only as reporters of patients' symptoms or as inexpensive care providers.

In the 1990s, more discussion arose about the political side of caregiving. Some governments formulated documents and national policies such as Caring about Caregivers: A National Strategy for Caregivers (United Kingdom), which emphasized the provision of information about and for caregivers, support for caregivers, and care for caregivers (Lloyd, 2000). Caregivers' organizations were actively involved in this process (Lloyd, 2000), making this group's needs visible.

The inclusion of the term *caregiver* in this chapter is in consonance with Ungerson's (2000) assertion that the development of benefits for caregivers is based on the identification, defining and naming of one as a caregiver. As Wallerstein (1995) suggests, groupism is at play here, defined as "the construction of defensive groups, each of which asserts an identity around which it builds solidarity and struggles to survive alongside and against another groups" (pp. 6–7). The campaigns by caregivers for recognition were essential to enabling them to develop a political voice, yet not all nations have caregiver lobbies and in some cases, those providing informal assistance to cancer patients do not so label themselves.

"WHAT I'M GONNA DO? SHE'S MY MOTHER": CARING IS NOT ALWAYS A CHOSEN DESTINY

Relatives and friends often take on the caring role without choice and may be unaware of the extent and nature of what the caring role implies (Ellis-Hill, 2001). Thus, they assume the role because they feel obligated to provide care, a situation defined primarily by the relationship they have with the patient. It is seen as embedded in the responsibility and duties that the bond imposes. For example, we identified female caregivers who had separated or divorced, yet still felt responsible for the care of ex-husbands. Most of these participants reported that the children they had in common was the reason: "He is the father of my kids, I cannot leave him alone"; "I'm doing this for my son. He is a good guy, with his own problems. He doesn't deserve it [to deal with]." Many caregivers are also motivated by reciprocity (Finch & Mason, 1993) because they know that at some point they may need to be cared for and hope that someone else will repay the services they have provided.

When someone is defined as a caregiver, he or she may come to feel they exist only in relation to the patient and not as individuals with his or her own needs (Ellis-Hill, 2001). Caring relationships are defined by pre-existing personalities and roles, which give sense and meaning to many decisions. For example, when staff and secondary caregivers insist on the hospitalization of a patient due to caregiver exhaustion and caregivers refuse to do so, even with the last quota of energy consumed, the decision is not irrational or obstinate. When reviewing their life story, partnership is an important factor: "he doesn't deserve it, he was always by my side." From the caregivers' perspective, hospitalization would mean *"abandonment."* Such a perspective renders understandable family decisions not to provide direct care. The caregiver subordinates his or her own needs to those of the patient.

Caregivers' Daily Dealings

A primary caring activity is medication administration. Metha, Cohen, Ezer, Carnevale and Ducharme (2011) found that many times relatives cannot decipher the exact type of suffering of the patient, so they give patients the wrong medicines. Or they do not give any medication because they think the complaints have to do with psychological or spiritual issues. At other times, they may respond to emotional issues by giving medication. For example, caregivers in our study talked about giving patients sleep medications because "*he's complaining too much,*" which might not be from pain but from the fear of death.

The labors caregivers perform are not only related to patient arrangements. Ordinary life with its routines and activities continues and caregivers must handle these responsibilities along with work outside the home and responsibilities to other relatives. Fulfilling the caring role and meeting the other demands on them can be difficult. Even the challenge of synchronizing competing demands can be difficult when certain routine activities are so attached to the caregiver's life and identity that they cannot be sacrificed. In this sense, there are social parameters that determine which activities are worth doing and which are not. For example, one respondent noted,

> My sister has kids. So, she only comes [to take care of her sick father] for a couple of hours, or less. And of course, nobody demands more of her time. I have lived with my parents for 35 years now. All my life I have spent running after them. But if I said that I'm going to a club they would accuse me of being selfish. Maybe it is true, but it is like the air, I need that time off for . . . nothing, nothing, just doing what I want, doesn't matter how stupid and irrelevant it might be for the others.
>
> (Matilde, daughter)

Most of the caregivers we interviewed ceased their leisure activities while caregiving at the patient's end of life. There were *more important issues* to think about. They felt ashamed of asking for time off because they wanted to laugh, relax or have fun. Many respondents considered whether others would think that their desires to take time off were legitimate or not, saying things like, "Do you think it is okay to visit my friend and have dinner with my husband dying?" "What will they think of me if I tell them I'm going shopping just in these moments?" Caregivers were consistently aware of social expectations and pressures upon them as they tried to perform the role.

Among caregivers who were still working, especially those working full-time, there were numerous challenges, particularly if the caregiving became long term. Employers were not always sympathetic, and absences from work sometimes resulted in job loss. Such loss impacted self-identity. As Rose (2001) noted, "the categories of experience are intimately linked to one another. Work affects not only time available for caring and finances, but also social relationships and a person's whole perception of self and position in society" (p. 70). Loss of income at a time when there is an increase of costs can be critical. Even when oncology treatment and palliative drugs are provided by the state, other costs caused financial strain: formal caregivers, other medication (not opioids), special needs and equipment. Arrosi et al. (2007) carried out a survey of 120 cervical cancer patients to measure the socioeconomic impact borne by patients and their relatives. Households of patients report a reduction in hours of work, work interruption and loss of family income. As a result these households reported a reduction in their daily food intake, delays in paying for essential services, the sale of properties and use of savings (p. 338).

Burden of Care

Participants discussed the lack of sun, freedom and peace as key burdens resulting from caregiving. Primary caregivers reported feeling left alone by relatives, friends, the healthcare system and society. It was not a problem of quantity, because it did not seem to matter how many people might be around them: "you close the door, and you are alone, I'm the only soul he [her husband] has to hear his complaints, to bear his discomfort and to smell his [bad] odors." The miseries associated with end-of-life care are intimately experienced by caregivers, often in isolation. Patients, moreover, perceived caregivers, especially spouses, as part of themselves, and relied heavily on them. However, for caregivers bearing this weight alone can be challenging:

> Fine? Oh, my God, I can't believe what I have just heard! Did you answer "fine" [after the nurse asked him how he felt]? The hell with you Alberto! I've spent the whole night without having a second of peace because you were bothering me with demands and demands, complaints and complaints, noises and yells, and when there is the person to tell all these things [the nurse] you just told her "fine"? Who the hell understands you?

Caregivers have to bear loneliness and isolation. As many authors have previously noted (Ellis-Hill & Payne, 2001), few secondary caregivers are involved in the day-to-day support of patients. When friends and relatives visit the patient, they often arrive at once, causing extra work for the primary caregiver (e.g., preparing coffees or meals and cleaning up the mess after their departure). Dozens of people might come and go, but most of the time, only one caregiver is by the patient's side all of the time. Everything depends upon a single person whose identity is limited by this temporary role.

Patients sometimes feel overwhelmed by constant visitors; they want to be calm and quiet and not feel forced to talk or smile in front of others. Thus, they try to avoid being with friends and relatives, except the closest ones. Caregivers' worlds are *eaten* by the needs of patients, who many times refuse to accept anyone else besides the primary caregiver (a wife or daughter, often) to look after them. As a participant stated: "The sick person finally digs the grave of the healthy one." And the caregiver feels helpless to change this absolute dependence.

The healthcare system has a role here as well. Ellis-Hill (2001) writes that the system expects that a single person will be involved in the patient's matters. When all expectations rely upon the primary caregivers other actors with important roles are blurred from the scene. Sheldon, Turner & Wee (2001) argued for the importance of attending to broader relationships among formal and informal systems.

Caregivers' narratives also highlight how difficult it is for them to ask for *favors* on behalf of the patient (e.g., someone to drive them to the doctor). Eventually, many caregivers tend to keep problems to themselves and have difficulty negotiating for assistance or cooperating with others. Their despair can lead to depression and feelings of invisibility. Sometimes, being able to talk about their roles as patient supports was the only relief these caregivers had (Linderholm & Friederichsen, 2010). Alternatively, younger caregivers were more likely to argue for their *right* to receive help and assistance from the palliative care staff and from the rest of the family.

The second issue analyzed within the burden of care is the feeling expressed in some narratives that caring for someone who is dying consumed the life of the caregiver, not metaphorically but literally. In this regard, a number of scholars (Kutner et al., 2009; Lee, 2001; Rose, 2001) have identified stressors that can negatively impact the physical, psychological and emotional health of caregivers. For example, Hudson, Zordan and Trauer (2011) found that 44% of the caregivers in their study had a probable anxiety and/ or depressive disorder, with 40% scoring more than the cutoff score for probable anxiety and 20% scoring more than the cutoff score for probable depression. Anderson (1988) reported that family members found it distressing to see their relatives dependent and restricted. Sleep disturbance also affects caregivers both physically and psychologically and results in feelings of isolation (Rose, 2001).

In addition, caregivers are challenged to perform tasks for which they may feel unprepared, or at least, are not used to doing (Rose, 2001). Docherty et al. (2008) reviewed the information needs of informal caregivers in palliative settings (1994–2006) and identified that in the 34 studies included (from eight different countries), there is weak evidence for caregivers' knowledge and information needs in relation to welfare and social support. Goldschmidt, Schmidt, Krasnik, Christensen and Groenvold (2006) argue that caregivers expect medical team members to have specialized knowledge in palliative care and to improve their sense of security being at home. Some academics have pointed out that the most important need for caregivers is psychological (Hudson, Thomas, Trauer, Remedios & Clarke, 2011). Others state that the most important need is practical, such as the need for information (Ellis-Hill, 2001; Rosenthal, Pituch, Greninger & Metress, 1993). There are enough studies to support each of them.

The family caregivers in this study describe themselves as bearing primary responsibility in caring for their dying relatives. They had many concerns about their own situation, especially in regard to what might happen after the death of the patient, but seemed to have few sources of support related to these concerns. Professional support was described as expected primarily for care-related tasks, although hopes were expressed about social and emotional support as well. The distinction between resources described as existing in theory and those used in practice were also apparent in the interviews (Wennman-Larsen & Tishelman, 2002). Caregivers reported living in conditions of uncertainty, as the patients' constant physical, emotional and cognitive changes were unpredictable. Sudden outbursts by caregivers telling their stories and crying out of control were not uncommon and illustrate the despair many caregivers feel when they have no support and are unsure of how to cope with patient needs.

Another impact is in the social life of the patient, so many times postponed, as this narrative expresses: "The whole day in my father's house, looking after him, talking with the doctors, preparing the food, going in the middle of the night when the [formal] caregiver called me because something is wrong . . . I have a family, **I had** my own family and I'm feeling it's lost just because I disappeared from their lives for the sake of my father's . . ."

Many times caregivers bear the weight of crucial decisions that involve others. They are the ones to tell daughters and sons living far away that it is time to come be with the parent who is dying. Caregivers reported waiting until the last days to do so, and living with the stress that such waiting and measuring of time caused, in order not to inconvenience the children. As someone commented during a post-bereavement interview:

> Carla arrived when her father was in agony. She couldn't say goodbye to him. Well, she did, but at a moment when he was unable to recognize anything. Before that, he was asking for her constantly . . . I tried to manage myself with everything until the last minute. Carla has her own kids, her job. But, but I think I knew that she could only be here for a couple of days, and preferred those days when she could help me with the death arrangements. I thought I wouldn't be able to do so.

Many caregivers as a result cared not just for the patient but for the whole family and became overprotective of children and older spouses. Thus the amount of emotional energy expended was even greater. They learned how to fake smiles, to relax their face as if nothing happened, to hide their worries. Such situations were magnified when patients and family members had a past history of negative experiences such as alcoholism, interpersonal violence or living with debts.

CAREGIVERS' SILENCES

Unconfessed Wishes

The first expectations and thoughts caregivers fear to recognize as their own have to do with wishing death to occur soon: "I'm ashamed to confess you, but it's either his life or will be mine," "You are not supposed to be expecting the death of the person you love, but lately . . . I realized that it has been my only thought, and I wonder what that 24-hours-sleepy-complaining- and-dependent man has to do with the one I once fell in love with."

We noticed that among hospice caregivers, there is a kind of permission granted for using the name of *God* frequently in their narratives: God's plans, God's will, God's sake, appeared much more often than in narratives of caregivers with patients in palliative care services. It is not that caregivers accompanied by the hospice staff were necessarily more religious, but that their discourses about and interpretations of their situation reverted more to religious justifications, because this was the hospice background. In fact, data showed that half of the families in hospice care were either atheist or did not care about religion. Among the other half, most were Catholic, and some of Jewish or Protestant faiths. Only 22% answered positively when they were asked if they were active practitioners of their religion, measured in terms of rituals and expected behaviors as stipulated by their own religious criteria and parameters (Luxardo, 2011). Within this religious framework, the reference to God sometimes served as a kind of *alter ego* for their own voices, as they knew it was not politically correct to say or to think something like that. Thus, "I don't know why God makes it last so much," "God's mercy is not working with my husband, he shouldn't be alive by now under these circumstances . . ." and so on are phrases associated with inner conceptions about the injustice of the situation, which may not be God's ideas nor intentions but those of the caregiver.

Caregivers in our study, however, did not only express hidden wishes for death. Sometimes they expressed direct desires to accelerate the process: "I could kill him and make his sufferings shorten," "I can't promise you I wouldn't be able to help her get rid of this once forever," or as jokes and sarcasms: "Alcohol in the wound? Oh yes, and then some fire and we are all done!" Neither euthanasia nor assisted suicide is legal in Argentina, but many times the dying are assisted into a faster death indirectly. Relatives sometimes press and push professionals to do so. In fact, in a survey conducted amongst private physicians, 26% noted having accelerated a patient's death through medication forced by pressure from a relative or patient request (Cohen Agrest, 2008). The Senate and House of Deputies of Argentina passed a law in 2012, locally known as the *Death with Dignity Law*, giving terminally ill patients and their families the right to make their own decisions at the end of life, such as the refusal of treatment to prolong life (either mechanically or through medication), anticipated directives that can be signed by the patient or decided by someone else authorized, among many other issues that do not include euthanasia nor assisted suicide.

Besides expressed thoughts and wishes, caregivers also expressed frustration and exhaustion with the role in less direct ways. One of these was through negligence in the provision of care, which might take the form of changing prescriptions, poor pain management, *forgetting* patients' requests, using boiling water to wash patients' hands instead of warm, leaving the patient for hours in the same position resulting in bedsores, or neglecting to change overflowing diapers.

When lucid, many patients expressed feelings of insecurity and vulnerability because they recognized that their caregivers were overstressed and in difficulty. In some cases, when the caregiver left the bedroom, they asked to be transferred either to the hospital or to the hospice. Nonetheless, ironically, even neglectful caregivers often resisted any attempt by the staff and the secondary caregivers to change the situation. Medical staff often wanted to neutralize the caregiver, but the caregivers interpreted this as a negative judgment about their own abilities and levels of dedication.

In some cases, caregivers became angry with patients and yelled at them, even in presence of others. Minor events could trigger emotional outbursts from overstressed caregivers such as not following caregivers' instructions or directives. In these situations, verbal and psychological mistreatment were at the extreme. Patients were blamed for being lazy, for *abandoning* themselves. Caregivers felt the need to shake the patients, because they felt patients considered themselves as already dead. Sometimes harsh words were spoken, as this sister stated:

> You will be rotting in a coffin soon, don't worry about that, but not now, not today, not in my house! For God's sake, do something, put energy at least in spending this last moments with your [11-years-old] kid. Day after day watching TV. You are hurrying your death with that zombie's attitude, and I won't be your accomplice. Either you change or I will leave you at the hospital to be cared for by nurses.

The pieces of narratives transcribed next clarified the last type of unconfessed wishes we identified among caregivers—the ones related to the *redemption* of the caregiver:

> He deserves it [what he is suffering now]. He never cared for anybody except himself, he will live the humiliation of depending on others for the more basic things, such as eating or going to the toilet, as I've been humiliated during the last three decades when I needed to implore to get some money to buy food for my kids and myself.
>
> (Nora, 64)

> Well, there must be a reason to explain why he is going through this. Everything is paid in life, everything, nothing you do is free, consequences sooner or later come, and it was too much what he did to me.
>
> (Graciela, 56)

> My husband has always been a difficult man. We have spent 54 years together. He yelled at me so many times, he insulted me for so many days that you cannot figure out how happy I felt when doctor said he

wouldn't be able to talk again [due to the throat cancer]. If God takes him away, I will be finally in peace. Otherwise, what I'm gonna do? I will endure him some other time, but God knows why I will never be the best nurse . . .

(Rosa, 82)

These narratives express that death will bring justice to the caregiver and family members and highlight the ambivalence that many feel providing care to people who have mistreated them in the past.

CAREGIVERS' WORDS AS A DEFINITION OF PATIENT WORLDS

Favret-Saada (1980), among others, has analyzed the ways in which ideas have the power to create or to destroy worlds. As McMullin and Weiner (2008) argue, "language, whether spoken or silent, often assists the creation or continuation of the universe. From this perspective, the idea or the word is the mother or father of the reality or the deed" (p. 13). Caregivers in this study felt that their last words and actions were charged with some special power that made them responsible for patient deaths. "I shouldn't have moved away from her side [the morning she died]." Or on the contrary, caregivers felt the patient might want to die but could not do so because the relatives would not allow it. "He's waiting us to be ready [to pass away]. But we will never be ready for that. Never. When I said 'dad, see you in the morning' it is like a promise I force him to keep for not leaving me during the night."

In situations such as this, being transferred to the hospital was suggested by health personnel; however, when that happened and the patient finally died in the hospital, other issues arose. Caregivers felt the urgent need to reconstruct the last moments of the patient's life. "Please help me to find out what happened at the end, how were his/her last moments?" Caregivers could not find peace until they knew exactly what happened in these last moments. Many expressed guilt for not having been by the dying, even when they had spent the whole illness trajectory together.

A challenge for those remaining in the home was palliative sedation, the responsibility for which rested with caregivers. The progressive increase of the medication (drops of morphine) in the presence of the patients' last symptoms was difficult to gauge. "If he can't move? If he is moving too much? But when exactly?" Many felt overwhelmed by these decisions, insecure of the directives, although secondary caregivers (usually children) and the staff shaped an alliance to insist that the primary caregiver medicate the patient. We observed primary caregivers who were offended and hurt by being responsible for palliative sedation near death. Some caregivers put it clearly and explicitly. "I feel I'm killing her," "No food, no water, they [palliative nurses] told me it's the best for him, otherwise he could choke or vomit, but it's terrible, terrible [outburst crying]. I wonder if he is feeling, dying of starvation, such cruelty . . . Oh, God! Not even dogs deserve to be treated like that." To make matters worse, patients often experienced an unexpected recovery, extending the agony of dying over days instead of the originally anticipated few hours. We observed caregiver anger and impotence in such moments.

In post-bereavement interviews, when the crises caused by the arrival of the last moments in the life was over and after the burial and immediate post-death arrangements had occurred, we observed a shift in perception of caregivers. What they did, what they said, what they thought about the patient was placed under scrutiny. No matter how events might have finally ended, each word, each thought and each silence was evaluated time and again. For those caregivers who had been forced into the decision to medicate at death or to send relatives to the hospital to die, this process of self-recrimination was intense, which suggests that the act of forcing caregivers to certain actions in the absence of social and emotional support is problematic for their long-term adjustment to the event.

Among our informants, Julio, a 78-year-old retired husband who took care of his wife for two years, was angry with his sons and the palliative staff, because at the last moments they convinced him to hospitalize his wife, where she finally died. After her death he felt an inner remorse because he had not been by her side. It did not matter that he had stayed by her side, day after day, as she went through chemotherapy, had cleaned her after vomiting, had listened to her prayers, cried by her side, prepared her food, shared her hopelessness. Now that all it was over, he remarked, "*I failed her.*" He felt weak because being outnumbered by staff and relatives, he had been unable to continue arguing to keep her at home in spite of the exhaustion everybody noticed in him. This led Julio to question what had happened. Did she suffer? Did anyone take her hand at the end? Did she feel lonely with no relatives close by? Many caregivers went through such self-examinations after death, wondering if they had failed in fulfilling their obligations to the deceased.

THE POLITICAL AND SOCIAL CONTEXT OF CAREGIVING

Familism and the Role of Gender

Our study raised questions about the assumed prevalence and homogeneity of *familism* among Latinos. The assumption that all Latinos are naturally family-oriented does not necessarily hold true for every situation. Sharing enjoyable moments can be different than sharing the care of someone about to die. Family members in our study stayed in touch with caregivers but were not necessarily involved in day-to-day care. They could also be controlling, judgmental, reproachful and critical of the decisions made by primary caregivers. Moral condemnation (e.g., for hospitalizing the patient, not caring for him or her properly, taking time away) was always a threat felt by caregivers. Our work suggests that at times familism can add to, rather than relieve, the stress and burden of caregivers.

As Lee (2001) remarks in her gender-based analysis of family caregiving, the home-based care of the dying is a responsibility that falls disproportionately on women. Researchers and policy makers tend to ignore the gender inequities, "which are perpetuated by an assumption that family caregiving is naturally the work of women" (p. 123). In our study, the majority of caregivers were women (usually spouses or daughters). It was assumed by society that these women would continue to fulfill all domestic duties to others in the household while also assuming care of the dying. In addition, women were expected to be better able to manage social and emotional issues than men and were so called upon frequently to mediate family disputes and listen to the patients' fears. This led to often overwhelming burdens on female caregivers resulting in sleep disturbances, emotional outbursts and depression.

Arber and Gilberts (1989) maintain that when the kinship is spousal, there are few differences between genders and that men are as involved as women in the caring commitment to the patient. Although we had fewer male caregivers in our study, we did find elderly male caregivers (spouses) were very vulnerable as they lacked the social capital to deal with caring; they were ashamed to ask questions when they did not understand what to do about prescriptions, they were unable to move up appointments, and they found it extremely difficult to juggle house responsibilities (e.g., cooking and cleaning) with the caring activities.

Social Policies

Families face increased pressure to provide care to their terminally ill or dying kin in the home. It is known that balancing care with other personal and social roles can adversely affect caregivers' health, yet access to supportive services that can mitigate caregiver burden is often inadequate. Hudson, Thomas, Traver, Remedios & Clarke (2011) and Thomas (2008) explored policies that include the context of caring, in order to identify whether or not these policies take into consideration families' needs and obstacles to health care services. They identified many barriers to the best possible health services inherent in bureaucratic structures. For example, although having patients remain in their homes with informal caregivers reduces financial costs, the costs to the caregivers and families are often extreme. When health systems such as the one in Argentina provide unequal access to medical care and support services, caregivers may not be able to perform their roles adequately. Moreover, when health systems do intervene to assist caregivers, these interventions often focus on improving the coping strategies of caregivers instead of improving the access to services or reducing costs of care.

As Lee (2001) writes, "The burden of caregiving is not insignificant, and there is a need for analyses and interventions that address issues of public policy rather than the individual woman and her personal ability to cope" (p. 123). The promotion of home care reduces expenditures at a public level but does not contribute to the closing of the gap of sociomedical disparity, reproducing or even expanding the social inequality in access to or utilization of healthcare services.

CONCLUSION: NOT SICK, OVERWHELMED

What we should be worried about, as we consider our disciplinary position as producers and consumers of knowledge in the global political economy, is the pressing question of "so what"?

(Janes & Corbett, 2010, p. 415)

Amelia has spent the last four months taking care of Pedro, her 74-year-old husband with pulmonary metastasis. She washes him, changes his diapers, prepares his food—tries to adapt to the multiple prescriptions that he requires now—asks for consultations, stands by him at night when nightmares and fear arise. Her husband suffers pain controlled by a strict regime of opioids every six hours, exhaustive fatigue which causes him to rely upon her to stand (he weighs almost 85 kilos). Amelia, 72 years old, is like a robot about to burn. She never complains, she never explodes in anger, it's not her style and from her perspective there would not be any justification. "Care in case of illness" she promised in front of God almost 50 years ago. "What am I'm gonna do, then?" she asked in resignation. However, it is clear that she's not really asking, there is no other option for her but the one she is involved in. There is nothing to do but to stand by him day after day, night after night, bearing everything alone, no matter her wishes, her wellness, herself. With the best facade in her face, doing what she had to do, until the end (hospice fieldnotes, July 2011).

Although my description of Amelia's sacrifice may be somewhat biased by my outsider perspective, it remains clear that she is in a vulnerable position and the system fails to support her. Vulnerability is measured by delays in attending to her own health, by her exhaustion after months without sleeping and eating well, by the sadness she is experiencing over the imminent loss of her partner, by her isolation from friends and relatives and by her abandonment of enjoyable activities since the caring began.

Yet, she did not openly complain or express frustration with knowing that nothing can be done to stop death. She did not make explicit demands of significant others in Pedro's life who might have been concerned about his situation but who were not involved in his daily care. When staff interventions address the burden of care, in the case of Amelia but also in others, they frequently offer psychological interventions to help caregivers cope, but they fail to offer her the practical support she clearly needs, but is unable to request.

If caregivers continue to be viewed as victims, interventions will continue to focus on psychological coping. There needs be a shift in the biomedical community from treating caregivers as sick to seeing them as overwhelmed and in need of concrete support for their daily labors. At the same time, it is important to recognize when concrete support is no longer enough and when caregiving needs to end. Negligence in the caring activities that leads to poor pain management, inability to manage the patient's daily activities and expressed wishes for the patient's death is a clue that something is dramatically wrong in the caring situation and that the caregiver is no longer able to function effectively. At that point, there needs to be a change in the situation itself. Dying at home is not always the best option, but hospitalization might not be either. In the first instance, the physical and emotional health of the caregiver can be compromised. In the second, the caregiver may feel extreme distress over not being present to assist with death and may suffer psychologically long after bereavement.

Current strategies in Argentina and in other systems where care of the dying is being shifted more and more to families fail to address the complex nature of caring relationships; there is too much emphasis on coping in lieu of providing the basic support services caregivers need in order to fulfill their roles. An ethnography of caring that considers caring not as a private issue, as many stakeholders insist, but a public one that requires public answers, is important at this juncture.

As social scientists who believe in the role of research in helping achieve social transformation, we are committed to making the complexity behind caregiving visible. The analysis of caregiver narratives helps make their issues and needs apparent. By addressing these issues, we hope to expand beyond individually focused interventions based on an assumption of victimhood. Most of the time, caregivers are not sick. They do not (necessarily) need more visits with psychologists, psychiatrists, social workers or counselors. The caregivers in this study require more daily assistance with the tasks they are being asked to perform on behalf of the health care system including training in how to manage cancer and administer medications, support with transportation and equipment needs, back up assistance to provide time for household duties and personal needs, and information on the process and stages of death itself. In addition, caregivers struggle in a system of fragmented care when physician directives are confusing and contradictory and where palliative care options are lacking. Palliative care began in Argentina in 1990 and has a low priority in the public health system compared with preventive and curative services (Wenk, 2009). There is no national health policy to implement palliative care, and its financing remains difficult. As a result, resources to aid with such care come from a diverse mix of sources including charities, volunteers or paid providers when available. At present there are 70 palliative care teams in Argentina, concentrated in large cities, and only a few of these have specific in-patient facilities as there are only 40 palliative care beds in the country (Wenk, 2009, p. 351). It has been estimated that less than 5% of the patients who need palliative care in Argentina receive it. The remainder relies on informal caregivers to minister to their needs at home or they receive aggressive medical interventions when in crisis in hospitals. Our data clearly illustrate the need for a coordinated national palliative care plan to provide services not just to patients in need but to empower and equip their caregivers to assist them at home. The development of more coordinated palliative care services in Argentina along with support teams for caregivers and patients with terminal conditions could help to alleviate many of the problems caregivers report in our study.

REFERENCES

Anderson, R. (1988). The quality of life of stroke patients and their carers. In R. Anderson & M. Bury (Eds.), *Living with chronic illness: The experience of patients and their families* (pp. 89–116). London: Unwin Hyman.
Arber, S., & Gilberts, N. (1989). Men: The forgotten carers. *Sociology, 23,* 111–118.
Arrosi, S., Matos, E., Zengarini, N., Roth, B., Sankaranayananan, R., & Parkin, M. (2007). The socio-economic impact of cervical cancer on patients and their families in Argentina, and its influence on radiotherapy compliance: Results from a cross-sectional study. *Gynecologic Oncology, 105,* 335–340.
Belmartino, S. (2000). Reorganizing the health care system in Argentina. In S. Fleury, S. Belmartino & E. Baris (Eds.), *Reshaping health care in Latin America: A comparative analysis of health care reform in Argentina, Brazil, and Mexico* (pp. 47–78). Ottawa, Canada: International Development Research Centre.
Cohen Agrest, D. (2008). *¿Qué piensan los que no piensan como yo? Diez controversias éticas.* [What think people that don't think as I do? Ten ethical controversies]. Buenos Aires: Editorial Sudamericana.
Davies, A. J. (1980). Disability, home-care and the care-taking role in family life. *Journal of Advance Nursing, 5,* 475–484.
Docherty, A., Owens, A., Asadi-Lari, M., Petchey R., Williams, J., & Carter, Y. H. (2008). Knowledge and information needs of informal caregivers in palliative care: A qualitative systematic review. *Palliative Medicine, 22,* 153–71.
Ellis-Hill, C. (2001). Caring and identity: The experience of spouses in stroke and other chronic neurological conditions. S. Payne & C. Ellis-Hill (Eds.), *Chronic and terminal illness: New perspectives on caring and caregivers* (pp. 44–63). Oxford: Oxford University Press.
Ellis-Hill, C., & Payne, S. (2001). The future: Interventions and conceptual issues. S. Payne & C. Ellis-Hill (Eds.), *Chronic and Terminal Illness. New perspectives on caring and caregivers* (pp. 155–166). Oxford: Oxford University Press.
Favret-Saada, J. (1980). *Deadly words.* Cambridge, MA: Cambridge University Press.
Finch, J. & Mason, J. (1993). *Negotiating family responsibilities.* London: Routledge.
Given, B. A., Gien C. W., & Kozachik, S. (2001). Family support in advanced cancer. *Cancer Journal for Clinicians, 51,* 213–231.
Goldschmidt, D., Schmidt, L., Krasnik, A., Christensen, U., & Groenvold, M. (2006). Expectations to and evaluation of a palliative home-care team as seen by patients and caregivers. *Supportive Care Cancer, 14,* 1232–1240.

210 *Natalia Luxardo*

Hayman, J. A., Langa, K. M., Kabeto, M. U., Katz, S. J., DeMonner, S. M., Chernew, M. E., . . . & Fendrick, A. M. (2001). Estimating the cost of informal caregiving for elderly patients with cancer. *Journal of Clinical Oncology, 19,* 3219–3225.

Heaton, J. (1999). The gaze and visibility of the carer: A foucauldian analysis of the discourse of informal care. *Sociology of Health and Illness, 21,* 759–777.

Hudson, P. L., Thomas, K., Trauer, T., Remedios, C., & Clarke D. (2011). Psychological and social profile of family caregivers on commencement of palliative care. *Journal of Pain Symptom Management, 41,* 522–534.

Janes, C. R., & Corbett, K. K. (2010). Anthropology and Global Health. In B. J. Good, M. M. Fisher, S. Willen & M. DelVecchio Good (Eds.), *Reader in medical anthropology: Theoretical trajectories, emergent realities* (pp. 405–421). Malden, MA: Wiley-Blackwell.

Kutner, J., Kilbourn, K. M., Costenaro, A., Lee, C. A., Nowels, C., Vancura, J. L., Anderson, D., & Keech, T. E. (2009). Support needs of informal hospice caregivers: a qualitative study. *Journal of Palliative Medicine, 12,* 1101–1104.

Lee, C. (2001). Family caregiving: A gender-based analysis of women's experiences. S. Payne & C. Ellis-Hill (Eds.), *Chronic and terminal illness: New perspectives on caring and caregivers* (pp. 123–139). Oxford: Oxford University Press.

Linderholm, M., & Friedrichsen, M. (2010). A desire to be seen: family caregivers' experiences of their caring role in palliative home care. *Cancer Nursing, 33,* 28–36.

Lloyd, L. (2000). Caring about carers: Only half of the picture? *Critical Social Policy, 20,* 136–150.

Luxardo, N. (2011). *Morir en casa. El cuidado en el hogar en el final de la vida.* [Dying at home. Homecare at the end of life]. Buenos Aires: Biblos Editorial.

Mattingly, C. (2010). The concept of therapeutic 'emplotment'. In B. J. Good, M. M. Fisher, S. Willen & M. DelVecchio Good (Eds.), *Reader in medical anthropology: Theoretical trajectories, emergent realities* (pp. 121–136). Malden, MA: Wiley-Blackwell.

McMullin, J., & Weiner, D. (2008). Introduction. In J. McMullin & D. Weiner (Eds.), *Confronting cancer: Metaphors, advocacy, and anthropology* (pp. 3–26). Santa Fe, NM: School of American Research Press.

Mehta, A., Cohen, S. R., Ezer, H., Carnevale, F. A., & Ducharme, F. (2011). Striving to respond to palliative care patients' pain at home: A puzzle for family caregivers. *Oncology Nursing Forum 1, 38,* 37–45.

Murray, S. A., Grant, E., Grant, A., Kendall, M. (2003). Dying from cancer in developing and developed countries: lessons from two qualitative interview studies of patients and their carers. *British Medical Journal, 326,* 1–5.

Nolan, M. (2001). Positive aspects of caring. In S. Payne & C. Ellis-Hill (Eds.), *Chronic and terminal illness: New perspectives on caring and caregivers* (pp. 22–43). Oxford: Oxford University Press.

Penchaszadeh, V., Leone, F., & Rovere, M. (2010). The health system in Argentina: An unequal struggle between equity and the market. *Italian Journal of Public Health, 7,* 350–359.

Rose, K. (2001). A longitudinal study of caregivers providing palliative care. In S. Payne & C. Ellis-Hill (Eds.), *Chronic and terminal illness. New perspectives on caring and caregivers* (pp. 64–82). Oxford: Oxford University Press.

Rosenthal, S., Pituch, M., Greninger, L., & Metress, E. (1993). Perceived needs of wives of stroke patients. *Rehabilitation, 18,* 148–167.

Schultz, R., & Sherwood, P. R. (2008). Physical and mental effects of family caregiving. *American Journal of Nursing, 1008,* 23–27.

Sheldon, F., Turner, P., & Wee, B. (2001). The contribution of carers to professional education. In S. Payne & C. Ellis-Hill (Eds.), *Chronic and terminal illness: New perspectives on caring and carers* (pp. 140–154). Oxford: Oxford University Press.

Thomas, C. (2008). Cancer narratives and methodological uncertainties. *Qualitative Research, 8,* 423–433.

Twigg, J., & Atkin, K. (1994). *Carers perceived: Policy and practice in informal care.* Buckingham: Open University Press.

Ungerson, C. (2000). Cash in carers. In H. Meyer (Ed.), *Care work, gender labour and the welfare state.* New York, NY: Routledge.

van Ryn, M., Sanders, S., Kahn, K., van Houtven, C., Griffin, J., Martin, M., Atienza, A., Phelan, S., Finstad, D., & Rowland, J. (2011). Objective burden, resources and other stressors among informal cancer caregivers: a hidden quality issue? *Psycho-Oncology, 20,* 44–52.

Wallerstein, I. (1995). *After Liberalism.* New York, NY: The New York Press.

Wenk, R. (2009). Cancer pain-progress and ongoing issues in Argentina. *Pain Research Management, 14,* 350–351.

Wennman-Larsen, A., & Tishelman, C. (2002). Advanced home care for cancer patients at the end of life: A qualitative study of hopes and expectations of family caregivers. *Scandanavian Journal of Caring Sciences, 16,* 240–247.

World Health Organization/ International Agency for Research on Cancer. World Cancer Report 2008. Ed. P. Boyle & B. Lewin (Eds.). Retrieved from http://www. iarc.fr/en/publications/pdfs-online/wcr/2008/

11 Suffering in Local Worlds
Oncological Discourses, Cancer and Infertility in Puerto Rico

Karen E. Dyer[1]

Camila was diagnosed with breast cancer at age 22 in San Juan, Puerto Rico. She had married her childhood sweetheart 18 months earlier and subsequently became pregnant with their first son. While breastfeeding, she found a large lump, which turned out to be an aggressive cancer. She immediately went into treatment with a physician she now declares was incompetent. She received chemotherapy, radiation, and surgery to remove the mass. These treatments, unbeknownst to her then, included a class of chemotherapies called alkylating agents, which are known to cause infertility in the men and women who take them.

Camila had grown up wanting and planning for a large family of six children. The possibility of infertility as a result of her cancer treatments was not discussed with her at the time of diagnosis. Instead, she learned about the risk from another oncologist one year after completing treatment. She was extremely angry about the failure of her first oncologist to disclose this information, especially since he had spent a great deal of time discussing the prospect of hair loss and nausea with her at the beginning of treatment. She maintained that if she had known about the risks of infertility, she would have been willing to pursue egg or embryo freezing in order to ensure her chances of having genetically related offspring. Fortunately, Camila did go on to have another baby a few years later, but she realized that her risk for premature menopause might mean that her second child would be her last. At the time of our interview, Camila remained angry with her oncologist— she believed that he neglected to tell her about the risks of infertility because she already had a child, and he thought it to be unnecessary.

This excerpt is taken from field notes written during an anthropological study of cancer survivorship in Puerto Rico between 2011 and 2012. It illustrates the dilemma of treatment-induced infertility that is all too common among young people suffering from cancer. Infertility can affect both men and women, and is caused by certain classes of chemotherapies, abdominal and pelvic radiation, surgery to the reproductive organs, and bone marrow/ stem cell transplants. Infertility can occur immediately following treatment or years later (Sklar, 2005). In most cases it is the cancer treatments themselves—rather than the disease processes—that create this effect, so it is an issue that crosscuts cancer diagnoses and has the potential to affect a large proportion of reproductive-aged people diagnosed with cancer.

A cohort of assisted reproductive technologies (ARTs) termed *fertility preservation techniques* is available in the United States and many Western countries. Fertility preservation allows newly diagnosed individuals to freeze their sperm, eggs, fertilized embryos, or—more experimentally—ovarian or testicular tissue before cancer treatment begins. They can then use those materials after treatment in order to create a genetically related pregnancy. Because these technologies are expensive and not usually covered by insurance, their use is rare, and much of the current literature in the United States and other Western countries has focused on barriers to access. Of these, patient-provider communication difficulties receive the most attention, because—as Camila's case illustrates—individuals are often not informed of the risks that cancer treatment poses to their reproductive capacities, nor do they receive information about or referrals for fertility-related services from their oncologists.[2]

One of the puzzling questions that arises from Camila's story is why her oncologist discussed hair loss and nausea with her at length but never mentioned the risk of infertility, a situation commonly reported in the academic literature on use of fertility preservation. This chapter argues that while providers themselves may lack knowledge of infertility risks and solutions for them, it is also likely that the goals and assumptions of professional oncology culture, embedded in a Western biomedical framework, direct practitioners to focus on certain issues and practices while ignoring others in response to the life-threatening nature of cancer. For example, Del Vecchio-Good, Good, Schaffer and Lind (1990) demonstrated that the goal of oncologists in America is to instill hope, and to encourage patients to pursue a cure above all else. Similarly, American oncologists in Balshem's (1993) study saw themselves as ultimately responsible for the life or death of the patient and, as a result, thought that patients should pursue all treatment options regardless of negative side effects or costs. These oncologists, moreover, valued patients who demonstrated a fighting spirit and submitted compliantly to medical authority, which suggests that they may fear that if a patient knows about infertility risks, he or she may choose to delay or forego certain curative treatments.

At the same time, the ways that biomedical discourses are appropriated within and shaped by national and regional contexts also influence how physicians communicate with patients about cancer and how patients respond. Del Vecchio-Good, Good, Schaffer & Lind (1990) point out that there "are 'local' (national, provincial, regional) variants of international biomedical culture which are powerfully influenced by societal and institutional contexts, traditional medical cultures, and the history of cosmopolitan medicine within those contexts" (p. 60). Puerto Rico is a particularly important site for a more in-depth examination of these interconnections because of its historic colonial status and ongoing dependency relationship to the United States. Many Puerto Rican physicians, including oncologists and fertility specialists, receive either all or part of their medical training in the United States and return to the island to practice. Thus, American discourses and assumptions related to cancer are incorporated by these medical professionals and shape the local context of cancer care and therapeutic expectations. Accordingly, this chapter examines the social and historical context of population policy and the use of reproductive technologies in Puerto Rico, arguing that the discourses produced through this colonial relationship have shaped the landscape of fertility preservation options open to cancer patients. Two discourses in particular link closely to cancer-related infertility: (1) that of Puerto Rico's "overpopulation problem," a product of the eugenics logic that pervaded public health and development programs throughout the course of the 20th century, and (2) the biomedical and oncological discourses of expert physician as gatekeeper/decision-maker who emphasizes survival from cancer at all costs. Consequently, these discourses are intimately tied to the ways in which patients suffer from the prospect of infertility as well as their (in)ability to make use of limited fertility preservation technologies.

A second implicit goal of this chapter is to illustrate the ways that an anthropological perspective can inform public health practice and policy. By combining an examination of the social and historical context with data from fieldwork conducted in San Juan and Ponce, Puerto Rico, between 2011–2012, this study situates the issue of cancer treatments and infertility risks within a broader context than is normally found in most public health studies. In addition, the use of in-depth interviews with reproductive-aged cancer survivors, oncologists and cancer advocates enables a closer analysis of how the differing goals, values and actions of patients and providers take shape in relationship to each other as a response to both international biomedical practice and national and regional histories. This holistic perspective enables a more nuanced consideration of how the issues surrounding cancer treatments for the young and for the poor are complex ones that are not easily resolved. In the examples to be discussed, both patients and providers struggle to make the right decisions when confronted with cancer and are often uncertain about their choices. Many Puerto Rican young people are particularly sensitive to issues of fertility control, whereas many oncologists see these as secondary to the more important goal of preserving life in the face of cancer. Oncologists sometimes assume that patients with poor prognoses will not live long enough to parent children or that patients who already have a child are not concerned with having more. Alternatively, patients who may be unable to afford or access reproductive technologies may themselves be more focused on a cure, not future childbearing. The ways these conflicts play out reveal a great deal about the complexities of new and emerging contexts of suffering associated with issues of uncertainty and risk that surround cancer and its treatment.

PUERTO RICO AND THE HISTORY OF DEPENDENCY

The archipelago of Puerto Rico lies in the northeastern Caribbean Sea. With a total population of nearly 4 million (US Census Bureau, 2010), it has existed as a colony in one form or another since 1508. The Spanish occupied Puerto Rico for nearly 400 years until 1898, when the colony was ceded to the United States after Spain's loss in the Spanish-American War. It has remained an unincorporated territory under American rule, and since 1952 has been a Commonwealth of the United States (or associated free state) (Cabán, 1993). Day to day, this means that Puerto Ricans are US citizens and subject to the federal laws of the United States, which supersedes territorial law. Yet, they cannot vote in federal elections such as the presidential election, there is no voting member of Congress, and the issue of legal status and relationship to the United States has remained an enduring national controversy (Cabán, 1993; Grosfoguel, 2003).

The lack of voting power means that Puerto Rico has no decisive voice in its own affairs at the federal level, and must rely on gaining the interest and commitment of lawmakers from other states and districts to raise or defend its case in Congress. The significance of this fact cannot be overstated: although structures, institutions and discourses have been imported from the United States into Puerto Rico—including those that create the kind of suffering this volume addresses—as a colony Puerto Rico has limited power to prevent or change those imported features. It can act to alleviate, manipulate or resist some of these features, but at the most basic level, it is not free to govern itself.

The health care situation in Puerto Rico is shaped by this territorial status (Mulligan, 2010). As mentioned earlier, many Puerto Rican physicians move back and forth between the United States and the island for study and work, drawing upon the same professional resources and materials as American doctors and gaining membership in the same associations and societies. Puerto Rico itself boasts a technologically advanced biomedical system that draws would-be patients from around the Caribbean region and, more recently, American "medical tourists" seeking lower-cost, high-quality health care (MTA, 2012). However, it has been challenged in recent years by neoliberal restructuring, the privatization of large parts of the health sector, the dismantling of many public health clinics and hospitals, and the ripple effects of the wide-reaching US recession, which has had exaggerated effects on the island economy (GAO, 2014; PAHO, 2007). Entitlement programs such as Medicaid and Medicare operate on the island; however, the federal government's financial contribution to Puerto Rico's programs is dramatically lower than what is given to states, leaving large gaps for the financially burdened territorial government to fill (Mulligan, 2010). Using the poverty-based calculation that is used for states, Puerto Rico should have received $1.7 billion in 2007 for its Medicaid program versus the actual reimbursement of $219 million (Hayashi, Finnegan, Shin, Jones & Rosenbaum, 2009).

A health care reform was implemented in the early 1990s in order to expand insurance coverage, and although this initiative has resulted in 93% coverage rates, recent evaluations have reported that both the infrastructure and quality of health care have been eroded (Hayashi, Finnegan, Shin, Jones & Rosenbaum, 2009; PAHO, 2007).

From a broader perspective, Puerto Rico's economy has been intimately tied to that of the United States since 1898. Rivera Ramos (2002) argues that the American occupation "set in motion a series of profound economic and social transformations that would eventually change the character of Puerto Rican society" (p. 59). The previously agriculture-based economy was deliberately dismantled in order to make way for industrialization, principally pharmaceutical and petrochemical production (Briggs, 2002; Grosfoguel, 2003; Rivera Ramos, 2002); proceeds from these industries were absorbed by international corporations rather than fed back into Puerto Rican society. Subsistence farmers were forced from their lands, faced impoverishment and starvation, and flooded the metropolitan areas to participate in the emerging wage economy. This extractive trend continues (GAO, 2014), and the nation remains highly dependent upon federal aid and imports (Grosfoguel, 2003; Rivera Ramos, 2002). Puerto Rico developed a high unemployment rate and significant income disparities, with approximately 50% of the population living below the federal poverty level (Rivera Ramos, 2002).

DEVELOPMENT PROGRAMS, POPULATION CONTROL AND BIOMEDICAL TESTING

According to Briggs (2002), the failure of the development programs described earlier to increase standards of living and decrease poverty was explained through the discourse of overpopulation. Capitalist expansion, industrialization and destruction of the agricultural sector generated rising urban poverty and crowding as people moved for wage jobs; however, officials ultimately attributed these problems to the over-fertility of the poor (Briggs, 2002; Colón Warren, 2003; Lopez, 2008). Lopez (2008) argues that, in many ways, the eugenics ideology of Social Darwinism that was then developing in the US mainland found reflection in the practices and policies of the colony. Neo-Malthusians maintained that the only way to solve the underdevelopment issue was through population reduction. Thus, both US and Puerto Rican government officials embarked on a two-pronged population control strategy that encompassed emigration as a temporary "relief" solution and fertility reduction through sterilization as the long-term measure (Lopez, 2008). Thus, the Puerto Rican diaspora began, marked by waves of migration (principally rural farmers) to fill the need for labor in the burgeoning factories of the American Northeast (Lopez, 2008).

While these first migration waves were taking place in the 1940s and 50s, officials embarked on a sterilization initiative to stem what was characterized

as a "rampant" tide of new births (Lopez, 2008). At the time, viable temporary forms of birth control were nonexistent for several reasons: the opposition of the Catholic Church (Colón Warren, 2003), the federal Comstock
Law that outlawed birth control, and the machinations of Clarence Gamble
(of Proctor and Gamble family fame) who "turned Puerto Rico into his own
personal birth control laboratory" (Lopez, 2008, p. 16) and experimented
with his ineffective contraceptive foams and jellies on thousands of women
while preventing the introduction of other effective temporary methods to
the island.[3] Puerto Rico has historically had one of the highest rates of sterilization in the world, reaching 39% of reproductive-aged women by 1982
(Vasquez-Calzada & Carnivalli, 1982).

Attention from both Puerto Rican and American officials to the so-called
overpopulation problem spanned decades (Briggs, 2002). However, Briggs
(2002) has argued that this attention was not rooted in demographic realities
of overpopulation. Puerto Rico possessed a very low population growth rate
in the early 1930s of 1.5% (Roberts, 1958, p. 129, as cited in Mass, 1977,
p. 67), whereas the population replacement rate in industrialized contexts is
2.1% (PRB, 2012). Rather, the overpopulation discourse was a tool deployed
to serve as a more acceptable excuse for the failure of the industrialization
program to improve economic and living conditions in Puerto Rico—a way to
deflect attention from colonialist economic policies that funneled money from
the island back to American corporations. Briggs (2002) notes: "in many ways,
overpopulation served as a reply to and encapsulation of this policy concern:
something was wrong in Puerto Rico, but it could not entirely be the fault of
the United States" (p. 87). Indeed, "overpopulation" seemed perhaps to be a
simpler and more "solvable" cause of Puerto Rico's continuing poverty, and
its solution fit perfectly the racist and eugenic underpinnings of this discourse.

Demographic numbers aside, the construction of a particular population
as overly fertile and a nation as overpopulated has implications for access to
health services. In Puerto Rico, as I have argued previously, a socially constructed discourse of overpopulation is directly related to access and nonac-
cess to specific health services. In past decades this connection has been clear
in terms of sterilization and birth control and in the present day, access to
assisted reproductive technologies (Dyer, Mitu & Vindrola Padros, 2012, p.
43). The few fertility clinics that operate on the island do offer both fertility
preservation and post-treatment parenthood options. However, numerous
barriers hinder widespread access to them, including lack of insurance coverage, high cost, geographic centralization of clinics in the capital city and
limited public/provider awareness of available fertility preservation services
(Dyer, 2013).

The Puerto Rican context, in which infertility clinics are few and far
between and the island has been portrayed as dangerously overpopulated,
is not necessarily unique. According to Inhorn (2003), it can be conceived
of as part of a general trend: in countries that have historically been viewed
as overpopulated, infertility is often not conceived of as a problem in need

of redress and is treated as a nonissue by funding agencies and government officials. Assisted reproductive technologies are not covered by insurance nor offered in public health systems, thus becoming available only to a country's most wealthy.[4] Indeed, one of the health care providers in this study referenced this idea: when asked if he knew of any financial assistance programs that helped cancer survivors access fertility preservation, he replied: "I don't see how the government can deal with all of that. On the contrary, they probably want to control the population somehow."

PATIENT PERSPECTIVES

Given the above history of reproductive control and colonial intervention in Puerto Rico, the question that follows is thus: how does this context actualize itself in the clinic and what are the implications for patients' lives? This chapter follows the assumption that biomedicine as a cultural system is intimately tied to colonialism and has often served to reinforce its own hegemony while depicting local ethnomedical practices as inferior and, in Puerto Rico, rendering women in particular vulnerable in relation to their bodies and health. For survivors in this study, the contours of suffering linked to cancer-related infertility and access to fertility preservation revolved around the deep importance of children and the role of parenting in Puerto Rican society. They spoke about how the desire for children and/or large families is a "cultural trait," something that is, at its essence, "Puerto Rican." Therefore, having babies was a strong social expectation for members of the society. As Magdalena,[5] a breast cancer survivor and divorced mother of two, explained: "It is part of our culture, of who we are. We are like that and the great majority of us want children." Juanita, a married mother of four who was 40 when she was diagnosed with breast cancer, spoke about this expectation:

> Our society is driven by the family. They get married, and if you have a couple that marries and has not had children, then people start to ask them for kids: 'where are the kids?' As a society, like we are driven by, it is grounded in, the family.

Some survivors referenced an infertility stigma—for example, Sofia, a divorced mother of two and breast cancer survivor, indicated:

> If you do not have children, people criticize you or say whatever atrocity. I have seen friends of mine who cannot have kids and people say—a really ugly word, like 'barren,' which they tell me. Things like that, culturally yes, when you are married everyone expects you to have kids.

Of the 23 reproductive-aged male and female cancer survivors interviewed for this study, approximately half could not recall a conversation about fertility or childbearing with their oncologist before treatment commenced. Thus, the way that cancer-related infertility was dealt with, or avoided, in the clinical encounter served to magnify some survivors' suffering. Several cases are instructive in this regard. For example, Camila, the woman referenced at the beginning of this chapter, learned about the risk of infertility one year after completing chemotherapy. She offered clues as to why she thinks the doctor did not tell her about infertility: as she already had a child, telling her about the infertility risks and available options was perhaps a moot point—one that she contested:

[I would have liked to find out about the fertility risks] immediately, because I was so young. I didn't want to be greedy or selfish. People would say, 'oh, but you already have one child.' But I don't think any child is replaceable with one another. You have children and they're totally different, and one can't replace the other one. He knew that I wanted to have more children. So it was frustrating . . . I was not even interested in learning whether or not my hair was going to fall out, because it was not important anymore. It was more important for me to know that I was going to be sterile than to know that my hair was going to fall out. Because I don't need my hair for anything; it just looks nice. So, I mean I got upset and I would have loved to find out even before I started the treatment, or the possibility of getting chemotherapy.

Camila cited recent media attention surrounding a Puerto Rican celebrity who had frozen her eggs prior to cancer treatment. Awareness of this option, discovered after the fact, magnified her anger and suffering:

I don't know exactly when I found out [the possible infertility], but I'm sure it was probably a year after I had taken the chemotherapy. And that's why I was really mad, because you see all the celebrities that come on the TV, and they immediately go and freeze their eggs, but I didn't have that chance, and they never gave me that chance.

Even survivors who were not planning on having additional children were angered at not having received information about this side effect. Inez, who had three children when she was diagnosed at age 38 with breast cancer, was upset that she was not informed, even though she had undergone tubal ligation prior to the treatment. She firmly believed that oncologists should always inform their patients about this whether or not that patient has children—or if they have previously been sterilized:

No, that subject was not addressed, because I had three [children] already, and I was operated on also. I had been sterilized. [He never talked about it.] No. Never. They never explained to me either that the chemo could make my ovaries stop functioning. If I would like to have more children? They did not orient me. [I feel] very sad, because although I had three already and I did not want more, I think that they should orient you about it, because if your plans are to have children or if you have one and you want to have another one—and I know of people that have done it—they should be oriented, of course, to save their eggs. So, the doctor, without knowing, should orient [the patient]. If you have children or not. They did not tell me anything; he did not ask me and did not orientate me. He went from the premise that I had three children and did not want any more.

PROVIDER PERSPECTIVES

Interviews with oncologists helped to elucidate their perspectives and their beliefs about the importance of fertility to cancer patients. Nearly all providers who worked directly in treating cancer patients believed that newly diagnosed patients should be informed about the possibility of infertility as a side effect and fertility preservation options. For example, Dr. Pedreira, an oncologist, outlined his strategy about deciding which patients to inform:

> Well, that is really easy. The best policy is not to judge anybody, so I tell everybody of childbearing age. Everybody. If they are a nun, I would say, 'Listen you can't get pregnant during chemotherapy, and you're at risk of infertility.' Because people change, you know, people make changes in their lives. So you pretty much have to tell everybody.

However, these same oncologists were of the opinion that the majority of their colleagues in Puerto Rico do not feel similarly. In their experience, discussions about infertility and fertility preservation are not a routine pretreatment topic of conversation, either because the oncologists are not aware of the options themselves or because they assume that it is not—or should not be—an important concern for patients in the face of diagnosis with a life-threatening disease. Even in their own practices, providers faced challenges in remembering to discuss it with their patients. As one oncologist noted, "Having said that we talk about it, we barely talk about it. Really, people only talk about it in terms of '[is she of] childbearing age? [Then] she's got to consider fertility preservation,' and then we forget about it."

Oncologists often stratified patients into those whom they considered "appropriate" or not for discussion about infertility and fertility preservation. This assessment was often related to the patients' age and treatment, but also to other social categories such as their financial situation and current family status. Oncologists frequently pointed to cost as the major deterrent to the utilization of fertility preservation, firmly believed that the vast majority of patients cannot afford it and implied that many colleagues only inform well-to-do patients. Presenting this information to low-income patients seemed to some providers to be causing them further anguish—knowing that there are options available that are completely unaffordable for them. Providers also explicitly referenced the very few fertility clinics available that offer preservation services, and how they are all located in the metropolitan area—thus, few people in the more rural, poorer areas of the island are able to travel for these services.

The oncological discourse of cure-at-all-costs was also incorporated into these providers' discussions about informing patients—in other words, the idea that physical survival and cure is the utmost goal when faced with cancer, and all other concerns are secondary. In this discourse, quality of life concerns can register as unimportant, even if patients themselves desire more of a balance between a quality-versus-quantity approach to life. Dr. Colón, a 42-year-old oncologist, explained:

> I don't think many oncologists have this type of conversation, unless it's obvious. Very young female with no children, or they are taking drugs that says right across the label 'this is very high risk for fertility problems.' . . . I think that we assume that maybe this is not as important as treating the cancer. It is like the utmost goal is to have you disease-free forever, no matter what the consequences. And this is a feeling, this is something that patients bring to the table, and other physicians also. They think that this [is a] war against cancer, and sometimes they don't think about the consequences of treatment. I don't think [that view] is changing . . . They feel like it is obligated, and they have to accept all consequences. And sometimes they don't think about long-term problems.

Oncologists spoke extensively about what they framed as "pressure from the patient"—in other words, their perceptions of patient priorities and anxieties to which they were obligated to respond. According to some providers, patients just wanted their treatment—they wanted "the cure," and they "do not care about anything else" at that point. They are so afraid of cancer and of dying that none of the other quality-of-life concerns take on any importance. Dr. Pedreira related how fear drives patients to seek treatment immediately:

> Another problem besides the economic is the fear. You tell somebody they have cancer; they don't want to wait until the gynecologist sees them and does procedures and tests. It's like "I want my chemo now." *(pounding desk)*

Sra. Benitez, an oncology nurse, reinforced the dichotomy of treatment-versus-everything-else in her comment about her patients who might face infertility:

> Some of these chemotherapies do give infertility, and those that do give infertility the doctor lets them know, so they can decide what they want

to do. . . . I don't know what these people do. I don't know if they decide simply not to have children and go ahead with the treatment. It depends on their priorities. If they decide that they want their health, it's their health, no children. You can live without children. . . . The young guy that had the bone cancer, he just had a kid. We knew he was going to be infertile, but he has one [already]. It's not necessary to have 2 or 3. It depends on their priorities.

Here, she describes the idea that patients must choose one or the other, implying that those who opt for a less-aggressive treatment in an attempt to spare their fertility may have skewed priorities and a damaging focus on having more children when they are not "needed." Through this perspective emerges the oncological discourse of cure-at-all-costs, where patients should merely be happy to be alive and not concerned about the other impacts of treatment.

The providers in this study generally believed that patients' first priority lay with their existing children and that they preferred to focus on them, rather than consider fertility preservation; thus, they did not need more children because they already had one or two. This reflects Camila's experience at the beginning of the chapter and the reason that she believed her oncologist did not inform her about egg freezing. Several providers and advocates assumed that because Puerto Ricans tend to marry and have children early, most of them already have the number of children desired when they are diagnosed with cancer, even though the general trend is towards later childbearing. Dr. Corzo, a 49-year-old male oncologist, described this idea:

Yes, I think that [fertility] is very important, but most don't want more children. In our culture—and I think in the States, it is different—people tend to marry very early. They have already children at 18, 19 years, so most of them have completed their families before [the cancer]. In my setting. I know in the pediatric hospital, they get patients that are adolescents or younger. But in my patients, most of them have completed their families. I remember two patients because one was going to get married, and the other wanted more children. But it's rare to see a patient not married with no children.

Oncologists also expressed personal difficulties about the complexities and ambiguities of fertility preservation, and thus informing patients about it. This happened most prominently in discussions with patients that were presumed to have poor prognoses. As one oncologist noted:

It's a big concern for most people, fertility after chemotherapy. But again, always, the bigger problem is the ones that are at higher risk of recurrence. Sometimes it's really hard to tell somebody, "Listen I wouldn't do this if I were you. Because you don't want to leave your kid without a mom or a dad if you don't have to." If you already have the kid and you get the disease, that's nobody's fault. But if you don't and you have a high chance of recurrence, it's rough.

Oncologists want their patients to undergo treatments that provide the best chance of survival, yet sometimes these treatments are the ones most likely to cause infertility. It was therefore an emotionally and professionally difficult situation for the oncologist if a patient expressed preference for a treatment that carried a lower risk of infertility but may be considered suboptimal therapy for that particular cancer. Patients with poor prognoses or aggressive disease thus presented an excruciating counseling dilemma for the oncologist, who often expressed uncertainty about which course to recommend.

DISCUSSION

This chapter has argued that discourses produced through the colonial relationship have shaped the landscape of fertility preservation options open to cancer patients, thereby shaping the context and mutual construction of suffering. In situating a discussion about suffering within the context of cancer-related infertility and fertility preservation, two layers are important to consider: first, the discourse of overpopulation and the resultant sterilization/population control initiatives in Puerto Rico, and second, the professional oncological discourse of expert physician as gatekeeper who emphasizes survival from cancer above all else.

The construction of the entire Puerto Rican population as overly fertile and the nation as dangerously overpopulated has had tragic consequences, paving the way for a massive migration push and acting as a justification for the unethical sterilization initiatives and birth control experimentation. Following Inhorn (2003), I argue that residue from this discourse has implications for the current restricted availability of infertility services in Puerto Rico and the lack of attention to infertility as a social or medical problem. Although clinics exist, they are few in number and geographically concentrated in the capital region. Infertility treatment and fertility preservation both cost more than the majority of Puerto Ricans can afford, leaving these technologies available only for the very wealthy.

The deep Puerto Rican cultural value on children and parenting espoused by the survivors in this study clashes with the 20th century discourse of overpopulation. In such a context, the concept of stratified reproduction is clearly evident (Ginsburg & Rapp, 1995). Infertility and assisted reproduction are an example "par excellence" (Inhorn, Ceballo & Nachtigall, 2009, p. 182) of stratified reproduction, reflecting social values about who is privileged enough to reproduce. The *cancered* body is devalued as a site of reproduction, and parenthood takes low priority in biomedical discourse; at the same time, Puerto Rican reproduction in general has been historically and institutionally devalued. Puerto Rican cancer patients are thus doubly devalued as potential parents. An interesting question is whether and how the quintessentially Puerto Rican value on children and large families has at some level been formulated and expressed as a challenge or resistance to the colonial legacy and the overarching emphasis on overpopulation and fertility control.

The ways in which cancer-related fertility are dealt with in the clinical encounter, in terms of disclosure about the infertility risks and the available fertility preservation options, can both produce and magnify suffering. The dominant discourse of the expert physician acting as paternalistic information gatekeeper and decision-maker has a long history in biomedicine; it has only been relatively recently that this model has been challenged by other approaches in the American context such as shared decision-making. Roter and Hall (2006) argue that there are two dominant perspectives on the withholding of medical information—in other words, why physicians withhold or give incomplete information. First, physicians "believe that most patients are unprepared to evaluate and comprehend the complex information they may receive . . . [and second], information is power, and an informed patient is a possible threat to the physician's professional status and control of the therapeutic situation" (p. 128). Further, they argue that "physicians and patients often disagree as to the likely outcome of the disclosure, and consequently what it is in the patient's best interest" (p. 128). The concerns of the oncologist quoted earlier, who outlined his discomfort with broaching the topic with patients who had poor prognoses, hint at the latter arguments. By not raising the topic, the oncologist avoids a potentially uncomfortable, ambiguous situation: a patient with a poor prognosis choosing a less-aggressive treatment in order to lessen the risk of infertility, something that the oncologist—on the other hand—regards as suboptimal. Whereas the patient may be balancing their need for cancer treatment with preserving their autonomy and ability to pursue life goals, the oncologist is often not trained to see this as a balance, viewing it instead in a more dichotomous fashion. By avoiding the conversation, they therefore avoid the challenge to their professional training and sense of purpose as a clinician.

Exportation of biomedical cultures of practice and technologies is uneven and the implementation and adoption of these is heavily influenced by the national and regional context. Structures, values and discourses are not merely accepted wholesale but clash and engage with existing values, culture and local histories. Puerto Rico, with its history of dependency and biological intervention from outside, is an area where individuals may be especially sensitive to issues of infertility; however, professional oncology practice, with its emphasis on treatment and disease management, is not focused on these matters. In addition, because many oncologists themselves are from the upper classes and educated within a Western medical paradigm, they may often make assumptions about the reproductive patterns of their patients that are similar to the ones made in the past by public health and pharmaceutical agencies seeking to use the island for research.

Physicians' cherry picking and assumptions about the financial positions of their patients are a product of what they see as their responsibility to protect patients psychologically from knowledge about options that they cannot afford. The power that oncologists wield to control the information and options available to patients takes shape in a similar manner to colonial power. Yet, at the same time, health care providers in this study expressed a deep value on time spent in discussions with their patients and took great pains to nurture healthy, trusting relationships.

In such situations, contexts of suffering are dynamic, mutually constructed and shifting. Patients and providers collectively share the burden of diagnosis, treatment and survival, yet they speak past each other and disagree to some extent on what is important, such as fertility and continued childbearing. Providers are presented with difficult decisions: either remain silent or inform patients about unaffordable technologies. They take the risk of either increasing patients' suffering or potentially pushing them to question undergoing the recommended cancer treatment. Physicians clearly challenged the assumptions behind the discourses of gatekeeping and cure-at-all-costs—voicing their own anguish about being stuck between a rock and a hard place—at the same time that these discourses were incorporated into their own practice and shaped interactions with their patients.

The collective burden sharing described in this chapter exists within a context of inequality. Solutions depend upon the exportation of biomedical technology from the developed world that is prohibitively expensive and beyond the reach of people requiring basic cancer care. Indeed, Puerto Rico is embedded within an interesting contradiction; although much of the emerging fertility preservation technology is being researched and developed in the United States, even within its own borders, steep disparities in access to these technologies are evident. This speaks to the idea that technology itself, introduced with the intention of reducing suffering and expanding therapeutic options, can itself create suffering and inequality—in this case, by the lack of ability to gain access to an option that exists (Livingston, 2012; Lock, 1997). If the U.S. situation is any indication, it is unlikely that the price of fertility preservation will drop in the near future or that insurance policies will voluntarily offer coverage. An honest and candid discussion with patients about what the side effects may be, and what options are available even if beyond financial reach, requires the oncologist to give up control and let patients decide their own courses of action. With increasing cancer incidence rates especially among young people, it is more critical than ever to formulate patterns of communication that minimize the suffering of all actors.

NOTES

1. The author wishes to acknowledge support from the Ponce School of Medicine—Moffitt Cancer Center partnership (NCI #U56 CA118809), the University of South Florida Dissertation Completion program, and the Brocher Foundation. A special thank you goes to all those who participated in this

226 Karen E. Dyer

study and shared their stories and experiences, and to this volume's editors and workshop organizers. Finally, thank you to Drs. Nancy Romero-Daza, Heide Castañeda, Gwendolyn Quinn, Federico Cintrón-Moscoso, Sarah A. Smith and Hannah Helmy for their guidance and critique.

2. For example, see Quinn et al. (2007), and Quinn, Vadaparampil, Bell-Ellison, Gwede and Albrecht (2008). Frequently cited studies in the United States have pointed to significant problems in disclosure about infertility and fertility preservation. In one study, only 51% of eligible male cancer patients were offered sperm banking as an option (Schover, Brey, Lichtin, Lipshultz & Jeha, 2002a). In another, while 91% of surveyed oncologists believed that sperm banking *should* be offered to all eligible men, only 10% reported that they in fact always did so (Schover, Brey, Lichtin, Lipshultz & Jeha, 2002b). From the patient perspective, Zebrack (2004) found that only half of the patients in his sample could recall a health care provider mentioning the fertility risks of their treatment.

3. Anthropologist Iris Lopez (2008) argues that the major reason why women were sterilized in such high numbers throughout the course of the 20th century was because it was the only *effective* birth control option available. Although Puerto Rico's sterilization campaign has often been framed in black-and-white terms as an example of scientific abuse, Lopez (2008) maintains that the issue is much more complex, demonstrated by the still-high rates of *voluntary* sterilization that take place among both island and mainland Puerto Ricans decades after the campaign ended.

4. This applies to the discourse in the United States as well, and popular constructions of Latina immigrants (as well as other ethnic minority groups) as overly fertile *hyperbreeders*. Chavez (2004) argues that "discourses that construct people with 'dangerous,' 'pathological,' and 'abnormal' reproductive behaviors are not simply of academic interest" (p. 173) but instead have serious ramifications. One such consequence was the "Save Our State" movement in California, which culminated in Proposition 187—this policy attempted to restrict the numbers of undocumented immigrants by denying them critical social services such as prenatal care and education (Chavez 2004) because of the perception that the population was increasing too rapidly. These groups are perceived to be in need of reproductive control rather than access for the reason that their over-fertility is threatening to squeeze the country's precious resources (Culley 2009)—especially welfare resources. Culley, Hudson and Van Rooij (2009) aptly observe that "the idea of fertility treatment in less developed countries of the world often evokes feelings of disbelief and discomfort, as the dominant image of such societies is that of 'over-population'. There are those who suggest that similar feelings pervade public perceptions of marginalized communities in Western societies and that a desire to limit the reproductive capacity of such groups has been more apparent than any effort to assist procreative choice" (p. 10).

5. Pseudonyms have been used to protect the privacy of the participants.

REFERENCES

Balshem, M. (1993). *Cancer in the community: Class and medical authority*. Washington, DC: Smithsonian Institution Press.

Briggs, L. (2002). *Reproducing empire: Race, sex, science, and U.S. imperialism in Puerto Rico*. Berkeley, CA: University of California Press.

Cabán, P. (1993). Redefining Puerto Rico's political status. In E. Melendez & E. Melende (Eds.), *Colonial dilemma: Critical perspectives on contemporary Puerto Rico* (pp. 19–40). Boston, MA: South End Press.

Chavez, L. R. (2004). A glass half empty: Latina reproduction and public discourse. *Human Organization, 63,* 173–188.

Colón Warren, A. E. (2003). Puerto Rico feminism and feminist studies. *Gender & Society, 17,* 664–690.

Culley, L. (2009). Dominant narratives and excluded voices: Research on ethnic differences in access to assisted conception in more developed societies. In L. Culley, N. Hudson, & F. Van Rooij (Eds.), *Marginalized reproduction: Ethnicity, infertility and reproductive technologies* (pp. 17–33). London: Earthscan.

Culley, L., Hudson, N., & Van Rooij, F. (Eds.). (2012). *Marginalized reproduction: Ethnicity, infertility and reproductive technologies.* London: Routledge.

Del Vecchio-Good, M. J., Good, B. J., Schaffer, C., & Lind, S. E. (1990). American oncology and the discourse on hope. *Culture, Medicine, & Psychiatry, 14,* 59–79.

Dyer, K. E. (2013). *Survivorship, infertility and parenthood: Experiencing life after cancer in Puerto Rico* (Doctoral dissertation). Retrieved from http://scholarcommons.usf.edu/etd/

Dyer, K. E., Mitu, K., & Vindrola Padros, C. (2012). The social shaping of fertility loss due to cancer treatment: A comparative perspective. In S. Earle, C. Komaromy, & L. Layne (Eds.), *Understanding reproductive loss: International perspectives on life, death and fertility* (pp. 37–50). London: Ashgate Publishing.

Ginsburg, F. D., & Rapp, R. (Eds.). (1995). *Conceiving the new world order: The global politics of reproduction.* Berkeley, CA: University of California Press.

Grosfoguel, R. (2003). The political economy of Puerto Rico in the twentieth century and Puerto Rican postnational strategies. In *Colonial subjects: Puerto Ricans in a global perspective* (pp. 43–77). Berkeley, CA: University of California Press.

Hayashi, A. S., Finnegan, B., Shin, P., Jones, E., & Rosenbaum, S. (2009). *Examining the experiences of Puerto Rico's community health centers under the government health insurance plan* (Policy Research Brief No. 8). Washington, DC: Geiger Gibson/RCHN Community Health Foundation Research Collaborative.

Inhorn, M. C. (2003). Global infertility and the globalization of new reproductive technologies: Illustrations from Egypt. *Social Science & Medicine, 56,* 1837–1851.

Inhorn, M. C., Ceballo, R., & Nachtigall, R. D. (2009). Marginalized, invisible and unwanted: American minority struggles with infertility and assisted conception. In L. Culley, N. Hudson, & F. van Rooij (Eds.), *Marginalized reproduction: Ethnicity, infertility and reproductive technologies* (pp. 181–197). London: Earthscan.

Livingston, J. (2012). *Improvising medicine: An African oncology ward in an emerging cancer epidemic.* Durham, NC: Duke University Press.

Lock, M. (1997). Displacing suffering: The reconstruction of death in North America and Japan. In A. Kleinman, V. Das, & M. Lock (Eds.), *Social suffering* (pp. 207–244). Berkeley, CA: University of California Press.

Lopez, I. (2008). *Matters of choice: Puerto Rican women's struggle for reproductive freedom.* New Brunswick, NJ: Rutgers University Press.

Mass, B. (1977). Puerto Rico: A case study of population control. *Latin American Perspectives, 4,* 66–82.

Medical Tourism Association (MTA). (2012). *Press release: Puerto Rico poised for medical tourism.* Retrieved from: http://www.marketwired.com/press-release/puerto-rico- poised-for-medical-tourism-1717917.htm

Mulligan, J. (2010). It gets better if you do? Measuring quality care in Puerto Rico. *Medical Anthropology, 29,* 303–329.

Pan American Health Organization (PAHO). (2007). *Health systems profile Puerto Rico.* Retrieved from: http://www2.paho.org/hq/dmdocuments/2010/Health_System_Profile-Puerto_Rico_2007.pdf. Washington, DC: PAHO/WHO.

Population Reference Bureau (PRB). (2012). *World population data sheet.* Retrieved from: https://www.prb.org.

Quinn, G. P., Vadaparampil, S. T., Gwede, C. K., Miree, C., King, L. M., Clayton, H. B., Wilson, C., & Munster, P. (2007). Discussion of fertility preservation with newly diagnosed patients: Oncologist's views. *Journal of Cancer Survivorship, 1,* 146–155.

Quinn, G. P., Vadaparampil, S. T., Bell-Ellison, B. A., Gwede, C. K., & Albrecht, T. L. (2008). Patient-physician communication barriers regarding fertility preservation among newly diagnosed cancer patients. *Social Science & Medicine, 66,* 784–789.

Rivera Ramos, E. (2002). The legal construction of identity: The judicial and social legacy of American colonialism in Puerto Rico. Washington, DC: APA.

Roberts, G.W. (1958). The Caribbean islands. *Annals of the American Academy of Political & Social Science, March,* 127–136.

Roter, D., & Hall, J.A. (2006). *Doctors talking with patients/patients talking with doctors: Improving communication in medical visits* (Vol. 2). Westport, CT: Praeger.

Schover, L. R., Brey, K., Lichtin, A., Lipshultz, L. I., & Jeha, S. (2002a). Knowledge and experience regarding cancer, infertility and sperm banking in younger male survivors. *Journal of Clinical Oncology, 20,* 1880–1889.

Schover, L. R., Brey, K., Lichtin, A., Lipshultz, L. I., & Jeha, S. (2002b). Oncologists' attitudes and practices regarding banking sperm before cancer treatment. *Journal of Clinical Oncology, 20,* 1890–1897.

Sklar, C. A. (2005). Maintenance of ovarian function and risk of premature menopause related to cancer treatment. *Journal of the National Cancer Institute Monographs, 34,* 25–27.

US Census Bureau. (2010). *State & county quickfacts: U.S.A.—median household income, 2008.* Retrieved from: http://quickfacts.census.gov/qfd/states/00000.html.

US Government Accountability Office (GAO). (2014). *Puerto Rico: Information on how statehood would potentially affect selected federal programs and revenue sources* [Publication GAO-14–31]. Retrieved from: http://www.gao.gov/assets/670/661334.pdf. Washington, DC: United States Government Accountability Office.

Vasquez-Calzada, J. L., & Carnivalli, J. (1982). *El uso de métodos anticonceptivos en Puerto Rico: Tendencias recientes.* Centro de Investigaciones Demograficás, Escuela de Salud Pública, Recinto de Ciencias Médicas. San Juan: Universidad de Puerto Rico.

Zebrack, B. (2004). Fertility issues for young adult survivors of childhood cancer. *Psycho- Oncology, 13,* 689–699.

12 Dying to Be Heard
Cancer, Imagined Experience and the Moral Geographies of Care in the UK

Fiona M. Harris[1]

INTRODUCTION

In a comparison of cancer experiences in Scotland and Kenya (Murray, Grant, Grant & Kendall, 2003), a key finding was that cancer narratives in Scotland focused on anger, distress and the fear of dying; whereas in Kenya narratives focus on physical pain and suffering in the absence of comfort and support that minimizes fears of dying or other forms of existential distress. The authors argue that although Scotland (unlike Kenya) provides no-cost access to specialist cancer and palliative care services, the inability to voice distress and fears around death and dying remains an important area of unmet need for most Scottish cancer patients. The authors then pose the question: "has the professionalization of palliative care and the medicalization of death [in the UK] taken away skills and power from families and communities so that they are no longer able to accommodate the distress of dying?" (Murray, Grant, Grant & Kendall, 2003, p. 4). This question is linked to the sociology and anthropology of death and dying more broadly and exploring this provides a key to understanding and situating the narratives of cancer patients in Scotland.[2]

How we talk about, manage and experience death and dying in the UK has changed dramatically over the last 50 years. For instance, the majority of deaths in the UK now occur in hospitals, hospices or nursing homes and only around 20% of people die at home (Taylor & Carter, 2004). Current UK policy supports the notion that dying at home is a hallmark of a "good death," however, whether dying at home reflects the wishes of patients and their families has been subject to debate (Thomas, Morris & Clark, 2004). For instance, one study found that those who have a terminal illness are more inclined to choose death outside the home, because of (for instance) fears around the final stages of dying, or the impact on families (Seymour, Payne, Chapman & Holloway, 2007). There is no doubt that dying bodies have become subject to a multidisciplinary professional scrutiny (Giddens, 1991): death is no longer the preserve of communities, but has become *invisible*, sequestered from everyday life by institutional practices (Aries, 1981).

The sequestration thesis argues that with modernity, processes of death and dying have become separated from everyday life and communities (Giddens, 1991; Mellor & Shilling, 1993). Dying has become inaccessible and perhaps incomprehensible to public view, thus "dying is hidden, and its meaning privatized" (Walter, 2009, paragraph 2.1). As Aries (1981) elaborates, bodies are no longer laid out at home, religious institutions are also on the wane in our largely secularized society, bereaved persons are no longer easily identified by black clothing or armbands, and grief too remains a largely private experience.

Formal participation in religious institutions (such as church attendance) is declining in the UK (Voas & Crockett, 2005). Religious institutions, once firmly embedded within communities and responsible for guiding our beliefs and practices around death and dying are now a relatively minor player for the majority of the population. Indeed, in discussing Aries's (1981) thesis about the denial of death, Green (2008) writes: "This cultural context presents death as less hidden, less explicitly religious, and more individualized" (p. 3). It may well be that our uncertainties and fears around death have grown along with the process of secularization, and this is explored with reference to research on cancer experiences in Scotland. I consider how our cultural expectations and constructions of cancer are implicated within contemporary cancer narratives and how they reflect the privatization of death and dying. I do this by bringing together a range of voices: from the media, from my own autobiography and from the voices of research participants. Through drawing explicitly on intersubjectivity, I attempt to illustrate how our experiences intersect and reveal some of the spaces occupied by unvoiced, other kinds of suffering that are often difficult to unravel in cancer narratives. This space of silence is filled with what Hallowell (2006) eloquently referred to as the "memory of others' suffering" (p. 23) and this is one that adds to what I have referred to elsewhere as the *imagined experience* of cancer (Harris, 2008). However, by listening to these voices and placing them alongside public/media-generated narratives of cancer experience, we begin to see a collapse in those dichotomies raised by Aries and others. I argue here that the public grief and mourning of the Victorians cannot simply be contrasted to a privatized, individualized death of contemporary society. Instead, we see a continuum of public expressions of death illustrated by media narratives of cancer (*see* Green, 2008; Seale, 2002, 2003) alongside hidden grief and private dying revealed by personal narratives. Instead, we might explore this notion of secularized death and the meaning of cultural scripts that are enacted around this.

PUBLIC CONSTRUCTIONS OF CANCER

If we are to think of the story of cancer experience, what springs to mind is a dichotomy of horror and hero: where one resides in the popular imagination and the other in the mass media. *Cancer heroics* as it has been so aptly named (Clarke & Everest, 2006; Dixon-Woods, Seale, Young, Findlay & Heney, 2003; Seale 2002) has been explored by sociologists in the UK at length, revealing the propensity for media representations of cancer sufferers to draw on metaphors of bravery, heroism and the stoic sufferer. At times this narrative has placed a burden of expectation on cancer sufferers as well as close family members that they will assume this *cultural script* (Seale, 2002) and enact a theatre of noble suffering and unconditional love. Writing of childhood cancer experiences, for instance, Dixon-Woods, Seale, Young, Findlay & Henry (2003) reveal the difficulties experienced by parents whose personal and family resilience might begin to unravel in the face of a child's illness and yet be muzzled by the rhetoric of heroics, unable to voice their own needs or unfairly judged if they pierce the bubble of sainthood upheld by the cancer narrative. Indeed another version of these narratives is to attribute a seemingly miraculous agency to cancer, where on diagnosis the sufferer is transformed from sinner to saint from one news release to the next (Walter, 2009, 2010).

This was illustrated by the story of Jade Goody, a former *Big Brother* contestant who gained minor celebrity status with regular print media coverage, TV appearances and lucrative advertising deals. Following a return to the Big Brother Celebrity House, Jade then received widespread condemnation for racist, bullying behavior that saw her removed from the series and the loss of media interest. Any subsequent media reports of Jade plunged into widespread condemnation of her behavior, which undoubtedly contributed to her return to nonentity; a nonentity that remained until her media profile was resurrected most cruelly by a diagnosis of cervical cancer that was to prove terminal. This unfortunate young woman then leapt onto our television screens once again, transformed from bigot to saint in one fell swoop, her cancer experience becoming the subject of another docu-soap that mapped her trajectory from home to hospice and the last hours of her life, her illness experience appropriated and yet sanitized for a very public dying (Walter, 2009, 2010).

Jade's story illustrated that the transformative power of a cancer diagnosis is one that is wrought through the collusion of a society that seems unable to embrace the reality face-to-face. As Stoller (2009) has written, the cancer patient is urged into the arena, cheered on by health professionals who provide advice and information that represent "guides for the battlefield." And yet, the smiling faces of the cheer squad mask a politics of *dread* (McMullin & Weiner, 2009), that have wider implications for how we approach the study of cancer.

Indeed the appropriation of cancer into narratives of the battleground, of heroics and sainthood has become so pervasive that it has infiltrated into psychiatry and psychology and studies of the psychological distress in cancer patients. For instance, a recent review of cancer-related distress found that prevalence was difficult to determine because previous studies assumed that any psychological distress experienced by couples where a cancer diagnosis was present must be related to the experience of cancer, when this might not, in fact, be justified. As the authors elaborate:

> Being diagnosed with cancer remains a threatening experience, but there is still some tendency in the literature to construe cancer in terms of trauma and catastrophe in a manner that may not be consistent with the contemporary experience of many persons with cancer, or their partners, or with the available data.
>
> (Hagendoorn, Sanderman, Bolks, Tuinstra & Coyne, 2008, p. 4)

In fact, a meta-analysis of studies included in this review found that distress was more strongly associated with female gender and the caregiver role than with the cancer diagnosis. The authors raised important questions about the need to go beyond the cancer diagnosis to explore the person in terms of age, gender and social circumstance (Hagendoorn et al., 2008, p. 4).

This suggests that the vision of researchers too may be clouded by cancer as battlefield, and nowhere is this more apparent when the cancer diagnosis is terminal and researchers wish to explore the views of the dying person. Here the metaphors are doubly multiplied, drawing on cultural scripts around death, dying and cancer that include profound silences around end-of-life issues. Furthermore, adding to these silences is a discourse of legitimacy that maps onto a moral geography of cancer. Anthropologists have used the term *moral geography* to link narratives and experiences of place or locality with moral discourses. Thomas (2002), for instance, writes: "As a structure of feeling, moral geography represents aspects of people's knowledge of their present situation . . . a domain of understanding and imagination that draws on a deeply emplaced identity and ancestral history" (p. 384). Rather than tie geography to place, instead I apply the term to a "space" created by cancer experience, thus a moral geography of cancer becomes a map of territories occupied by silence, by heroics or by other representations of dying.

I draw on a study of research methods and challenges to research the views of persons who have terminal cancer. The analysis synthesizes interviews with cancer researchers, cancer sufferers approaching the end of their lives, partners of cancer patients and cancer survivors, along with autobiographical narrative. The chapter explores what cancer and the process of dying means in contemporary British society and how this is mediated by the power of imagined experience (Harris, 2008), which is fuelled by the prevailing metaphors of dread and heroism alongside the sequestration of death and dying. I draw on my own experience of caring for a family member who had cancer and how this influenced my own reaction to recruiting and talking to hospice patients. I explore the deeply embodied nature of cancer representations and the difficulty of cancer realities to be heard above these. I argue that cancer as it is imagined constructs the patient in such powerful ways that it is difficult for their voices to be heard above this. As with other illnesses, cancer patients may struggle to assert their personhood beyond the disease (Sontag, 1978), and when those voices may wish to talk about dying, they may encounter profound deafness in their loved ones, health professionals and even among researchers seeking to explore their experiences and needs.

ENTERING THE FIELD

I brought to the study of research methods in palliative care the personal experience of caring for my father until his death from pleural mesothelioma, a cancer of the lining of the lungs caused by asbestos exposure. His illness trajectory included a gradual decline subsequent to his diagnosis, followed by his death eight months later. He had one episode of extreme pain that led to his admittance to hospital for assessment. The following day he showered, went back to bed and quietly died.

Some weeks later I received a letter of invitation to attend a bereavement support group from a local cancer charity. Although I might have benefited from this, I declined the invitation as I felt that my story of loss would not measure up to what I imagined must be the grim experience of other members of the group. I convinced myself that my father's comparatively *good death* was an extraordinary one for which I could be thankful, but did not lend legitimacy to my experience of cancer-related grief and loss. Thinking back to this experience I began to realize that this quest for legitimate experience was a part of a moral geography surrounding cancer.

Sinding and Wiernikowski (2008), for instance, identified a tendency for their research participants to evaluate and assign legitimacy (or not) to potential narratives of their cancer experience, editing out and silencing those thoughts and feelings that might cause a burden on relatives or caregivers. This process is one that they called *foreclosure* of Bury's (1982) disrupted biographies, where cancer experience is situated within the wider contexts of difficult lives. This study was based in Canada rather than the UK, which then raises the question: does the sequestration of death and dying associated with modernity also connect with moral geographies of cancer that render particular experiences, thoughts or emotions muted?

Writing this chapter 10 years after my father's death, it seems incredible that despite an experience of cancer that did not support the horror or hero narratives, I hardly slept the night before a job interview for a research post within a multidisciplinary palliative care research group. I tossed and turned with anxiety, worrying about what interviewing terminally ill cancer patients might mean and whether I could bear the exposure to such dreadful suffering.

THE RESEARCH PROJECT

I conducted semi-structured interviews (n = 30) with researchers from a range of disciplinary backgrounds who worked in cancer and palliative care. I also facilitated three focus groups: one with a group of men who attended a day hospice, another group of cancer survivors (all female) and finally a gender-mixed group of spouses of terminally ill cancer patients. As important as the recorded and transcribed interview material was, I also brought an ethnographic perspective to bear on this experience, and some observations made during this research became key to my understanding of cancer experience as a moral geography.

Interviews with researchers focused on the methodological challenges of engaging in palliative care research and were reported previously in an overview of the study (Kendall et al., 2007). Many of these challenges have been written about elsewhere, such as in recruitment of participants (Ingleton, Skillbeck & Clark, 2001), attrition due to uncertain prognoses and death or deteriorating health (Addington-Hall, 2002), issues around gatekeeping, the emotional burden on researchers (Hallowell, 2006) and frustrations around the bureaucratic hurdles associated with gaining research approval from Ethics and Research Governance Committees (Kendall et al., 2007).

TALKING TO CANCER SURVIVORS AND SPOUSES OF THE TERMINALLY ILL

I met with three women who had been treated variously for breast, colorectal cancer and melanoma and showed every sign of living well with no outward signs of treatment. Given the concerns in the literature around the vulnerability of persons with cancer, I asked them how they would have felt about a researcher coming to speak to them when they were ill and receiving treatment. All three of them spoke emphatically of how they would have valued this. Indeed, one of them had taken part in a qualitative interview when she was in treatment and she said, "When I spoke to [researcher's name] it really helped me. Because I felt that it was somebody listening, and I know it helped me."

Another woman spoke angrily of hospital staff who continually spoke in metaphors, referring to the very language of the battlefield written about elsewhere (McMullin & Weiner, 2009; Stoller, 2009). She lamented the fact that giving in to despair or expressing negative emotion was frowned upon and that no one ever engaged with her as a person with emotion. Indeed, she said, "No one ever asks how you feel." Health professionals effectively demonstrated the power to legitimize narratives, for instance by showing approval for "positive thinking" and foreclosing any attempt to present alternative narratives.

This propensity for listeners to silence particular narratives adds to the self-censure that some cancer patients may assume. However, as the research project continued, it became clear that a lack of talk around fear of death or other potentially negative emotions did not indicate the lack of this inner experience. Indeed this was illustrated by the second focus group that I convened with help from a community palliative care service. The value of a research interview in providing a willing, nonjudgmental listener was illustrated for me by this group of four women and one man who were the primary informal caregivers of their partners who were receiving palliative care.

This group displayed an emotional fragility that resulted in several participants bursting into tears during the session as they spoke about their experiences. One of the women commented that she had felt able to attend because receiving a letter of invitation containing the hospital logo made her feel less guilty about leaving the house, and another commented, "I actually feel quite good that I had to do my hair today and had to make an effort." Realizing that they rarely had time for themselves and that at least two of them were showing signs of deep fatigue, I worried that I was using time that was for them a scarce resource. However, in no uncertain terms they spoke about how talking to each other was therapeutic and how they felt that they gained strength from being with a group in a similar situation to themselves. Indeed, very early on in the discussion, the meeting was appropriated by the participants who drew on it for their own purposes, supporting each other as they told their stories, wept or expressed their fears or concerns.

The focus group became a space that was itself sequestrated from the everyday; it became a place out of the ordinary where they could talk about their own needs and emotions without having to addressing moral claims to narrative legitimacy. Thus, through appropriating the space of the focus group, the biographic foreclosure of their everyday lives became transformed into reinstated biographies of their own personal stories. *Space* figured in their discussion about being able to talk about how they were feeling.

> Space is a problem. Unless you live in a very big house . . . but space is a problem, you know, to sit and to speak to somebody . . . and you don't want the patient to hear things that you are saying in case it upsets them and everything . . .

Not upsetting the patient was something that constrained them and prevented the expression of their own pain or fears for the future. They referred to their lives as an "emotional rollercoaster," and as one woman elaborated: "it is such a crazy mixture of emotions that the likes of we go through, that I don't think there are two days when you feel the same, you know."

One final heartbreaking story from this group was that of the woman whose husband was told that he had a terminal cancer and would only live for two years. When we met it was over 15 years later and she lived in fear that he would find the credit card bills that she intercepted each time they came through the letterbox. Tragically, his survival long beyond that initial prognosis had set off a spending spree beginning with "the holiday of a lifetime" to be enjoyed as his life drew (supposedly) to a close. This led to enduring debts that the woman was unable to pay off and their precarious financial situation was a constant source of anxiety to her. Nevertheless, she strove to hide this from her husband, shouldering the burden silently, her story remaining within illegitimate territory.

The final focus group with day hospice users provided an extraordinary example of the subtle processes inherent in the flow between foreclosed biographies that adhere to a cultural script and how we as listeners can so easily demand that script to be reenacted.

TALKING TO THE DAY HOSPICE USERS

Four men with advanced cancer who attended a day hospice on a weekly basis agreed to take part in a focus group discussion. It swiftly became clear that the men enjoyed the opportunity to take part in a discussion and I found myself thinking that if I had had time I would have liked to have put something in place so that they could continue to meet to discuss a range of issues. However, we did agree to meet for a second time so that I could provide them with a summary of what I had learned from them and to get them to reflect on this further.

When we met again three weeks later, one of the men did not attend as he had been referred into respite care and the others showed signs of deterioration in the few short weeks since we had last met. One participant actually attended our meeting in his pajamas and dressing gown, dragging a drip and assorted medical equipment with him from his bed in the hospice ward. The nurse who had helped me to recruit the group spoke to me after I walked two of the men out to their cars. She said that Bob had been admitted to the hospice in crisis and had not been expected to survive. However, after several blood transfusions, he regained consciousness a few days later. She whispered, "His first words . . . his first words, mind, were—have I missed it?" That illustrated how important it was to him to take part in the discussion.

I sat on with Bob chatting while we waited for the nurse to come back and help him back to bed. He told me that he was being discharged and would be getting home the following day to which I responded with something to the effect that I was glad that he was feeling better. But then something quite extraordinary happened. He smiled gently at me and told me that he was not going to get better and that he was going home to die. I then simply did not respond to his cue that he wanted to talk about his impending death. It was not a conscious decision on my part, in fact, it was not until later that evening that the conversation came back to me and I finally admitted to myself what had happened. I heard him, convinced myself that I had not heard correctly, and used that as an excuse to avoid carrying on that discussion. I had effectively foreclosed his attempt to talk about his impending death.

This I will always remember as a moment of profound deafness on my part. It was a moment of hearing without listening. And as I continued working on that project and interviewed other researchers I learned that some of them (those who, like me, were new to the palliative care field) had done something similar. One researcher told me that her research supervisor pointed out the cues that kept appearing in interview transcripts that she continued to ignore and, in a similar way to me, had simply not heard the voices of those who wished to talk about dying.

SEQUESTRATION AND THE MORAL GEOGRAPHIES OF CANCER

This journey from a personal experience of cancer through to researching the views of cancer patients became a powerful lesson in the politics of dread. Even though I had been up close and personal with a *good death*, I nevertheless was deeply indoctrinated by an *imagined* cancer experience fuelled by media representations. Cancer's publics had constructed a moral geography around cancer experiences that left no space for my own, which I had judged as illegitimate and unrepresentative of the vast majority of cancer experiences. Through analyzing these processes however it has become apparent that this moral geography is one that is inherently contradictory. My father's good death should have offered a positive narrative that fitted with the prevailing moral code, but in fact this was a narrative that called into question the prevailing dichotomy of cancer heroics. A death that came easy thus undermined the cancer hero. Although public deaths like those of Jade Goody remained sanitized for public viewing, the careful manipulation of silence around the actual, lived experience ensured that the viewing public was left to imagine only the very worst kind of suffering, which allowed for the hero to emerge.

I remained tied to an illegitimate grief linked to a death without dread. I was left as a bereaved person with a biography disrupted (Bury, 1982) by loss, with a narrative foreclosed by ambiguity. Whereas others have drawn on Mary Douglas's classic work on *matter out of place* (Douglas, 1966) to explore the notion of cancer and *dirty dying* (Lawton, 2001), here I find a new use for the concept, for mine was a story *out of place*. Thus the moral geography of cancer is populated by these articulations of spaces that gain legitimacy by media and cancers' publics working in collusion. The dichotomy of hero and horror remains legitimate, with the hero remaining public and the horror-filled death imagined and relegated to the space of individualized death and dying. As a result, the public and the private become confused and populate similar spaces within the moral geography of cancer, while foreclosed biographies, particularly my illegitimate grief and the emotion expressed by family caregivers, inhabit the ambiguous territory of a landscape all too often never visited.

As postmodern publics then, we have hidden cancer realities behind a dichotomy of fear and adulation, motivated by media reports and tempered by an imagined experience that has no room for the multiple and disparate cancer realities. My narrative of loss remained ambiguous and a story foreclosed. In contrast, the focus group participants subverted the morally acceptable narratives of positive coping for their cancer heroes and heroines with alternative stories of their own pain and suffering. However, they remained true to one prevailing cultural script: they revealed their own suffering within the context of cancer, their own exhaustion pointing to the unspoken suffering of loved ones approaching the end of life.

When the imagined experience of cancer is combined with a terminal diagnosis, the reality becomes even further submerged under the *loneliness of dying* (Elias, 1985). During my time at the hospice, one of the men who took part in the focus group spoke at length about the fact that he was an elderly man (in his 70s) who lived alone. His loneliness was mediated by his cancer diagnosis in unexpected and positive ways. Of his weekly visits to the day hospice, he said, "It's the highlight of my week!" He saw it as an opportunity to get out of the house and enjoy contact with others. He spoke proudly of learning silk scarf painting in the art therapy group. Thus, allowed to speak beyond prevailing narratives, he invited me to see beyond his disease and to reclaim his voice from the popular imagination of cancer.

CONCLUSION

My initial research with persons who have cancer was deeply entwined with those widely known cultural scripts that left little room for personhood and the variation that is at the root of what it means to experience illness. By exploring these cultural scripts and the narratives that remain outside these, I was able to reveal other scripts that struggle to assert themselves above the powerful and prevailing moral geography associated with cancer narratives. However, as the cultural blinkers were peeled off, my ears remained shut to a lone voice who wished to talk to me about dying.

Persons who have terminal cancer may struggle to assert their identity and to tell a story that strays into new countries, into a land that remains largely unmapped by prevailing moral geographies of cancer. They may indeed be heroes, some of them. They may run marathons and collude in the acceptable (public) face of cancer that remains juxtaposed to the darker side of terminal illness. This dark side may only be alluded to, feared by cancer's publics, but cannot be given its own voice. The fear of dying and narrating this fear remain scripts that both arise from the politics of dread and yet remain within illegitimate territory for public consumption. The foreclosing of narratives related to fears of death and dying appears to perpetuate the widespread inability of postmodern selves to engage with this talk. Ill equipped to provide comfort and make sense of the incomprehensible in our secularized world, we simply do not hear those voices who wish to embark on new scripts.

Whereas Kenyans narrate the pain and suffering of cancer experiences, in Scotland our voices are muted by a sense that we must bear our suffering silently. When cancer sufferers or their families are permitted to enter that space of foreclosed narratives, the stories may not be so very different for some. Hallowell (2006), for instance, writes of the fear of the dying process spoken about by her participants and how for many years she was unable to read whole interview transcripts as, in her words, "I could not face revisiting the anguish they contained" (p. 11). Perhaps Murray et al. (2003) were right to highlight the narratives of physical suffering in contrast to our more emotion-laden, existential narratives. But the silences occupied by horror may perhaps speak for themselves of a more multicultural, shared land that remains a part of the moral geography of cancer.

NOTES

1. The study referred to in this chapter was funded by Macmillan Cancer Support. The research team included Marilyn Kendall, Scott Murray, Aziz Sheikh, Nora Kearney, Alison Worth, Kirsty Boyd, Duncan Brown and Ian Mallinson.
2. This chapter partially draws on the following chapter where the concept of *imagined experience* was first introduced in brief: Harris, F.M. (2008). Cancer the bogeyman and me: Reflexivity and emotion in 'end of life' research. *Anthropology in Action*, (Special issue) *15*, 5–13.

REFERENCES

Addington-Hall, J. (2002). Research sensitivities to palliative care patients. *European Journal of Cancer Care, 11,* 220–224.
Aries, P. (1981). *The hour of our death*. London: Penguin.
Bury, M. (1982). Chronic illness as biographical disruption. *Sociology of Health & Illness, 4,* 167–182.
Clarke, J., & Everest, M. M. (2006). Cancer in the mass print media: fear, uncertainty and the medical model. *Social Science & Medicine, 6,* 2591–2600.
Dixon-Woods, M., Seale, C., Young, B., Findlay, M., & Heney, D. (2003). Representing childhood cancer: accounts from newspapers and parents. *Sociology of Health & Illness, 25,* 143–164.
Douglas, M. (1966). *Purity and danger: An analysis of concepts of purity and taboo*. London: Routledge & Kegan Paul.
Elias, N. (1985). *The loneliness of the dying*. Oxford: Blackwell.
Giddens, A. (1991). *Modernity and self-identity*. Oxford: Polity.
Green, J. W. (2008). *The anthropology of modern dying*. Philadelphia, PA: University of Pennsylvania Press.
Hagedoorn, M., Sanderman, R., Bolks, H.N., Tuinstra, J., & Coyne, J. C. (2008). Distress in couples coping with cancer: A meta-analysis and critical review of role and gender effects. *Psychological Bulletin, 133,* 1–30.
Hallowell, N. (2006). Varieties of suffering: Living with the risk of ovarian cancer. *Health, Risk & Society, 8,* 9–26.
Harris, F. M. (2008). Cancer the bogeyman and me: Reflexivity and emotion in 'end of life' research. *Anthropology in Action, 15,* 5–13.

Ingleton, C., Skilbeck, J., & Clark, D. (2001). Needs assessment for palliative care: Three projects compared. *Palliative Medicine, 15,* 398–404.

Kendall, M., Harris, F., Boyd, K., Sheikh, A., Brown, D., Mallinson, I., Kearney, N., & Worth, A. (2007). Key challenges and ways forward in researching the 'good death': Qualitative in-depth interview and focus group study. *British Medical Journal, 334,* 521.

Lawton, J. (2001). Contemporary hospice care: the sequestration of the unbounded body and 'dirty dying.' *Sociology of Health & Illness, 20,* 121–143.

McMullin, J., & Weiner, D. (2009) Introduction: an anthropology of cancer, In J. McMullin & D. Weiner (Eds.), *Confronting cancer: Metaphors, advocacy and anthropology* (pp. 3–26). Santa Fe, NM: School for Advanced Research Press.

Mellor, P. & Shilling, C. (1993). Modernity, self-identity and the sequestration of death. *Sociology, 27,* 411–431.

Murray, S., Grant, E., Grant, A. & Kendall, M. (2003). Dying from cancer in developed and developing countries: Lessons from two qualitative interview studies of patients and their carers. *British Medical Journal, 326,* 368–372.

Seale, C. (2002). Cancer heroics: A study of news reports with particular reference to gender. *Sociology, 36,* 107–126.

Seale, C. (2003). Health and media: an overview. *Sociology of Health & Illness, 25,* 513–531.

Seymour, J., Payne, S., Chapman, A., & Holloway, M. (2007). Hospice or home? Expectations of end-of-life care among white and Chinese older people in the UK. *Sociology of Health and Illness, 29,* 872–890.

Sinding, C., & Wiernikowski, J. (2008). Disruption foreclosed: Older women's cancer narratives. *Health, 12,* 389–411.

Sontag, S. (1978). *Illness as metaphor.* New York, NY: McGraw-Hill.

Stoller, P. (2009), Remissioning life: Reconfiguring anthropology. In J. McMullin & D. Weiner (Eds.), *Confronting cancer: Metaphors, advocacy and anthropology* (pp. 27–42). Santa Fe, NM: School for Advanced Research Press.

Taylor, D. G. & Carter, S. (2004). *Valuing choice: Dying at home.* London: Marie Curie Cancer Care. Retrieved from http://www.mariecurie.org.uk/campaign/downloads/valuingchoice.pdf

Thomas, C., Morris, S.M., & Clark, D. (2004). Place of death: Preferences among cancer patients and their carers. *Social Science and Medicine, 58,* 2431–2444.

Thomas, P. (2002). The river, the road, and the rural-urban divide: A postcolonial moral geography from Southeast Madagascar. *American Ethnologist, 29,* 366–391.

Voas, D., & Crockett, A. (2005). Religion in Britain: Neither believing nor belonging. *Sociology, 39,* 11–28.

Walter, T. (2009). Jade's dying body: the ultimate reality show. *Sociological Research Online, 14.*

Walter, T. (2010). Jade and the journalists: Media coverage of a young British celebrity dying of cancer. Social Science & Medicine, 71, 853–860.

Afterword
Cancer Enigmas and Agendas[1]

Lenore Manderson

For a medical anthropologist, to borrow from Lévi-Strauss, cancer is good to think with. As Mathews and Burke emphasize in their introduction to this volume, cancer is both one and many conditions—over 100 different cancers exist in humans in diverse organs and tissues. These cancers are characterized by abnormal cell growth—cells failing to die, or growing when they are not needed, replicating, acquiring mass, invading other tissue and spreading to other parts of the body. With cancer, the normal process of cell regeneration is out of control; cancer is invasive and corrosive. Without effective intervention, cancers are fatal, hence the fear around them.

Although media reports, health promotional material, medical advice and personal experience mean that we are familiar with some of the diversity of cancer types, their etiologies, presentation and prognosis, we are surprisingly imprecise in the ways in which we group so many diseases under one frightening banner. In the north, in the global language of biomedicine and in its adaptations into vernacular nosology, we pay little attention to difference: to different kinds of cancers; in different organs, tissues and fluids; with different presentations and techniques of diagnosis; different treatments, management and prognosis. For although the pathological process is the same in the broadest sense, there are very different kinds of cancer. Carcinomas begin in the skin or in tissues of internal organs; sarcomas begin in bone, cartilage, fat, muscle, blood vessels, or other connective or supportive tissue. Carcinomas and sarcomas are discrete cancers, therefore, capable of excision. Leukemia, in contrast, originates in blood-forming tissue such as the bone marrow, and from there enters the blood stream, penetrating the entire system. Lymphoma and myeloma are cancers that originate in the cells of the immune system; central nervous system cancers begin in the tissues of the brain and spinal cord: here, the sites of origin and the types of cells involved make intervention difficult. Further, although many cancers are identified and described as tumors, not all tumors are cancers, and the signs and symptoms of cancer may also be signs of other diseases. New lumps or moles, abnormal bleeding or blood in any other body fluid or from any orifice, prolonged cough, chest pain or breathlessness, unexplained weight loss, constipation or diarrhea—any of these symptoms might indicate cancer.

They might equally be signs of another condition, however, some easily treated and others insidious, slow to treat but not necessarily pernicious.

This lack of differentiation contrasts with the precision by which typically, in lay and specialist language, we speak of other diseases that present or develop in ways similar to each other. We distinguish between Alzheimer's disease, Parkinson's disease, multiple sclerosis and motor neurone disease rather than speaking globally of neurological conditions, for instance; we treat as discrete—and make a point of establishing the difference—between a 'common cold' and other respiratory tract infections. Yet cancer is cancer at first moment of diagnosis, and in the telling. The differentiation comes later, to a smaller community, when clinicians, patients, family and friends all try to make sense of its emergence, determine intervention and assess the outcome.

Cancer is dense with metaphor, with English language metaphors spilling into other languages in which biomedical talk might be communicated. The most common metaphors are those of war, embattlement, struggles and victories—points well made by Mathews and Burke in the introduction to this volume, as by others (Garrison, 2007; Lerner, 2001). But metaphors of stealth and victimhood are no less common. Cancers sneak up on people, attack innocent children, kill people in the 'prime of life' and rob others of shared history. Metaphors of war rally the troops to fight a common enemy—they are the victory metaphors in the face of tropes of agony and defeat. The fear of cancer informs and follows from these tropes. Fear is always part of any explanation, regardless of cultural setting, for people's reluctance to participate in screening, follow up on screening results and respond to call-back notices. Stigma explains people's reluctance to tell others of a diagnosis, deal comfortably with its occurrence in others, or address questions of death and dying for those with terminal disease (Bennett, 1999; Kaufert, 1999). Fear and stigma are two sides of a coin, one fixing the other.

Because this is known, there is an extensive literature on cancers, virological, clinical and epidemiological, sociological and cultural. Although anthropologists' contributions to this literature are still limited, much of it is simply hidden. The present volume, and the conference which preceded it, brings to light some of the important anthropological work on cancer being done by researchers in regions outside the global north, both to explore the possibilities for collaboration and to consider the insights from their work for rethinking global cancer agendas.

In writing of a hidden literature, I am mindful of two particular domains. The first is the work of applied and practicing anthropologists, working within ministries and departments of health, cancer support organizations and foundations, and in research groups, often within multidisciplinary teams, to gather empirical data to inform policies and programs in relation to screening, health education, counseling, treatment support and palliation. Some of this work is published in anthropology journals or books (Constant, Winkler, Bishop & Palomino, 2014; Manderson, Kirk & Hoban, 2001; McMichael, Manderson, Kirk, Hoban & Potts, 2000; Wood et al.,

2014; Wood, Jewkes & Abrahams, 1997; Wood, Flynn & Stockdale, 2013), but other articles appear in public health and oncology journals, and more often, the work is presented in reports to commissioning agencies, largely lost to a wider audience in a voluminous grey literature. This is not unique to cancer, of course; it is a feature of much medical and other applied anthropology. A second domain that is increasingly difficult to capture is doctoral and master's research. Many excellent dissertations are lost to an audience outside the home department in which the work was produced because little or none of the work is published. In writing this, I am mindful of the work of some of my own students: Karen Thurecht (2000) on abnormal smears, colposcopy and stigma; Natalie Wray (2004) on gynecological cancer diagnosis, treatment and support (Markovic, Manderson, Wray & Quinn, 2004, 2006; Wray, Markovic & Manderson, 2007); Sarah Drew (2003) on identity among young cancer survivors; Keely Macarow (2006) on the creative arts, image and representation for HIV and cancer. Susan Peake (2004; see also Manderson & Peake, 2005), writing on embodied loss, disability and identity, provides a compelling contemporary example of the presentation of self in everyday life, in her account of a woman who had lost her nose from cancer. Lorraine Yap (1998) explains the reasons for and effects of diagnostic and treatment delay in the Philippines; Elizabeth Bennett (2001) provides a superb ethnography of death and dying in northeast Thailand. Many of the rich ethnographies of various cancers remain bound volumes, unpublished.

Beyond that, there is a marked difference in the concentration of research, as reflected in this volume. Half of all chapters included herein are concerned solely with breast cancer (Gibbon, Armin, Burke, Macdonald, Bright and Aureliano), of which only one addresses questions of risk or screening—Gibbon's on breast cancer genetics in Brazil. Of the remaining six chapters (excluding the introduction), three discuss breast cancer by way of example (Luxardo, Dyer, Mulemi). Two others are concerned with etiology, causality and responsibility (Sarradon-Eck, Lora-Wainwright) and one with palliative care (Harris), so all are arguably applicable to breast cancer as to other types of disease. This visibility of breast cancer is replicated publicly—the size and success of its advocacy, screening programs, support organizations and fund raising, memoirs, journalism and creative arts (Manderson, 2011; Bell, 2014). Breast cancer captures the imagination in ways that other dominant organ cancers—prostate and colorectal cancers, for instance—do not.

But there is also a structural explanation for the preeminence of research on breast cancer. Many of the contributors, particularly those working in Latin America, have been funded by the Susan G. Komen Breast Cancer Foundation. Other researchers have been interested in replicating programs on breast cancer support, or have been involved in or followed the search for a Latina BC gene and genetic testing (Patel, 2010; Gibbon, 2013). In countries where resources for cancer are limited, breast cancer provides the best option for funds for research.

The most prevalent cancer among women is breast cancer—25% of all cancers in women—but again, these are cancers. We tend to elide differences in genetics, the presence or absence of hormone receptors, stage of development, and histology and cell type, although these various features of biology, pathophysiology and development of disease have different implications in terms of treatment and outcome, and so are of social as well as biomedical significance. Worldwide, breast cancer does not usually result in death, either in the global south or north. Other cancers—of the lung and bronchus especially, and of the liver, colon and rectum, and stomach are no less common, with higher fatality rates because of delays in diagnosis and less effective treatments.

* * * *

In 2012, there were an estimated 14.1 million new cancer cases, more men than women. The same year 8.2 million people died from cancers, with somewhat fewer than 60% of new cases and 65% of deaths occurring in low- and middle-income countries. These are of course rough estimates, and in many countries, no data exist or national data are extrapolated from regional data. Further, in the poorest countries, cause of death is most often proximate and the presence of cancer is never detected; in other places, low life expectancy mitigates incidence and prevalence of cancer. While cardiovascular diseases (ischemic heart disease and stroke), lower respiratory infections and chronic obstructive lung disease contribute most to deaths globally, cancers continue to rank among the top 10 causes of morbidity and death. We are only beginning to map out what this means as social researchers. The depth and breadth of the contributions of anthropologies of cancers in this volume provide an entry point to reflecting on future agendas for research in both global north and global south settings. In the following, I sketch out a research agenda that, with vicissitudes of scientific discovery, may extend even further. These agendas relate to different kinds of cancers; screening, diagnostic and treatment processes; the workforces and material cultures of cancer in both clinical and scientific settings; the overlapping of these fields; and the challenges of public health in different social and economic settings and systems of health.

DIFFERENTIATING CANCERS AND THEIR SOCIAL IMPACT

As I have noted earlier, we have paid disproportionate attention to breast cancer. Many other cancers are as important, because of greater mortality rates, challenges in diagnosis, their social and psychological impact, and their stigmatizing effects. Here, on the one hand, I am reflecting on the work that needs to be done on common cancers with high survival rates, where factors of stigma and disgust influence screening and diagnosis, and govern our own willingness to inquire into them and encourage others to speak of them.

Colorectal and bladder cancers are instances here, despite their high prevalence and the roll-out of public health initiatives to encourage regular fecal screening and colonoscopies, surgery, radiation and the management of colostomies (Manderson, 2005, 2011). Lung cancer, prostate cancer and stomach cancer are rarely written about from a social perspective, and research on cancer of the cervix had until recently focused more on Pap smears and screening programs than on colposcopy, radiotherapy, surgery and chemotherapy. We have paid very little attention to rare and cruel cancers—of the eyes and noses, mouth and ears, testes, penis and vulva. My own work on organ and tissue cancers, particularly sarcomas, that stripped men and women of limbs, bowels and bladders as well as breasts, highlights how such extensive excisions force people to reinvent themselves to maintain a semblance of an ordinary life. There are, as I have described briefly earlier, cancers that silently and perniciously creep through bodies, cancers that exude and seep and shock as they disfigure, horrendous teratomas that confront both parents and their clinicians (Stacey, 2013 [1997]). Many of these are discrete—cancers of the cervix, bladder, esophagus, liver, pancreas. Other cancers are difficult to conceptualize because they are pervasive cancers of the blood, bone marrow and lymphatic system. There are cancers that spread rapidly and are hallmarked by pain; precancers that are not yet, but might be, cancers; cancers that are good or bad depending on usual age at diagnosis, progression, treatment efficacy, survival rates and prognosis. We need an anthropological lens on all of these to better understand how 'cancer' comes to be.

TECHNOLOGIES IN AND BEYOND THE CLINIC

The Pap Smear (Papanicolaou test) was introduced in the 1940s and facilitated the early detection of atypical cells and lesions, leading to a dramatic decline in serious morbidity and mortality from cervical cancer from this time on. Since its introduction, there has been growing interest in developing and introducing early screening and diagnostic methods, including self-examination (for testes and breasts), internal examinations, stool and urine tests, blood assays and tissue biopsies. There has, in parallel, been a sustained interest among virologists to identify the etiology of cancers, so to develop effective vaccines. The established link between certain types of HPV (Human Papillomavirus) and certain cancers—cervical, anal, penile and oropharyngeal cancer—has opened up major areas of enquiry. This includes the characterization of (all) cervical cancer as sexually transmitted, proving women's moral culpability. But this raises questions also round the roll-out, in different settings, of vaccines to young women (and less often to men) (Lillvis, Kirkland & Frick, 2014). People understand, and misunderstand, vaccines. And although we know that the HPV vaccine will not prevent all gynecological cancers, that cervical cancers already are deeply stigmatizing, and that vaccines that link infection to cancers are likely to be stigmatizing for women and so resisted by target populations, we need to examine this closely in local contexts.

Medical anthropologists have increasingly turned to science studies for inspiration, as we interrogate the technologies; the established and emerging literature on assisted reproduction technologies is an example of the directions such enquiry might take. Karen-Sue Taussig and colleagues (2013) highlight the need for anthropological studies of technologies and disciplines within the life sciences. At every point from diagnosis of a cancer, people necessarily engage with technology and must (ideally) gain some comprehension of the instruments, the data that they generate and the work that they do. Vaccines and screening tests are only part of the story, therefore. People's engagement with instrumentation and technologies extends from screening and its equivocal reports, to diagnostic testing and biopsy, ultrasound and CAT scans (the scans increasingly transmitted as email attachments to smartphones for easy reference). And after screening and testing follow presurgical mark-ups, the insertion of dye for sentinel node biopsy, anesthesia, surgeries and surgical revisions, radiotherapy and chemotherapy, medication to counter the side effects of these, reconstructive surgery, more assays and ultrasound to monitor progress, and so on. People at the center of the dramas that unfold around cancer must come to terms with the lexicon of the clinic—for example, men with prostate cancer speak with their oncologists of PSA readings and da Vinci surgery. Much of this is both frightening and surreal, yet also reassuring: sophisticated technologies offer a semblance of confidence, hence people's bitter disappointment when the interventions fail and the possibility of survival, let alone cure, contracts. Further, familiarity with and the reassurance derived from the clinic, its specific vocabulary and its instrumentation are largely shaped by class, both in terms of education and income. Wealthier people have access to better care and timely treatment whereas poor people may have no access to care at all. Educated people in the global north have the capacity to master the language around a disease and its management, and access to internet to rehearse the alternatives and clarify the side effects. They can afford the care, for treatment and palliation. People with limited or no formal education and no way of accessing information are stripped of agency as they surrender their bodies to their physicians, if they have access to physicians and care at all.

THE CANCER WORKFORCE

Screening, diagnosis and treatments require various professionals and other workers to be involved: postal workers who deliver stool test kits to homes and the smeared cards to pathology laboratories, couriers who transport vials of bloods and tissue samples from collection points to laboratories, radiographers, pathologists, anesthetists, nurses, ward clerks, chaplains, pharmacists, geneticists and counselors, psychologists, wig makers and tattooists, prosthetists, physical and occupational therapists, NGO administrators and volunteers, the clowns in pediatric oncology wards, the undertakers at funeral parlors or the mourners in the village. We have been surprisingly uncurious about the training and roles of different health professionals, the production of the science of cancers, the growth of advocacy, and the ways in which experiences of cancer propel individuals to act in particular ways. Cancer provides multiple ways to understand social and technical structures and authority, and the economics of resources, and provides particular insights into the roles, and the habitus, of different kinds of professionals and support workers, as Aureliano, Dyer, Harris and Mulemi illustrate forcefully in their contributions to this volume. Studies with children and young people with cancer, for instance, highlight the "emotion work" of nursing staff (Hochschild, 1983; Rindstedt, 2013). Pediatric cancers lend themselves to this analysis, of course, as fund-raisers well know, but the emotional and ethical complexities of working on oncology wards extend to patients, their families and all health providers (Heinze & Nolan, 2012; Pavlish, Brown-Saltzman, Jakel & Rounkle, 2012). Again, Harris and Dyer both make this point in this volume.

These complexities extend also to the ethnographers themselves, as Sky Gross (2012) describes in relation to the shifts that occurred in her relationship from a person with brain cancer to a brain and its tumor. In an extraordinary article, she writes of her uneasy awareness of her own capacity (and perhaps need) to objectify the brain, over time and in the most controlled clinical environments, as she moved from being an ethnographer friend to a true observer of Omer's seizures, the bulging tumor, the decision-making in the Intensive Care Unit, his surgery and the "hours (that) went by as the surgeons methodically vacuumed tumour tissue and carefully sealed blood vessels" (p.1176). Her work is a pioneering ethnography of brain cancer not only because of the diversity of actors and events—patients and their families, neuro-oncologists, nurses, social workers, neuropsychologists, and radiologists; and observations of consultations, doctors' rounds and weekly professional meetings. It is pioneering too because the work steps away from exploring the social meanings of cancer and moves instead to the materiality of the disease. As might be anticipated from my earlier comments about stool samples and blood, the (absent) physicality of a sarcoma and the pervasive invisibility of lymphoma, we need to continue to interrogate cancers as embodied experiences within and outside of the body, intra- and interpersonal, objective and subjective. Depending on the kind of cancer, doctors and patients necessarily mediate tissue and exudate, the frankly visible and palpable, the invisible revealed through CT scans.

ANTICIPATING THE FUTURE

In her chapter in this volume, Sahra Gibbon attends to Brazilian cancer genetics, and the involvement of women in such research programs because of the access they gain to breast cancer services. Nurses and geneticists work to ensure that once a family member has been identified as carrying a mutation and so is at heightened risk of developing breast cancer, then extra screening is provided to other family members; the scientists involved emphasize the cost–benefits of genetic screening over treating those who develop breast cancer. The cost of such interventions is comparatively high, however, and in expanding on this, Gibbon illustrates the disproportionate confidence in the science of genetics, and the consequent misunderstandings of genetic screening as a way to prevent cancer. Despite that proportionately few breast cancers can be linked to genetic history, there has been increasing demand for genetic screening and advice about risk, globally; there is evidence also in studies of the genetics of other cancers, where authors almost invariably conclude with the need for health education and genetic counseling (Plaetke et al., 2002). Gibbon's chapter therefore illustrates the general enthusiasm (of scientists) for genetic research to prevent and cure cancers, and their advocacy for more translation of social science research for the public health applications of their work (cf. McBride et al., 2010; Schully et al., 2010. More work, however, is needed to explore what genetics means in social and political economic terms in relation to understandings of biology, prevention action, family and inheritance (see Finkler, 2000; Gibbon et al., 2010; Gibbon, Kampriani & zur Nieden, 2010; Gibbon, 2013).

In a recent article on "potentiality," Karen-Sue Taussig and colleagues (2013) highlight the imagined advantages of genetic testing, and of gene therapy and pharmacogenomics, driven by the hubristic claim that "doctors" will be able to cure cancer and other life-long degenerative diseases. Umbilical cord blood and adult stem cell harvesting, and the establishment and maintenance of biobanks, are predicated on this potentiality. Potentiality, the authors suggest, "suffuses conceptualizations of life everywhere in biomedicine: in the lab, in the clinic, in social policy, among the public at large, and in the politics at work across all of these domains" (Taussig et al., 2013, S3-S4). Yet, enthusiasm for biobanking is equivocal, and many publics are uneasy about the use of biomaterial for incidental research (Zubin, et al., 2013).

The importance of genetics in the future to the prevention of various cancers—and the prevention of other medical conditions—is fueled by a confidence in science and innovation and the continued directing of resources to enable research in this area. But the investment in the genetics of cancer creates false expectations of what 'science' might or can deliver. At the same time, it directs resources away from addressing the social, personal and health systems challenges related to cancer, and the inequalities that exist even in the distribution of the simplest oncology resources, as a number of the authors in this volume, including Mulemi, Gibbon and MacDonald, illustrate. Like the particular focus on breast cancer, the globalization of genomic research, and the hype around its potentiality, continues to efface the risks for and experiences of cancers in low-resources settings and for most people worldwide.

CAUSALITY AND THE ENVIRONMENT

I have left causality until last despite the extraordinarily obvious need for anthropological engagement in the relationship of the environment to etiology, as well as the complex political and legal economies that surround different cancers. Populations in much of the poor world, in the global north and south, live and work under conditions where exposure to carcinogens is unavoidable, where many risks are unknown and where other risks cannot be controlled. People who live on the margins have limited options to avoid exposure to toxins. Illegal mining and the use of heavy metals to extract gold; indoor air pollution from cooking with fossil fuel; exposure to asbestos and the associated high risk of mesothelioma and lung cancer; exposure to aluminum, radium, arsenic, chromium and other carcinogens; and industrial accidents occur at multiple points in everyday life. Agricultural development programs for decades have encouraged the use of pesticides, herbicides and fungicides, so fanning exposure to carcinogens. Poor people everywhere are most likely exposed to toxic waste sites. The challenge for anthropologists is to work alongside epidemiologists, with political activists and others. The challenge too is to negotiate or step around the resistance of governments, multinational corporations and local industries, eager to avoid accusations of their role in creating carcinogenic environments and so also avoiding individual litigation and class action (Petryna, 2002).

Cigarette smoking and exposure to side smoke too continues to place people at risk. In 1999, in introducing an article by Garrett Mehl and colleagues (1999), I drew attention to the need for more anthropological work on the uptake of, dependence on and quitting smoking, and the importance of context (Manderson, 1999). The single most effective step to reduce cancer from all causes, now as it was then, is to stop cigarette smoking, but in achieving this, there is wide disparity in country policies and the will to take steps to discourage smoking for political and economic reasons (Benson, 2012; Singer, 2001; Stebbins, 1991).

* * * *

Cancers are, after cardiometabolic diseases, the major causes of illness and death worldwide. Few of us will escape close encounters. I, and several of my friends, have had breast cancers of various types, and post mastectomies and reconstructions; we are in good health. We are annoyed by the indelibility of our histories, that people still say to us on the side, in whispers, How *are* you? We are fine. But others are not. In 2014, this past month, I have lost and mourned two people, one from brain cancer, one from pancreatic cancer. Two more—one with lung cancer, one with esophageal cancer—are coming to terms with shocking, unexpected diagnoses as they learn also of metastases, the guerrilla troops in an unwinnable war. The military metaphors are apt. And these are all people in their mid 50s to 60s, who never smoked, for whom risk would have been very low. Epidemiology is one thing, a friend once said to me, luck's another.

In 2010, Paul Farmer and colleagues (2010) announced in *The Lancet* the establishment of a Global Task Force on Expanded Access to Cancer Care and Control in Developing Countries (GTF.CCC) to develop global and regional initiatives for affordable drugs and innovative service delivery models. In framing this initiative, the authors drew attention to the lack of attention to cancer, as a global health problem, by private, government and multilateral donors; they noted specially its exclusion from key global health targets such as the Millennium Development Goals (MDGs). In elaborating on an agenda for action, the authors emphasized the need for appropriate, affordable and accessible strategies for cancer prevention and control, and for treatment and palliative care for people with cancer, including through the provision of affordable drugs and vaccines. Proposing a focus on cancers that could most readily be prevented or cured (such as breast, cervical and colorectal cancers), they argued for demonstration programs with new infrastructure, increased numbers of trained health professionals, and the effective use of telecommunications; the development of pricing and procurement systems to ensure affordable drugs and services; and the implementation of financing mechanisms to meet the costs associated with preventing and treating cancer. In a subsequent published comment, Felicia Marie Knaul and colleagues (2013) noted the challenges of preventing cancer, and providing treatment and palliation, where health systems were inadequate. But at the same time, they argued for a straightforward three-point approach to cancer control in poor countries: HPV vaccines and the use of various off-patent medications using global financing mechanisms, "harnessing" telecommunication infrastructure, and "using established health system platforms through a diagonal approach with primary and secondary caregivers" (p. 2239).

These recipes for cancer control, concerned with bridging the 'cancer divide' of north and south, seem to simplify the complex social, political, economic and cultural factors that pattern inequality within and between nations, and that shape risk, defer screening, delay detection and reduce the effectiveness of treatment, care and palliation. The omissions of local challenges, and the ways in which these impact on people's lives, are important. I am reminded of two powerful instances of cancers to argue this point. One concerns Antonina, a woman interviewed by Lorraine Yap in the Philippines. She speaks of a lump that was diagnosed, belatedly, as breast cancer:

> My lump started a long time ago . . . it was small and there was no pain . . . I became worried then it grew big, became red just like a tomato, and hard. But it was not painful . . . although I experienced some pain in my breast, I thought it was just a boil . . . this time it was big, red and hard and I felt that it was cancer . . . what I know is that cancer comes from inside the body, if not treated, the cancer will burst inside the body and poison it.
>
> (Yap, 1998, p. 85)

Antonia was one of dozens of women with the same story, always troubled by lack of access of transport, money and services as well as fear of disease, pain, surgery and death. The second example is from Elizabeth Bennett, who conducted research in Isaan (northeast Thailand), where cholangiocarcinoma (bile duct cancer; from a fluke infection, opisthorchiasis) was (and is) the most prevalent in the world (Bennett, 2001). Isaan people who are diagnosed with terminal disease are usually discharged from hospital without pain relief. Hospitals can only provide morphine by injection; nurses resist the idea of oral morphine because of problems of supply and fear of addiction. As a result, people with end-stage disease return home with paracetamol. In the study village, the only option was for people to make a half-hour trip to the nearest hospital, usually on the back of a pick-up truck, for a single dose of intramuscular morphine, which might provide them with four hours of relief. By the time they had returned home, the pain had often returned with a brutal edge (p.102).

The transnational approach of the chapters in this volume asks that we consider local understandings of cancers, the ethnocentric nature of biomedical and public health assumptions about and their approaches to the disease. In drawing attention to such complexities of different cancers, and to complications related to prevention, diagnosis and care, the authors contributing to this volume illustrate the importance of measured approaches that respond to and incorporate local circumstance and exigency. Through attending to ethnographic detail, health policies and interventions might be developed that best address local need, while allowing also for relations between local and global forces. Without attending to local reality, the particular needs of populations living in highly diverse political, social and economic systems, and the shifting contexts of suffering and uncertainty, such interventions have little hope of success (Whiteford & Manderson, 2000).

NOTE

1. I dedicate this chapter to Anthony, Janine, Jocelyn, Katie, Maureen, Mike, Olivia, Sue and Susan.

REFERENCES

Bell, K. (2014). The breast-cancer-ization of cancer survivorship: Implications for experiences of the disease. *Social Science & Medicine, 110*, 56–63.

Bennett, E. (1999). Soft truth: Ethics and cancer in northeast Thailand. *Anthropology and Medicine, 6*, 395–404.

Bennett, E. (2001). *The severed heart. Dying and death among the Isaan of rural northeast Thailand*. Unpublished PhD dissertation, The University of Melbourne, Melbourne, VIC, Australia.

Benson, P. (2012). *Tobacco capitalism: Growers, migrant workers, and the changing face of global industry*. Princeton, NJ: Princeton University Press.

Constant, T. K. H., Winkler, J. L., Bishop, A., & Palomino, L.G.T. (2014). Perilous uncertainty: Situating women's breast-health seeking in northern Peru. *Qualitative Health Research, 24*, 811–823. doi: 10.1177/1049732314529476

Drew, S. (2003). *'Stranger in the community': Long-term survival following cancer in childhood*. Unpublished PhD dissertation, The University of Melbourne Melbourne, VIC, Australia.

Farmer, P., Frenk, J., Knaul, F. M., Shulman, L. N., Alleyne, G., Armstrong, L., . . . et al. (2010). Expansion of cancer care and control in countries of low and middle income: a call to action. *The Lancet, 376*, 1186–1193.

Finkler, K. (2000). *Experiencing the new genetics family and kinship on the medical frontier*. Philadelphia, PA: University of Pennsylvania Press.

Garrison, K. (2007). The personal is rhetorical: War, protest, and peace in breast cancer narratives. *Disabilities Studies Quarterly, 27*, 114–118.

Gibbon, S. (2013). Ancestry, temporality, and potentiality engaging cancer genetics in Southern Brazil. *Current Anthropology, 54*, S107-S117.

Gibbon, S., Joseph, G., Kalender, U., Kampriani, E., Mozersky, J., zur Nieden, A., & Palfner, S. (2010). Special section: Perspectives on globalising genomics: The case of 'BRCA' breast cancer research and medical practice. Introduction. *Biosocieties, 5*, 407–414.

Gibbon, S., Kampriani, E., & zur Nieden, A. (2010). BRCA patients in Cuba, Greece and Germany: Comparative perspectives on public health, the state and the partial reproduction of 'neoliberal' subjects. *Biosocieties, 5*, 440–466.

Gross, S. (2012). Biomedicine inside out: An ethnography of brain surgery. *Sociology of Health & Illness, 34*, 1170–1183. doi: 10.1111/j.1467-9566.2012.01462.x

Heinze, K. E., & Nolan, M. T. (2012). Parental decision making for children with cancer at the end of life: A meta-ethnography. *Journal of Pediatric Oncology Nursing, 29*, 337–345. doi: 10.1177/1043454212456905

Hochschild, A. (1983). *The managed heart: The commercialization of human feeling*. Berkeley, CA: The University of California Press.

Kaufert, J. M. (1999). Cultural mediation in cancer diagnosis and end of life decisionmaking: The experience of Aboriginal patients in Canada. *Anthropology and Medicine, 6*, 405–421.

Knaul, F. M., Atun, R., Farmer, P., & Frenk, J. (2013). Seizing the opportunity to close the cancer divide. *The Lancet, 381*, 2238–2239.

Lerner, B. H. (2001). *The breast cancer wars: Hope, fear, and the pursuit of a cure in twentieth-century America*. Oxford: Oxford University Press.

Lillvis, D. F., Kirkland, A., & Frick, A. (2014). Power and persuasion in the vaccine debates: An analysis of political efforts and outcomes in the United States, 1998–2012. *The Milbank Quarterly, 92*, 475–508.

Macarow, K. (2006). *Disturbance: Bodies, disease, art*. Unpublished PhD dissertation. The University of Melbourne, Melbourne, VIC, Australia.

Manderson, L. (1999). Introduction. New perspectives in anthropology on cancer control, disease and palliative care. *Anthropology and Medicine, 6*, 317–321.

Manderson, L. (2005). Boundary breaches: The body, sex and sexuality post-stoma surgery. *Social Science & Medicine, 61*, 405–415.

Manderson, L. (2011). *Surface tensions: Surgery, bodily boundaries, and the social self*. Walnut Creek, CA: Left Coast Press.

Manderson, L., Kirk, M., & Hoban, E. (2001). Walking the talk: Research partnerships in women's business. In I. Dyck, N., Lewis, D. & McLafferty, S. (Eds.), *Geographies of women's health* (pp. 177–194). New York and London: Routledge.

Manderson, L., & Peake, S. (2005). Men in motion: The performance of masculinity by disabled men. In Auslander, P. and Sandahl, C. (Eds.), *Bodies in commotion: Disability and performance* (pp. 230–242). Wisconsin, MI: University of Michigan Press.

Markovic, M., Manderson, L., Wray, N., & Quinn, M. (2004). "He is telling us something": Women's experiences of cancer disclosure in Australia. *Anthropology and Medicine, 11*, 325–339.

Markovic, M., Manderson, L., Wray, N., & Quinn, M. (2006). Complementary medicine use by Australian women with gynaecological cancer. *Psycho-Oncology, 15*, 209–220.

Master, Z., Claudio, J. O., Rachul, C., Wang, J. C. Y., Minden, M. D., & Caulfield, T. (2013). Cancer patient perceptions on the ethical and legal issues related to biobanking. *BMC Medical Genomics, 6*, doi 10.1186/1755-8794-6-8.

McBride, C. M., Bowen, D., Brody, L. C., Condit, C. M., Croyle, R. T., Gwinn, M., . . . et al. (2010). Future health applications of genomics priorities for communication, behavioral, and social sciences research. *American Journal of Preventive Medicine, 38*, 556–565.

McMichael, C., Manderson, L., Kirk, M., Hoban, E., & Potts, H. (2000). Breast cancer among Indigenous women. *Australian and New Zealand Journal of Public Health, 24*, 515–519.

Mehl, G., Seimon, T., & Winch, P. (1999). Funerals, big matches and jolly trips: 'contextual spaces' of smoking risk for Sri Lankan adolescents. *Anthropology and Medicine, 6*, 337–358.

Patel, T. A., Colon-Otero, G., Hume, C. B., Copland, J. A., III, & Perez, E. A. (2010). Breast cancer in Latinas: Gene expression, differential response to treatments, and differential toxicities in Latinas compared with other population groups. *Oncologist, 15*, 466–475.

Pavlish, C., Brown-Saltzman, K., Jakel, P., & Rounkle, A. (2012). Nurses' responses to ethical challenges in oncology practice: An ethnographic study. *Clinical Journal of Oncology Nursing, 16*, 592–600. doi: 10.1188/12.cjon.592-600

Peake, S. (2004). *Embodying disability: Self, sexuality and body capital in Australian society*. Unpublished PhD dissertation. The University of Melbourne, Melbourne, VIC, Australia.

Petryna, A. (2002). *Life Exposed: Biological citizens after chernobyl*. Princeton, NJ: Princeton University Press.

Plaetke, R., Thompson, I., Sarosdy, M., Harris, J. M., Troyer, D., & Arar, N. H. (2002). Genetic fieldwork for hereditary prostate cancer studies. *Urologic Oncology, 7*, 19–27.

Rindstedt, C. (2013). Pain and nurses' emotion work in a paediatric clinic: Treatment procedures and nurse-child alignments. *Communication & Medicine, 10*, 51–61.

Schully, S. D., Benedicto, C. B., Gillanders, E. M., Wang, S. S., & Khoury, M. J. (2010). Translational research in cancer genetics: The road less traveled. *Public Health Genomics, 14*: 1–8.

Singer, M. (2001). Toward a bio-cultural and political economic integration of alcohol, tobacco and drug studies in the coming century. *Social Science & Medicine, 53*, 199–213.

Stacey, J. (2013 [1997]). *Teratologies: A cultural study of cancer*. London: Routledge.

Stebbins, K. R. (1991). Tobacco, politics, and economics: Implications for global health. *Social Science & Medicine, 33*, 1317–1326.

Taussig, K., Hoeyer, K., & Helmreich, S. (2013). The anthropology of potentiality in biomedicine An introduction to supplement 7. *Current Anthropology, 54*, S3-S14. doi: 10.1086/671401

Thurecht, K. (2000). *Barriers to cancer screening and treatment in contemporary Australia: "Good girls keep their legs together."* Unpublished PhD dissertation, The University of Queensland, Brisbane, QLD, Australia.

Whiteford, L. M., & Manderson, L. (2000). *Global health policy, local realities: The fallacy of the level playing field*. Boulder, CO: Lynne Reiner.

Wood, B., Burchell, A. N., Escott, N., Little, J., Maar, M., Ogilvie, G., & Zehbe, I. (2014). Using community engagement to inform and implement a community-randomized controlled trial in the anishinaabek cervical cancer screening study. *Frontiers in oncology, 4*, 27–27. doi:10.3389/fonc.2014.00027

Wood, K., Jewkes, R., & Abrahams, N. (1997). Cleaning the womb: Constructions of cervical screening and womb cancer among rural Black women in South Africa. *Social Science & Medicine, 45*, 283–294. doi: 10.1016/s0277-9536(96)00344-9

Wood, M. E., Flynn, B. S., & Stockdale, A. (2013). Primary care physician management, referral, and relations with specialists concerning patients at risk for cancer due to family history. *Public Health Genomics, 16*, 75–82. doi: 10.1159/000343790

Wray, N. (2004). *'Under the knickers': Uncertainty, the body and gynaecological cancer.* Unpublished PhD dissertation, The University of Melbourne, Melbourne, VIC, Australia.

Wray, N., Markovic, M., & Manderson, L. (2007). Discourses of normality and difference: Responses to diagnosis and treatment of gynaecological cancer of Australian women. *Social Science & Medicine, 64*, 2260–2271.

Yap, L. (1998). *A map of the human breast. An anthropological inquiry into the management of female breast cancer in la Union, Philippines.* Unpublished PhD dissertation, The University of Queensland, Brisbane, QLD, Australia.

Contributors

Julie S. Armin is in the Department of Anthropology, University of Arizona. She is a medical anthropologist with an interest in social inequality and health in the United States, and recently completed her dissertation, which examines the role of public policies in shaping cancer disparities.

Waleska de Araújo Aureliano is Professor in the Social Sciences Department of State University of Rio de Janeiro. She holds degrees in Social Anthropology and Sociology. She studies the anthropology of health, with particular interest in breast cancer, social movements in health, and rare genetic diseases.

Kristin Bright is Assistant Professor in the Department of Sociology and Anthropology, Carleton College. Her research over the past decade has focused on cultural and political configurations of gender, labor, capitalism, modernity, and other axes of social meaning and power in the ways people think about medical knowledge and practice in South Asia and North America.

Nancy J. Burke is Associate Professor of Medical Anthropology at the University of California, San Francisco, in the Department of Anthropology, History and Social Medicine and the Helen Diller Family Comprehensive Cancer Center. Her research in Cuba and the United States concerns chronic disease management, cancer prevention, treatment and survivorship, therapeutic subjectivity, bioethics, technologies of cancer care, and social inequality.

Karen E. Dyer is a postdoctoral fellow at Virginia Commonwealth University at the NCI-designated Massey Cancer Center Cancer Prevention and Control Research Fellowship. She completed her PhD in medical anthropology with a concentration in NGO/Non-Profit at the University of South Florida.

Sahra Gibbon is a Lecturer in the Anthropology Department at University College London, UK. She has a PhD in social anthropology and was a Wellcome Trust Research Fellow. Her research interests include genomic knowledges/technologies and public health in comparative cultural arenas (especially Latin America), breast cancer and "BRCA" genetics, and biosocialities and communities of health activism.

Fiona M. Harris is a Senior Lecturer in Health Sciences at the University of Stirling. She earned her doctorate in social anthropology from the University of Edinburgh. She now leads research on the mental health and well-being of cancer survivors and their families.

Anastasia Karakasidou is Professor of Anthropology at Wellesley College. She received her PhD from Colombia University and studied ethnicity, national consciousness and agrarian transformations. Since 2001, she has conducted multi-sited ethnographic research on cancer, the environment and social experiences of illness.

Anna Lora-Wainwright is Associate Professor in the Human Geography of China at the University of Oxford. She holds degrees in anthropology and in Chinese studies (SOAS and Oxon). Her research concerns development, health and environmental issues in rural China.

Natalia Luxardo is Research Associate at the National Scientific and Technical Research Council (Conicet) and Associate Professor at the University of Buenos Aires (UBA) in Argentina. Her research focuses on cancer phenomena and end-of-life issues. She holds a degree in Social Sciences (UBA) and an MA in Social Sciences specialized on Health (Flacso).

Alison Macdonald is a teaching fellow in the Department of Anthropology, University College London. She has carried out ethnographic research on the rise of breast cancer activism in India since 2008. She received her PhD in anthropology from University College London in 2013.

Lenore Manderson, PhD, is Professor of Public Health and Medical Anthropology at the University of the Witwatersrand (South Africa) and Visiting Distinguished Professor, Institute for the Study of Environment and Society, Brown University (USA). She has worked as an applied anthropologist with immigrant and indigenous Australians in relation to cervical and breast cancer screening, treatment and care, and has conducted research on the impact of cancers also with Anglo-Australian men and women.

Holly F. Mathews is Professor of Anthropology at East Carolina University in Greenville, NC, and a Fellow in the Leo Jenkins Cancer Center at the Brody School of Medicine. She received her PhD from Duke University and has research interests in medical anthropology, breast cancer, health disparities and barriers to mammography and cervical cancer screening.

Benson A. Mulemi is Senior Lecturer in the Department of Social Sciences at the Catholic University of Eastern Africa in Nairobi, Kenya. Mulemi holds a Master's degree in anthropology from the University of Nairobi, Kenya, and a PhD in medical anthropology from the University of Amsterdam. His research interests include hospital ethnography, ethnographies of the health and well-being, human albinism and livelihood in East Africa.

Aline Sarradon-Eck, PhD and MD, is a researcher at the Centre Norbert Elias (UMR 8562, Marseille, France). Her research interests include representations of the body, the cultural social construction of the illness experience, the anthropology of health systems, and cancer and mental health.

Index

For Product Safety Concerns and Information please contact our EU
representative GPSR@taylorandfrancis.com
Taylor & Francis Verlag GmbH, Kaufingerstraße 24, 80331 München, Germany

www.ingramcontent.com/pod-product-compliance
Ingram Content Group UK Ltd.
Pitfield, Milton Keynes, MK11 3LW, UK
UKHW021428080625
459435UK00011B/203